W9-BKB-223

AN
ATLAS OF NORMAL
RADIOGRAPHIC
ANATOMY

Also by Dr. Richard Snell

Clinical Anatomy for Medical Students

Clinical Embryology for Medical Students,
Second Edition

AN ATLAS OF NORMAL RADIOGRAPHIC ANATOMY

RICHARD S. SNELL, M.D., Ph.D.
Professor and Chairman,
Department of Anatomy, The George Washington University
School of Medicine and Health Sciences,
Washington, D.C.

ALVIN C. WYMAN, M.D.
Clinical Professor of Radiology,
The George Washington University
School of Medicine and Health Sciences,
Washington, D.C.

LITTLE, BROWN AND COMPANY
BOSTON

To
Our Students and House Officers
Past, Present, and Future

PREFACE

This atlas of normal human radiographic anatomy has
been prepared for medical students and house officers.
The authors have observed in the course of teaching
anatomy and the elements of diagnostic radiology
that physicians in training have a constant need
for constructive reinforcement of their knowledge of
normal anatomic relationships. Of particular
importance is the development of their ability to
relate their knowledge of three-dimensional
gross anatomy to the two-dimensional radiograph.
This book is designed to provide the fundamental
anatomic information based on radiographic views
commonly used in clinical radiologic practice.
Included are sections on the more specialized areas
of diagnostic radiology, such as angiography,
mammography, and computerized axial tomography.
It is not intended to be an encyclopedia of normal
radiographic anatomy, nor is it intended to demonstrate
the many variations of normal organ systems. We
leave this more detailed demonstration of radiographic
anatomy to the larger, comprehensive, classic textbooks
of radiology, which may be consulted if it becomes necessary.

Each radiograph is followed by a fully labeled diagram
enabling the reader quickly to identify the important
major structures demonstrated on the film. Below
each diagram is a line drawing showing the position
of the body area being x-rayed. For simplicity, no
attempt has been made to relate these diagrams
to the age or sex of the patient. The absence of a
written text makes this book a reference
instrument of easily available information.

We are most grateful to the following colleagues in
radiology who have assisted us in the compilation of
examples of normal studies: Christian V. Cimmino,
Stanley V. Perl, Olcay S. Cigtay, Massoud Majd,
Paul G. Harsanyi, Charles M. Citrin, Bruce L. McClennan,
Thomas L. Lawson, David O. Davis, Sigmund Mittler,
and William J. McSweeney; to our dental colleagues:
Joseph J. Eanet and Lee M. Sackett; and to
Joanne P. Coffee, R.T., and Carol G. Albin, R.T.
for their devoted technologic work.

We wish to thank the staff of the Audiovisual Services
of The George Washington University Medical Center
for their patience and skill in preparing suitable
photographic prints of the radiographs for publication.

We also extend our most sincere appreciation to
Mrs. Terry Dolan, our artist, for her careful interpretation
of the tracings of the radiographs and for her skillful
execution of the final artwork and to Miss Maryanne
Budd for her care in typing the many anatomic labels.

Finally, the authors wish to express their gratitude to
the staff of Little, Brown and Company for their great
assistance in the preparation of this atlas.

R. S. S.
Washington, D.C.   A. C. W.

CONTENTS

PREFACE
page ix

1
THE HEAD AND NECK
page 1

2
THE UPPER LIMB
page 41

3
THE THORAX
page 87

4
THE ABDOMEN
page 121

5
THE PELVIS
page 169

6
THE LOWER LIMB
page 193

7
THE VERTEBRAL COLUMN
page 269

8
PREGNANCY
page 315

9
ARTERIOGRAPHY AND VENOGRAPHY
page 323

10
LYMPHANGIOGRAPHY
page 365

11
THE CENTRAL NERVOUS SYSTEM
page 379

12
MAMMOGRAPHY
page 413

INDEX
page 419

AN
ATLAS OF NORMAL
RADIOGRAPHIC
ANATOMY

1

THE HEAD AND NECK

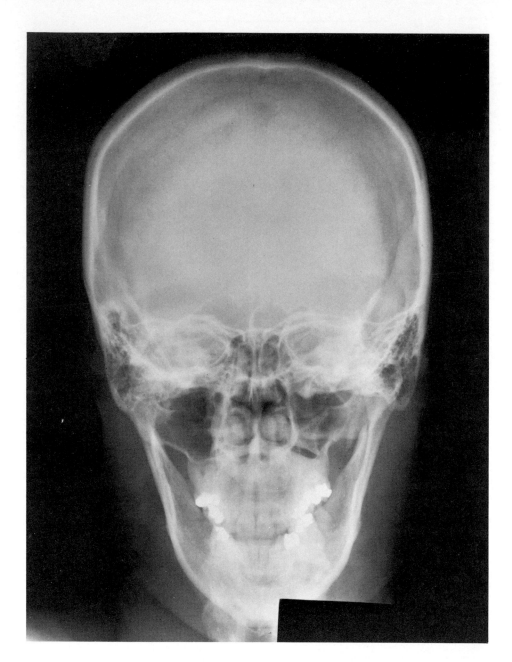

Figure 1

Posteroanterior radiograph of skull
(female aged 27 years).

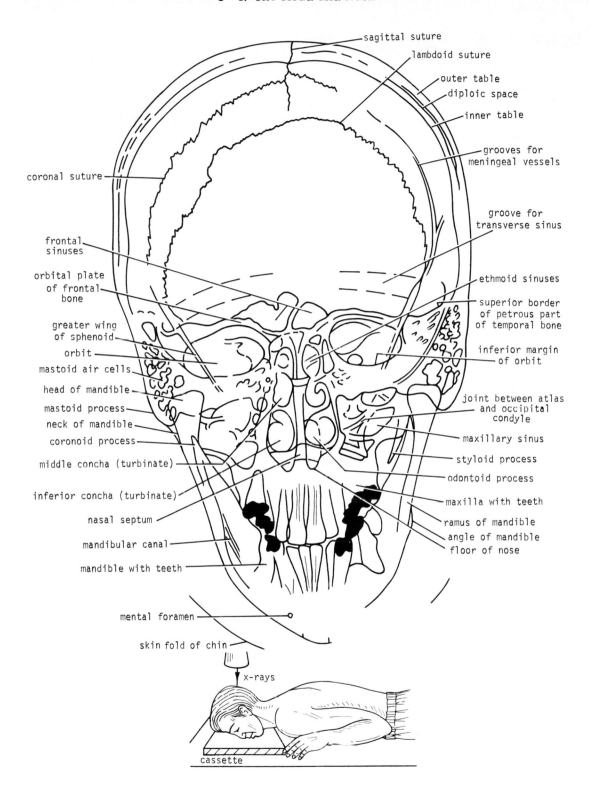

sagittal suture

lambdoid suture

outer table

diploic space

inner table

grooves for
meningeal vessels

groove for
transverse sinus

coronal suture

ethmoid sinuses

superior border
of petrous part
of temporal bone

inferior margin
of orbit

frontal
sinuses

orbital plate
of frontal
bone

greater wing
of sphenoid

orbit

mastoid air cells

head of mandible

mastoid process

neck of mandible

coronoid process

middle concha (turbinate)

inferior concha (turbinate)

nasal septum

mandibular canal

mandible with teeth

joint between atlas
and occipital
condyle

maxillary sinus

styloid process

odontoid process

maxilla with teeth

ramus of mandible

angle of mandible

floor of nose

mental foramen

skin fold of chin

x-rays

cassette

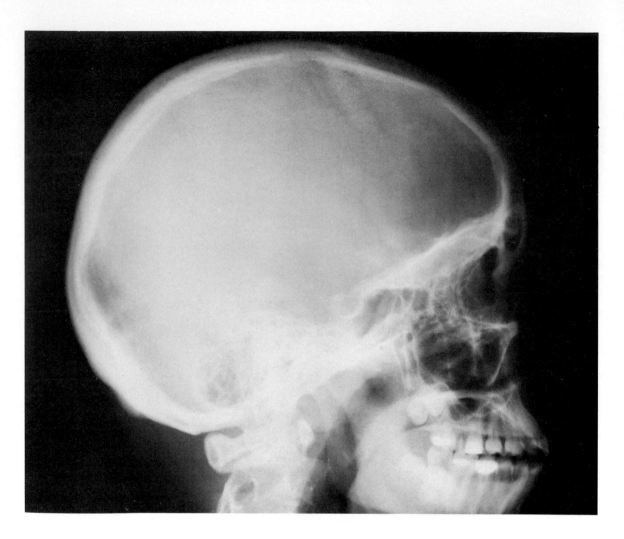

Figure 2

Lateral radiograph of skull
(female aged 17 years).

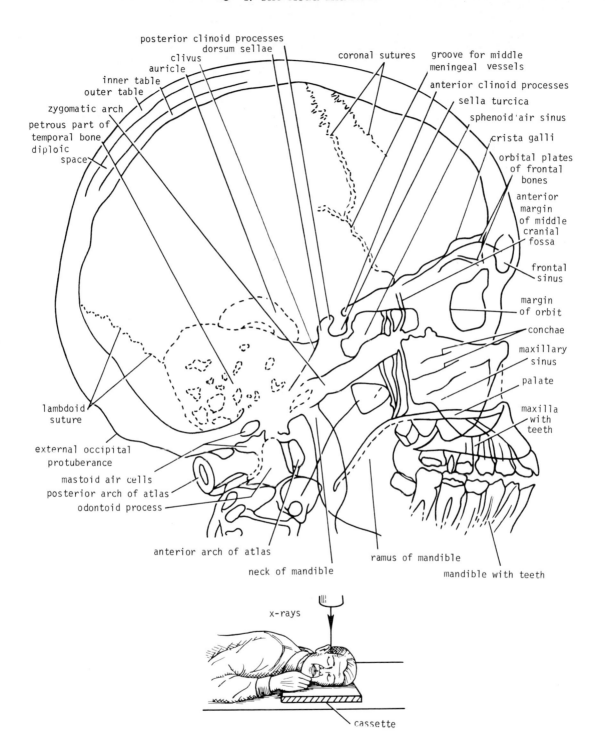

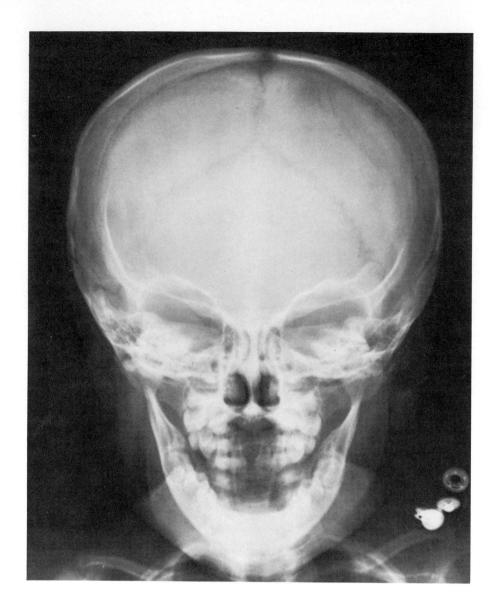

Figure 3

Posteroanterior radiograph of skull
(female aged 7 years).

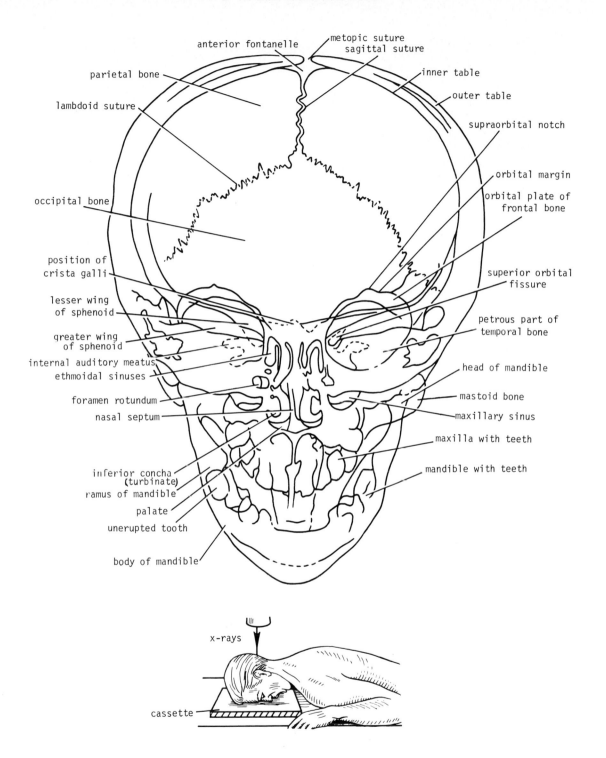

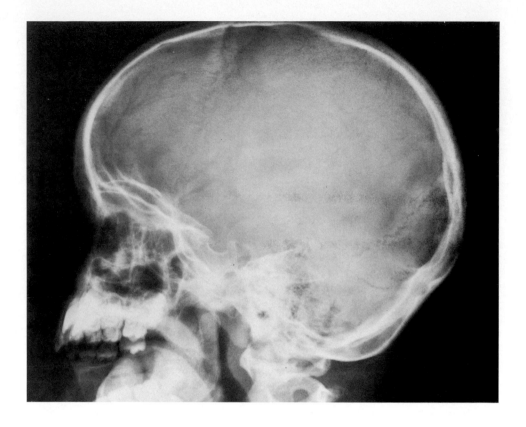

Figure 4

Lateral radiograph of skull
(male aged 6 years).

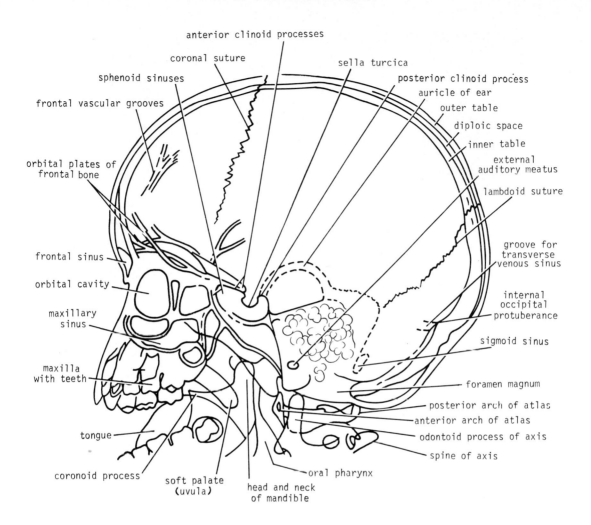

anterior clinoid processes

coronal suture

sphenoid sinuses

sella turcica

posterior clinoid process

frontal vascular grooves

auricle of ear

outer table

diploic space

inner table

external auditory meatus

orbital plates of frontal bone

lambdoid suture

frontal sinus

groove for transverse venous sinus

orbital cavity

internal occipital protuberance

maxillary sinus

sigmoid sinus

maxilla with teeth

foramen magnum

posterior arch of atlas

anterior arch of atlas

tongue

odontoid process of axis

spine of axis

coronoid process

soft palate (uvula)

head and neck of mandible

oral pharynx

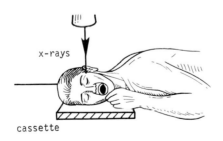

x-rays

cassette

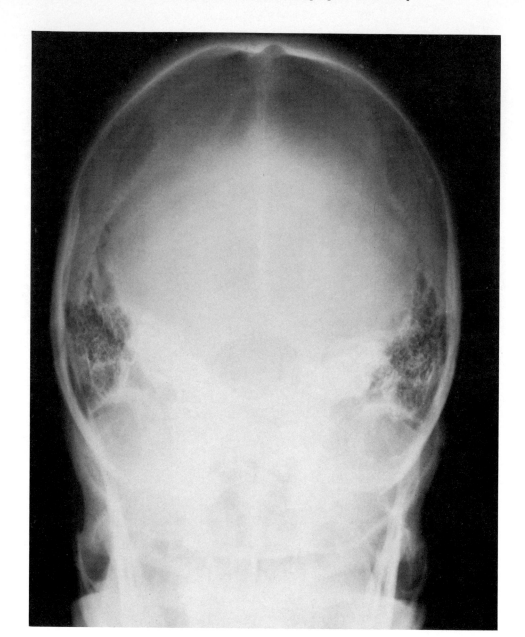

Figure 5

Anteroposterior angled
(Towne) radiograph of skull
(female aged 44 years).

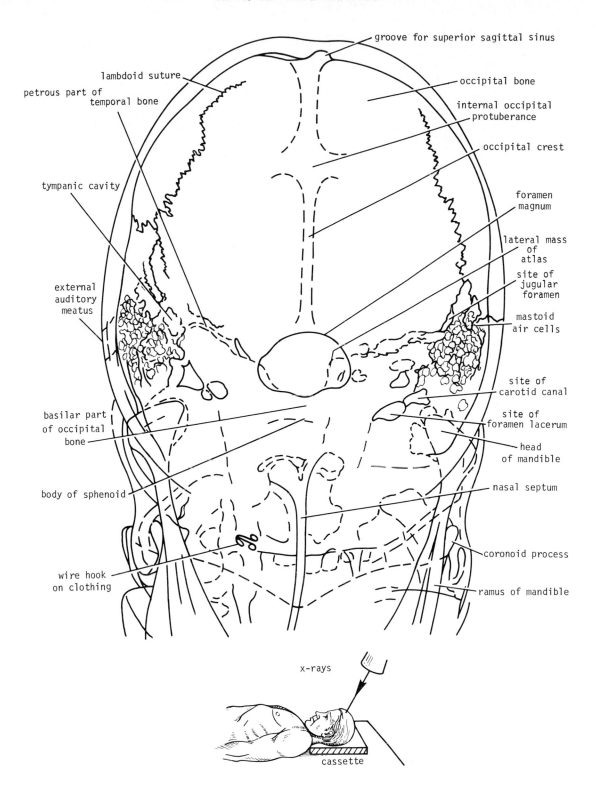

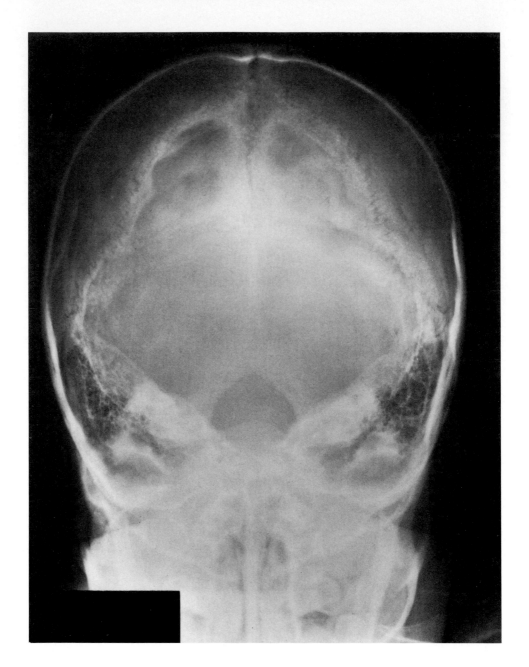

Figure 6

Anteroposterior
(Towne) radiograph of skull
(male aged 6 years).

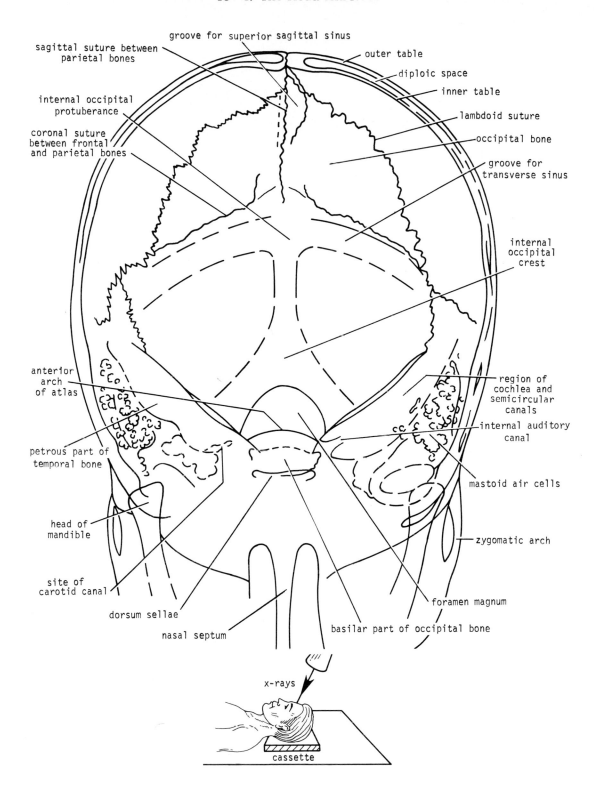

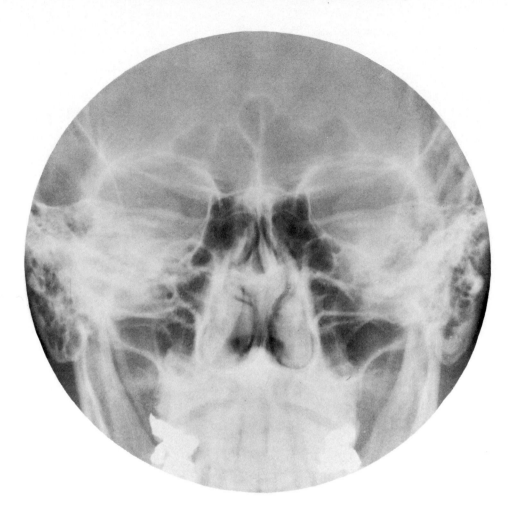

Figure 7

Posteroanterior
radiograph of paranasal sinuses
(male aged 36 years).

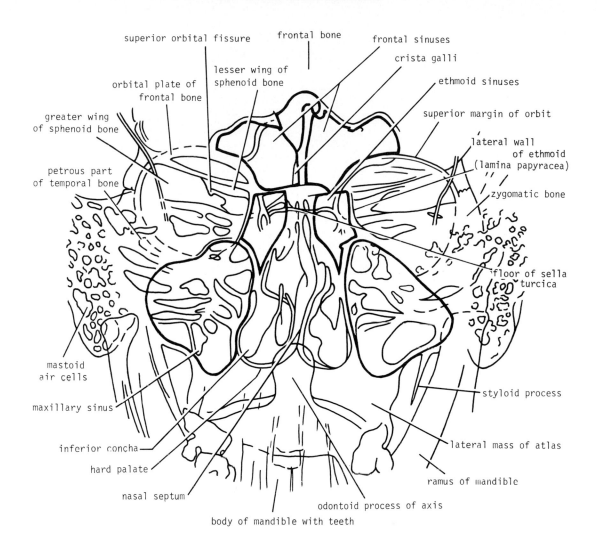

superior orbital fissure — frontal bone — frontal sinuses

crista galli

lesser wing of sphenoid bone

orbital plate of frontal bone

ethmoid sinuses

greater wing of sphenoid bone

superior margin of orbit

lateral wall of ethmoid (lamina papyracea)

petrous part of temporal bone

zygomatic bone

floor of sella turcica

mastoid air cells

maxillary sinus

styloid process

inferior concha

lateral mass of atlas

hard palate

ramus of mandible

nasal septum

odontoid process of axis

body of mandible with teeth

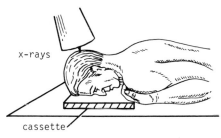

x-rays

cassette

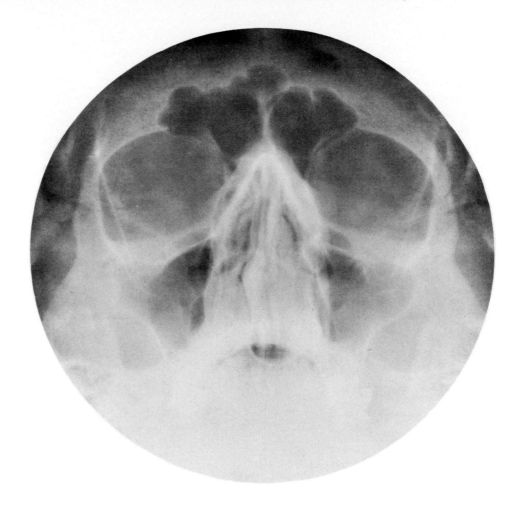

Figure 8

Posteroanterior (Waters)
radiograph of paranasal sinuses
(male aged 36 years).

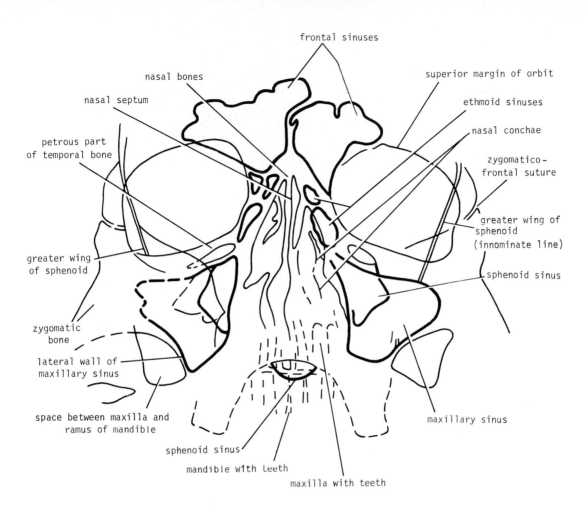

frontal sinuses

nasal bones

nasal septum

superior margin of orbit

ethmoid sinuses

nasal conchae

petrous part
of temporal bone

zygomatico-
frontal suture

greater wing of
sphenoid
(innominate line)

greater wing
of sphenoid

sphenoid sinus

zygomatic
bone

lateral wall of
maxillary sinus

space between maxilla and
ramus of mandible

maxillary sinus

sphenoid sinus

mandible with teeth

maxilla with teeth

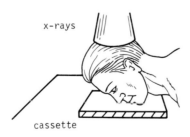

x-rays

cassette

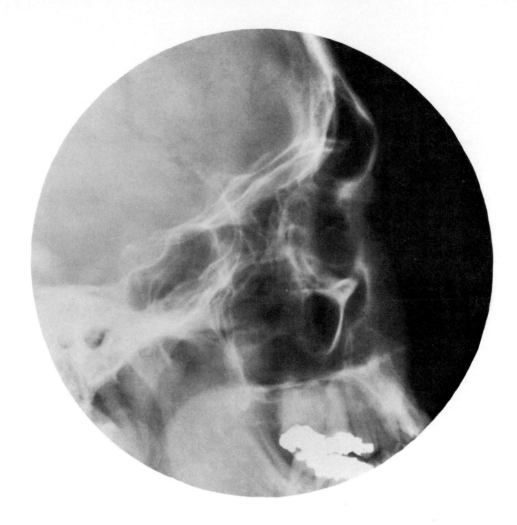

Figure 9

Lateral radiograph of paranasal sinuses
(male aged 36 years).

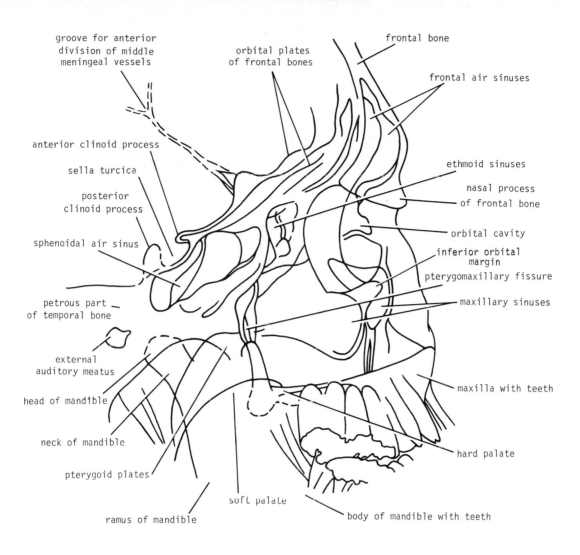

groove for anterior
division of middle
meningeal vessels

orbital plates
of frontal bones

frontal bone

frontal air sinuses

anterior clinoid process

ethmoid sinuses

sella turcica

nasal process
of frontal bone

posterior
clinoid process

orbital cavity

sphenoidal air sinus

inferior orbital
margin

pterygomaxillary fissure

petrous part
of temporal bone

maxillary sinuses

external
auditory meatus

head of mandible

maxilla with teeth

neck of mandible

hard palate

pterygoid plates

soft palate

ramus of mandible

body of mandible with teeth

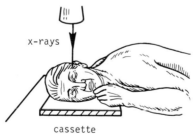

x-rays

cassette

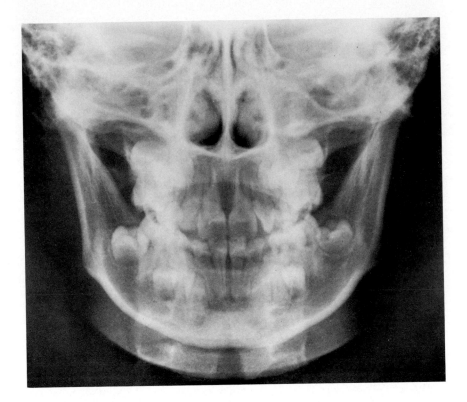

Figure 10

Posteroanterior
radiograph of mandible
(female aged 8 years).

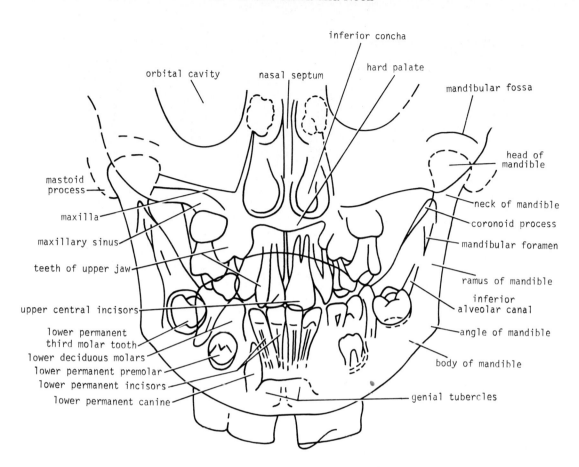

inferior concha

orbital cavity   nasal septum   hard palate

mandibular fossa

head of mandible

mastoid process

maxilla

maxillary sinus

teeth of upper jaw

upper central incisors

lower permanent third molar tooth

lower deciduous molars

lower permanent premolar

lower permanent incisors

lower permanent canine

neck of mandible

coronoid process

mandibular foramen

ramus of mandible

inferior alveolar canal

angle of mandible

body of mandible

genial tubercles

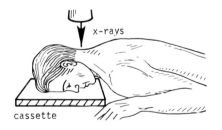

x-rays

cassette

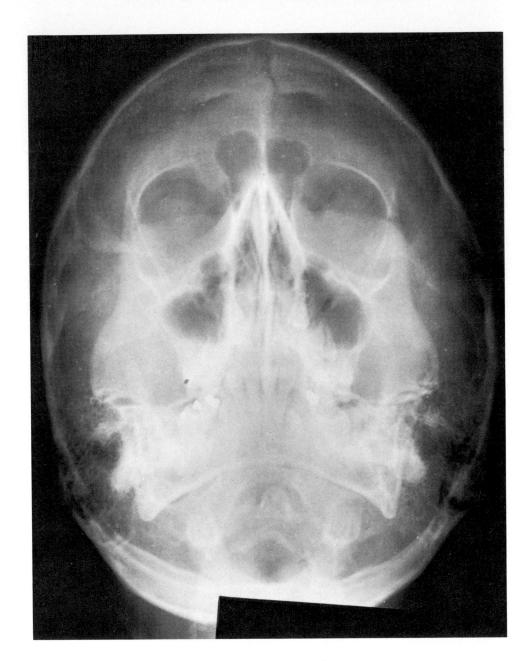

Figure 11

Posteroanterior (Waters)
radiograph of paranasal sinuses
(female aged 9 years).

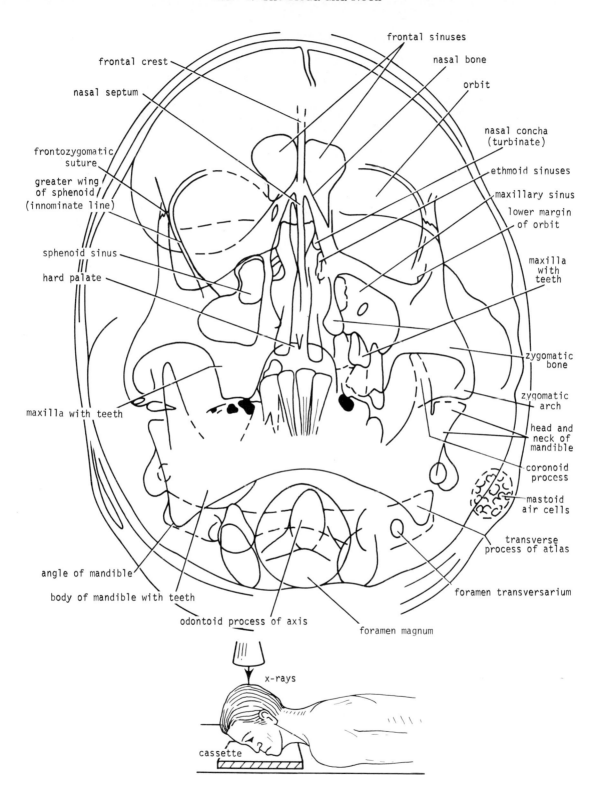

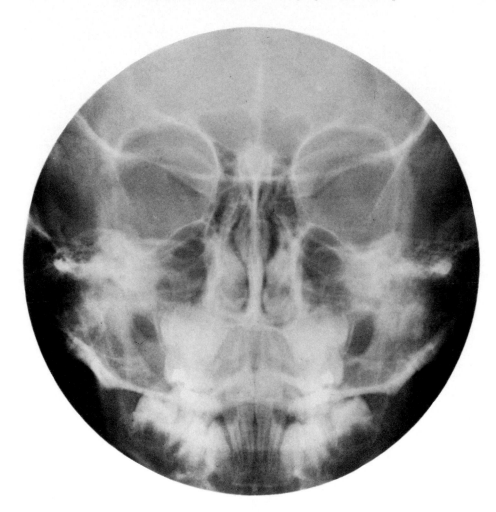

Figure 12

Posteroanterior (Caldwell)
radiograph of paranasal sinuses
(male aged 8 years).

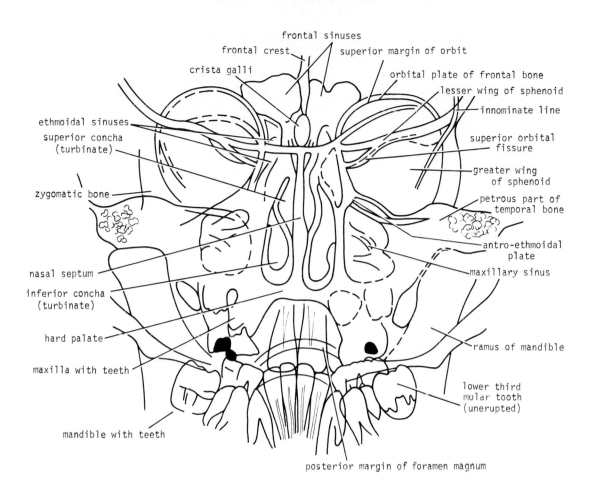

frontal sinuses
frontal crest
crista galli
superior margin of orbit
orbital plate of frontal bone
lesser wing of sphenoid
innominate line
ethmoidal sinuses
superior concha (turbinate)
superior orbital fissure
greater wing of sphenoid
zygomatic bone
petrous part of temporal bone
antro-ethmoidal plate
nasal septum
maxillary sinus
inferior concha (turbinate)
hard palate
ramus of mandible
maxilla with teeth
lower third molar tooth (unerupted)
mandible with teeth
posterior margin of foramen magnum

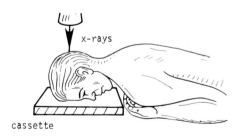

x-rays

cassette

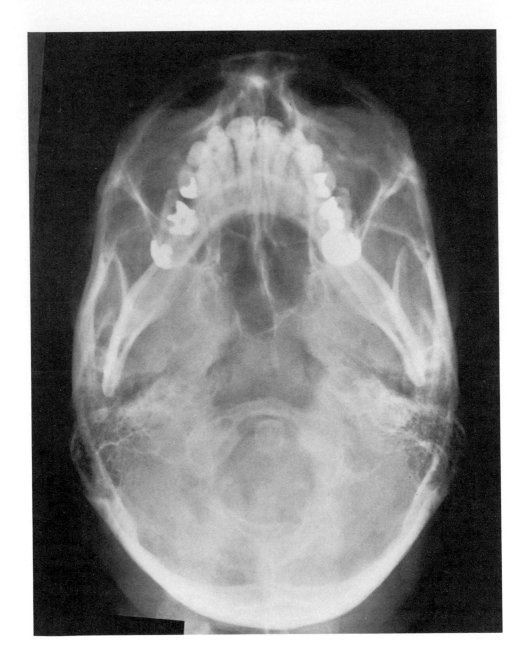

Figure 13

Submentovertical radiograph of skull
(female aged 31 years).

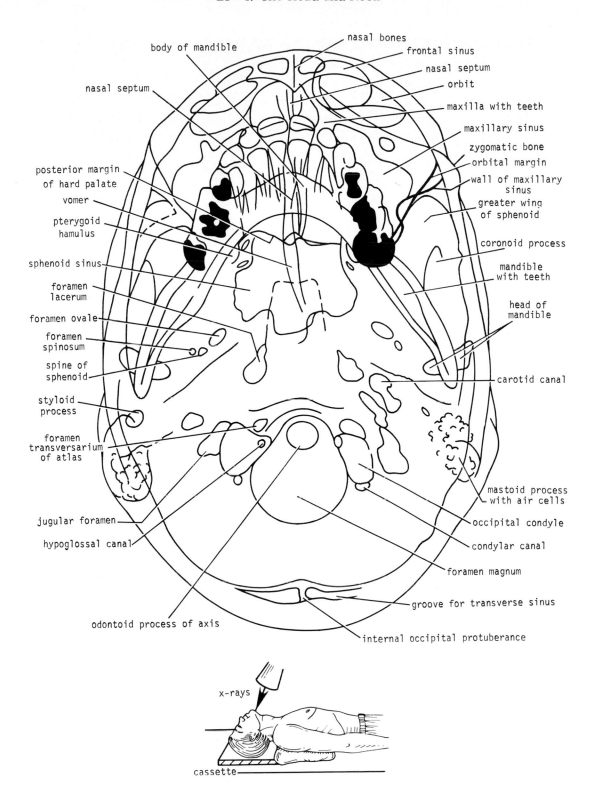

body of mandible

nasal bones

frontal sinus

nasal septum

orbit

maxilla with teeth

maxillary sinus

zygomatic bone

orbital margin

wall of maxillary sinus

greater wing of sphenoid

coronoid process

mandible with teeth

head of mandible

carotid canal

nasal septum

posterior margin of hard palate

vomer

pterygoid hamulus

sphenoid sinus

foramen lacerum

foramen ovale

foramen spinosum

spine of sphenoid

styloid process

foramen transversarium of atlas

jugular foramen

hypoglossal canal

odontoid process of axis

mastoid process with air cells

occipital condyle

condylar canal

foramen magnum

groove for transverse sinus

internal occipital protuberance

x-rays

cassette

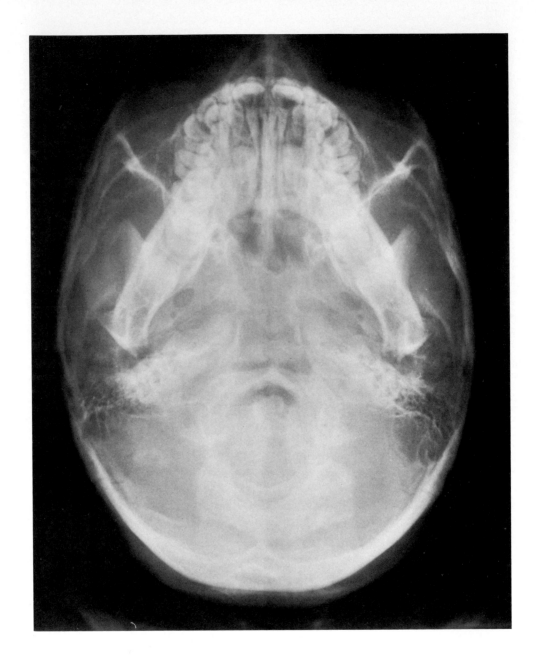

Figure 14

Submentovertical radiograph of skull
(male aged 6 years).

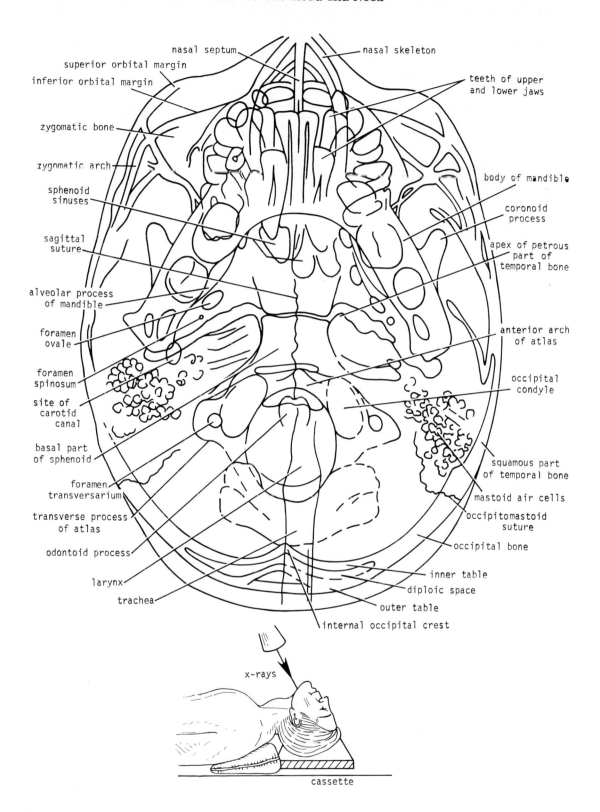

nasal septum

nasal skeleton

superior orbital margin

inferior orbital margin

teeth of upper and lower jaws

zygomatic bone

zygomatic arch

body of mandible

sphenoid sinuses

coronoid process

sagittal suture

apex of petrous part of temporal bone

alveolar process of mandible

anterior arch of atlas

foramen ovale

foramen spinosum

occipital condyle

site of carotid canal

basal part of sphenoid

squamous part of temporal bone

foramen transversarium

mastoid air cells

transverse process of atlas

occipitomastoid suture

odontoid process

occipital bone

larynx

inner table

trachea

diploic space

outer table

internal occipital crest

x-rays

cassette

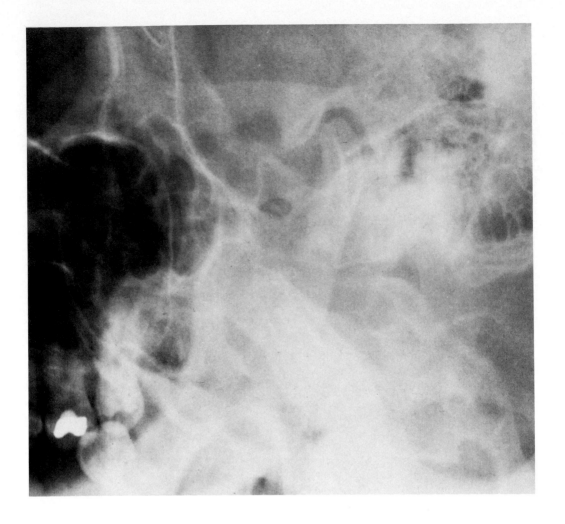

Figure 15

Lateral radiograph of temporomandibular
joint with mouth closed
(male aged 29 years).

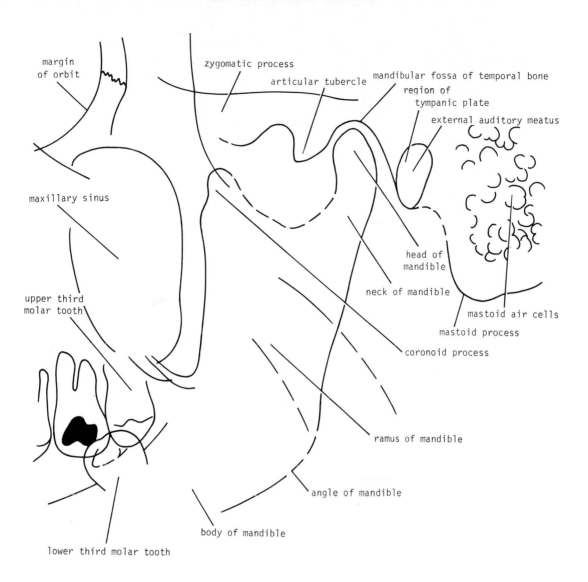

margin
of orbit

zygomatic process

articular tubercle

mandibular fossa of temporal bone

region of
tympanic plate

external auditory meatus

maxillary sinus

head of
mandible

neck of mandible

mastoid air cells

mastoid process

upper third
molar tooth

coronoid process

ramus of mandible

angle of mandible

body of mandible

lower third molar tooth

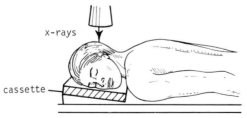

x-rays

cassette

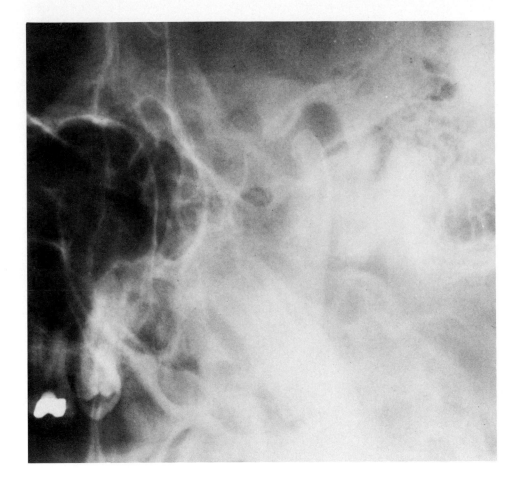

Figure 16

Lateral radiograph of temporomandibular
joint with mouth open
(male aged 29 years).

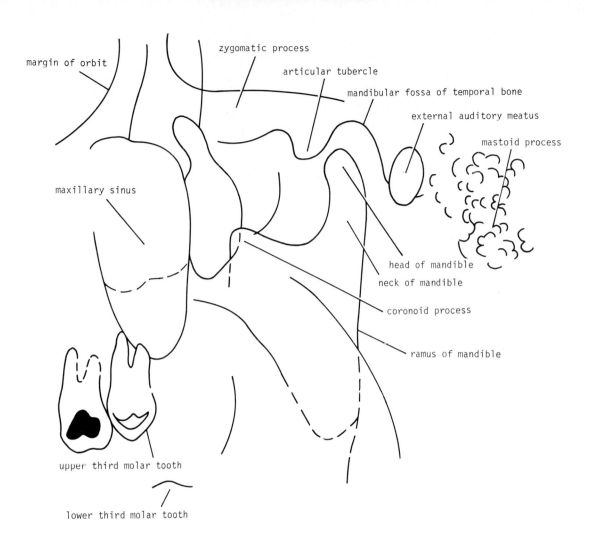

margin of orbit

zygomatic process

articular tubercle

mandibular fossa of temporal bone

external auditory meatus

mastoid process

maxillary sinus

head of mandible

neck of mandible

coronoid process

ramus of mandible

upper third molar tooth

lower third molar tooth

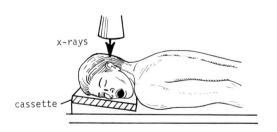

x-rays

cassette

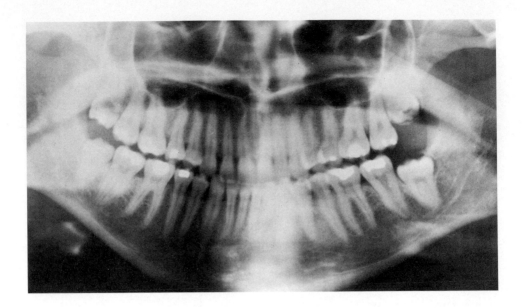

Figure 17

Panorex dental film of teeth
(female aged 20 years).

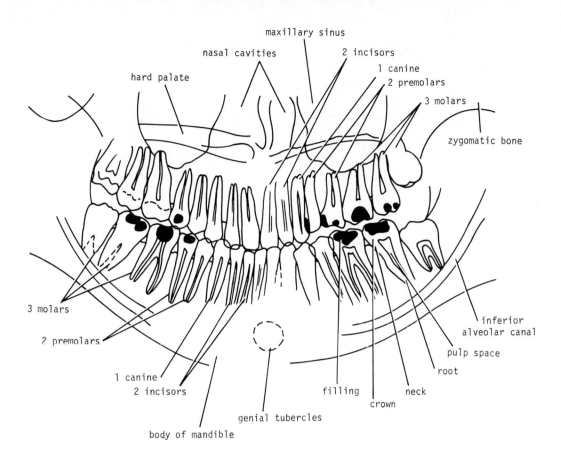

maxillary sinus

nasal cavities

2 incisors

hard palate

1 canine

2 premolars

3 molars

zygomatic bone

3 molars

2 premolars

1 canine

2 incisors

body of mandible

genial tubercles

filling

crown

neck

root

pulp space

inferior alveolar canal

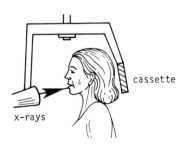

cassette

x-rays

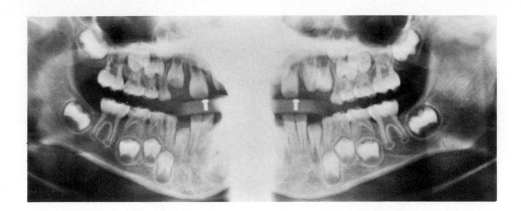

Figure 18

Panorex dental film of teeth
(male aged 9 years).

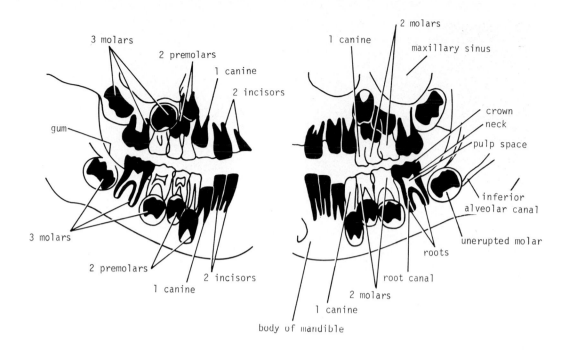

3 molars
2 premolars
1 canine
2 incisors
gum
3 molars
2 premolars
1 canine
2 incisors

1 canine
2 molars
maxillary sinus
crown
neck
pulp space
inferior
alveolar canal
unerupted molar
roots
root canal
2 molars
1 canine
body of mandible

permanent teeth = ■

deciduous teeth = □

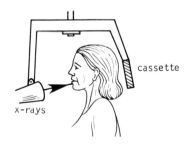

cassette
x-rays

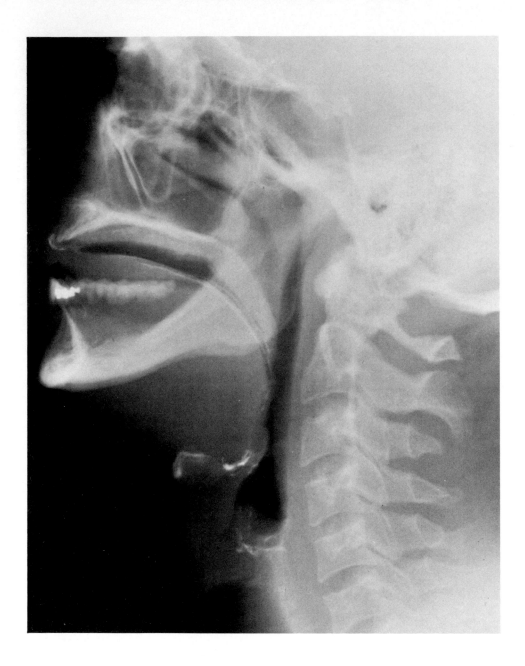

Figure 19

Lateral radiograph of the head and neck
showing the nose and pharynx
(female aged 45 years).

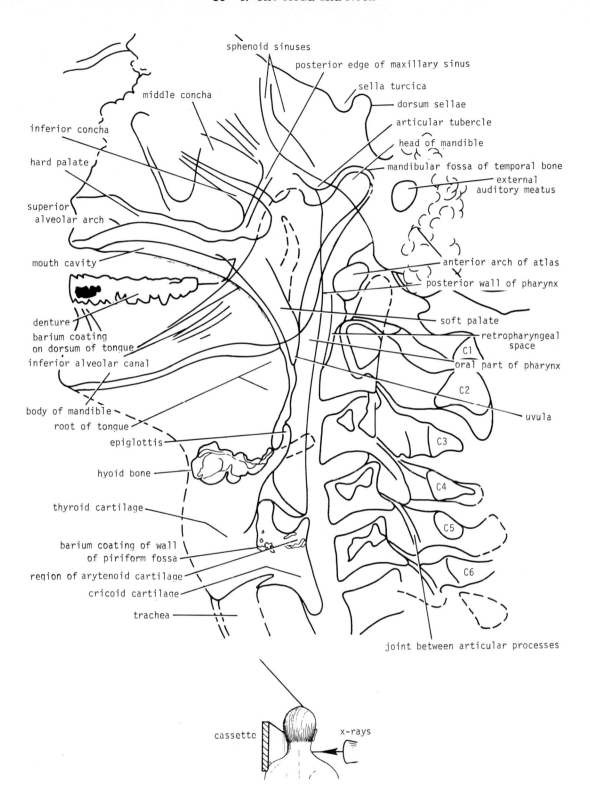

sphenoid sinuses

posterior edge of maxillary sinus

sella turcica

middle concha

dorsum sellae

articular tubercle

inferior concha

head of mandible

mandibular fossa of temporal bone

hard palate

external auditory meatus

superior alveolar arch

anterior arch of atlas

posterior wall of pharynx

mouth cavity

soft palate

retropharyngeal space

denture

C1

barium coating on dorsum of tongue

oral part of pharynx

inferior alveolar canal

C2

body of mandible

uvula

root of tongue

epiglottis

C3

hyoid bone

C4

thyroid cartilage

C5

barium coating of wall of piriform fossa

region of arytenoid cartilage

C6

cricoid cartilage

trachea

joint between articular processes

cassette   x-rays

THE UPPER LIMB

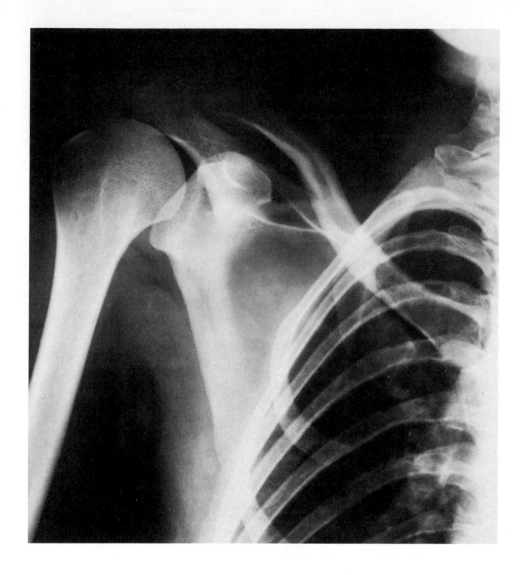

Figure 1

Anteroposterior
radiograph of shoulder region
(female aged 30 years).

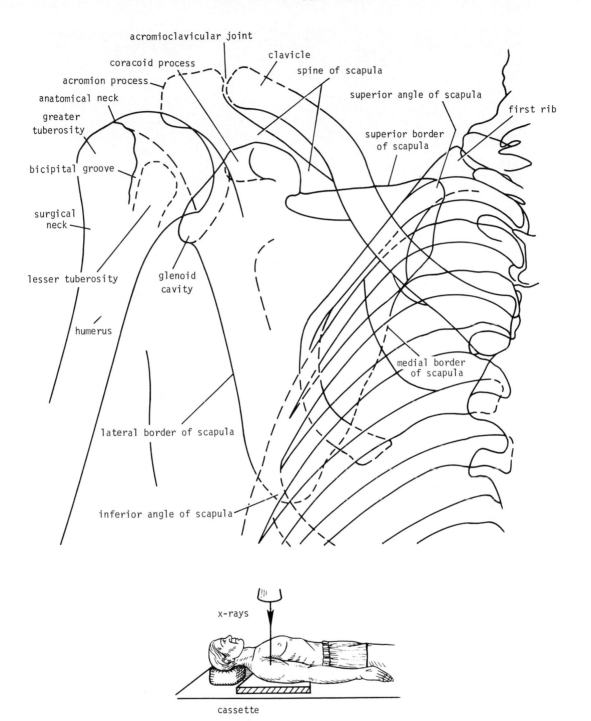

acromioclavicular joint

coracoid process

clavicle

spine of scapula

acromion process

anatomical neck

superior angle of scapula

greater
tuberosity

first rib

superior border
of scapula

bicipital groove

surgical
neck

lesser tuberosity

glenoid
cavity

humerus

medial border
of scapula

lateral border of scapula

inferior angle of scapula

x-rays

cassette

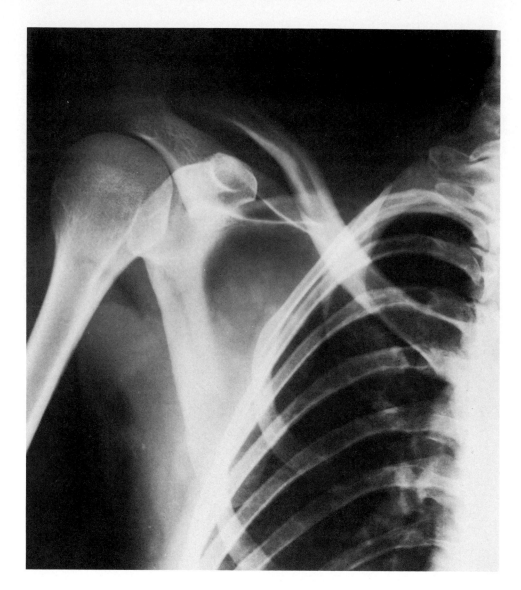

Figure 2

Anteroposterior
radiograph of shoulder region with
medial rotation of the humerus
(female aged 30 years).

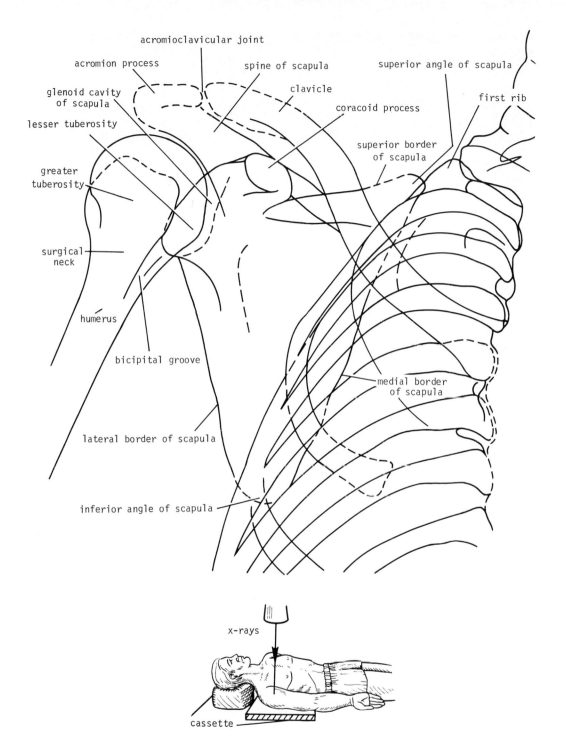

acromioclavicular joint

acromion process

glenoid cavity
of scapula

spine of scapula

clavicle

superior angle of scapula

first rib

lesser tuberosity

coracoid process

superior border
of scapula

greater
tuberosity

surgical
neck

humerus

bicipital groove

medial border
of scapula

lateral border of scapula

inferior angle of scapula

x-rays

cassette

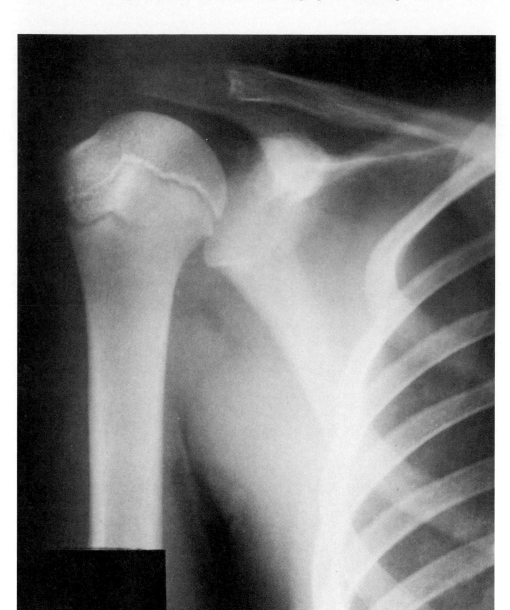

Figure 3

Anteroposterior
radiograph of shoulder region
(female aged 11 years).

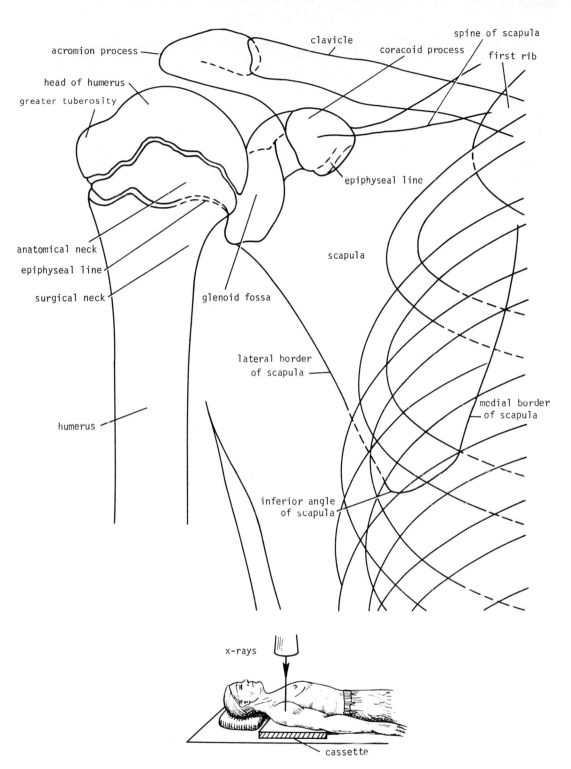

acromion process

head of humerus

greater tuberosity

clavicle

coracoid process

spine of scapula

first rib

epiphyseal line

anatomical neck

epiphyseal line

surgical neck

glenoid fossa

scapula

humerus

lateral border
of scapula

medial border
of scapula

inferior angle
of scapula

x-rays

cassette

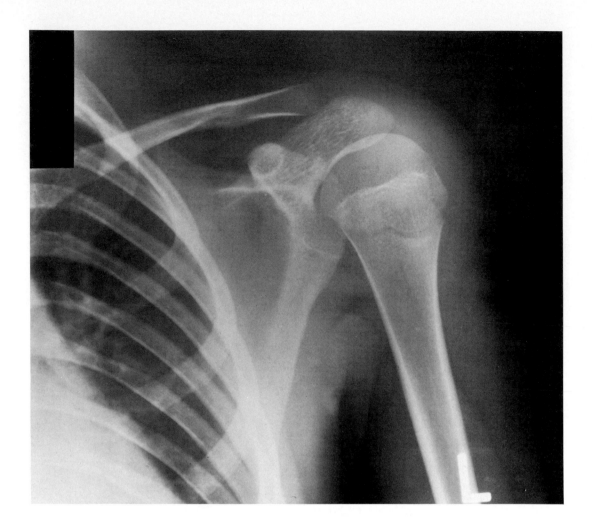

Figure 4

Anteroposterior
radiograph of shoulder region with
medial rotation of the humerus
(female aged 12 years).

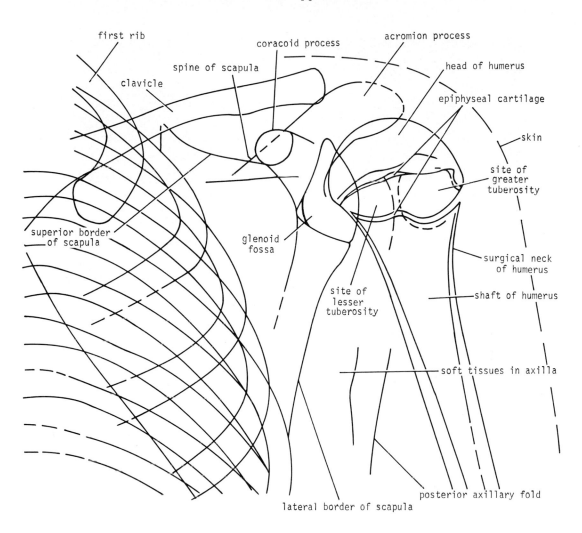

first rib

clavicle

spine of scapula

coracoid process

acromion process

head of humerus

epiphyseal cartilage

skin

site of greater tuberosity

superior border of scapula

glenoid fossa

site of lesser tuberosity

surgical neck of humerus

shaft of humerus

soft tissues in axilla

posterior axillary fold

lateral border of scapula

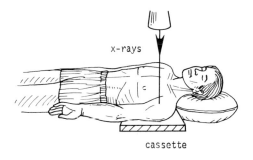

x-rays

cassette

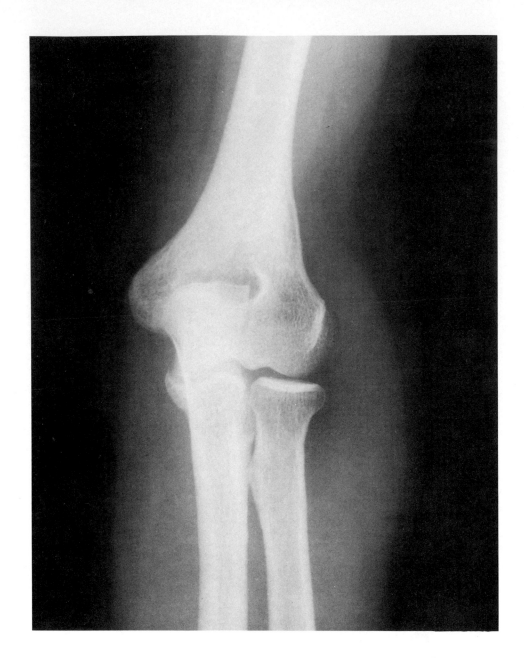

Figure 5

Anteroposterior
radiograph of elbow region
(female aged 49 years).

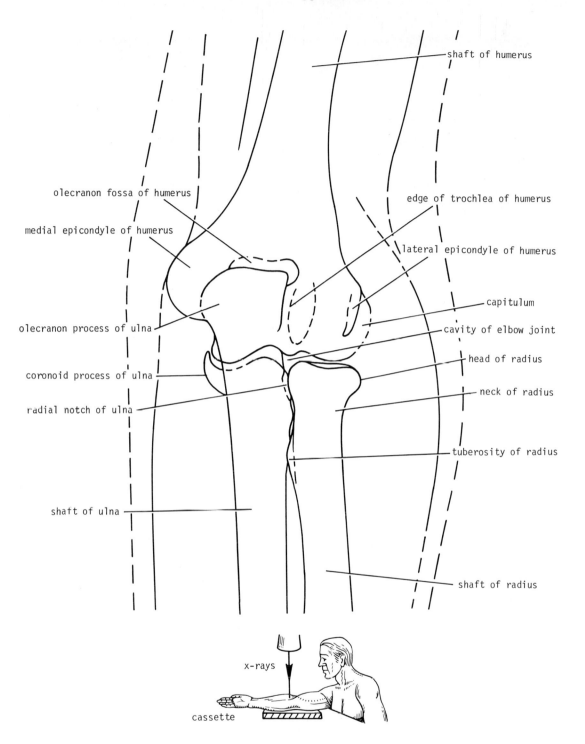

shaft of humerus

olecranon fossa of humerus

medial epicondyle of humerus

edge of trochlea of humerus

lateral epicondyle of humerus

capitulum

olecranon process of ulna

cavity of elbow joint

head of radius

coronoid process of ulna

neck of radius

radial notch of ulna

tuberosity of radius

shaft of ulna

shaft of radius

x-rays

cassette

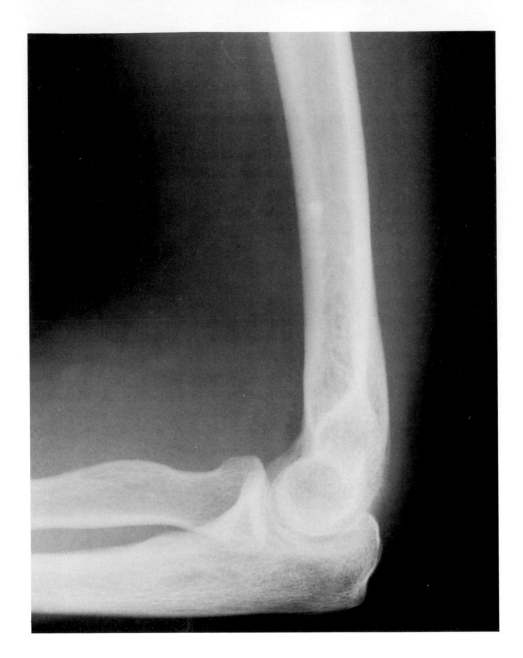

Figure 6

Lateral radiograph of elbow region
(female aged 49 years).

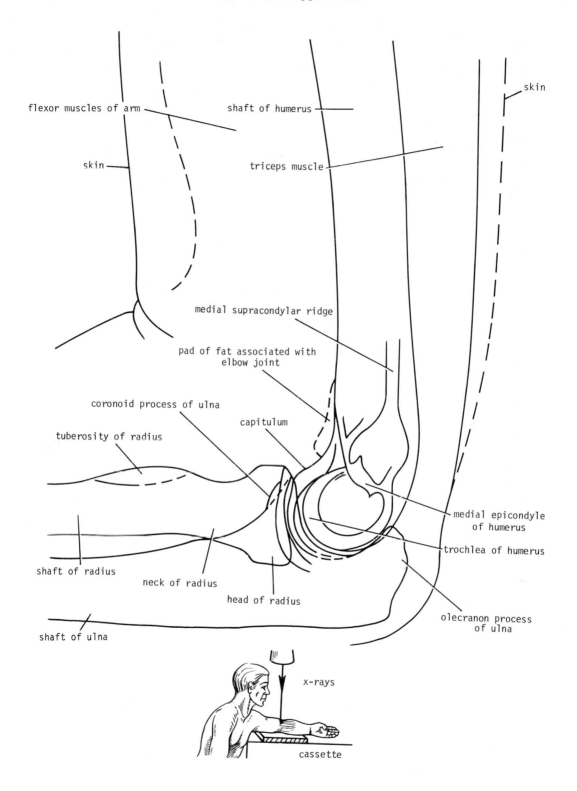

flexor muscles of arm

shaft of humerus

skin

skin

triceps muscle

medial supracondylar ridge

pad of fat associated with
elbow joint

coronoid process of ulna

capitulum

tuberosity of radius

medial epicondyle
of humerus

shaft of radius

trochlea of humerus

neck of radius

head of radius

olecranon process
of ulna

shaft of ulna

x-rays

cassette

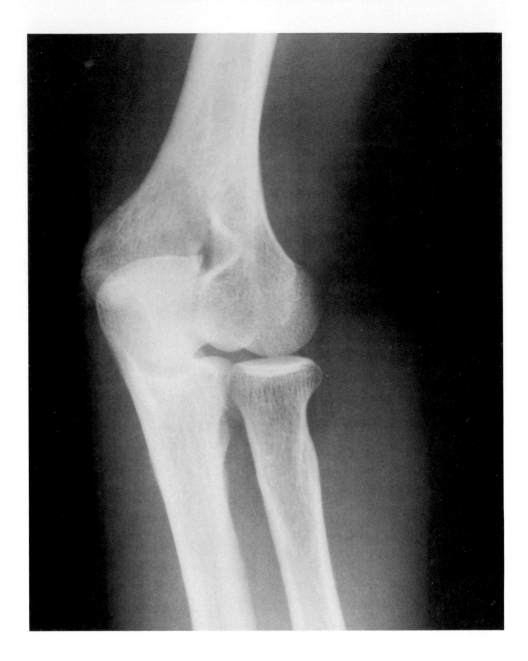

Figure 7

Oblique radiograph of elbow region
(female aged 49 years).

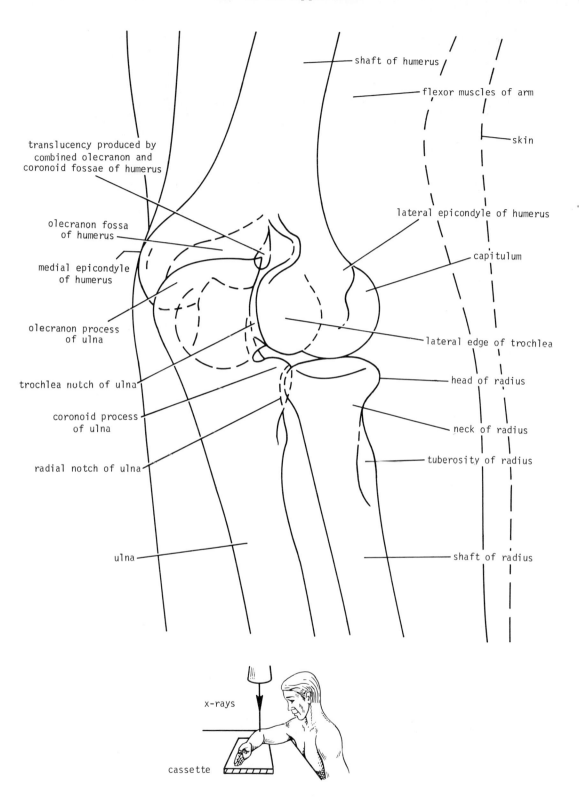

shaft of humerus

flexor muscles of arm

skin

translucency produced by combined olecranon and coronoid fossae of humerus

lateral epicondyle of humerus

olecranon fossa of humerus

capitulum

medial epicondyle of humerus

olecranon process of ulna

lateral edge of trochlea

trochlea notch of ulna

head of radius

coronoid process of ulna

neck of radius

radial notch of ulna

tuberosity of radius

ulna

shaft of radius

x-rays

cassette

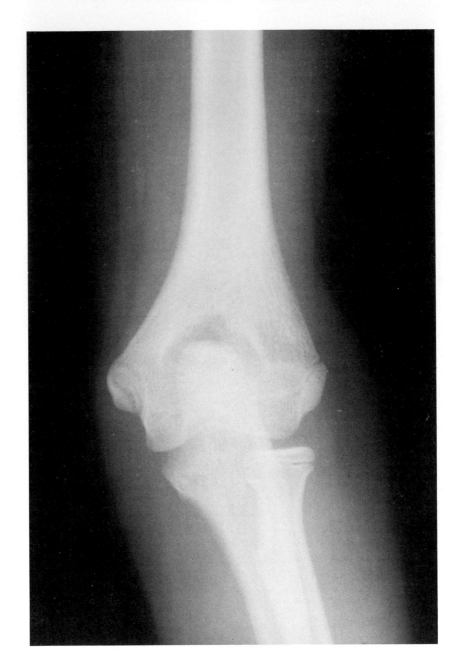

Figure 8

Anteroposterior
radiograph of elbow region
(female aged 11 years).

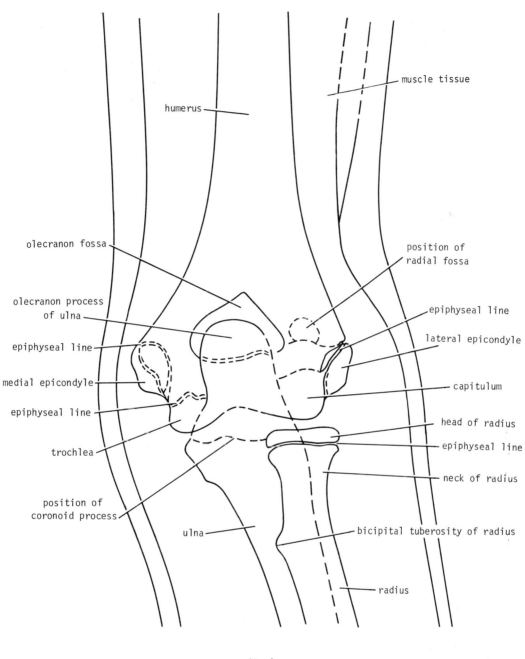

muscle tissue

humerus

olecranon fossa

position of
radial fossa

olecranon process
of ulna

epiphyseal line

epiphyseal line

lateral epicondyle

medial epicondyle

capitulum

epiphyseal line

head of radius

epiphyseal line

trochlea

neck of radius

position of
coronoid process

ulna

bicipital tuberosity of radius

radius

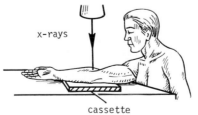

x-rays

cassette

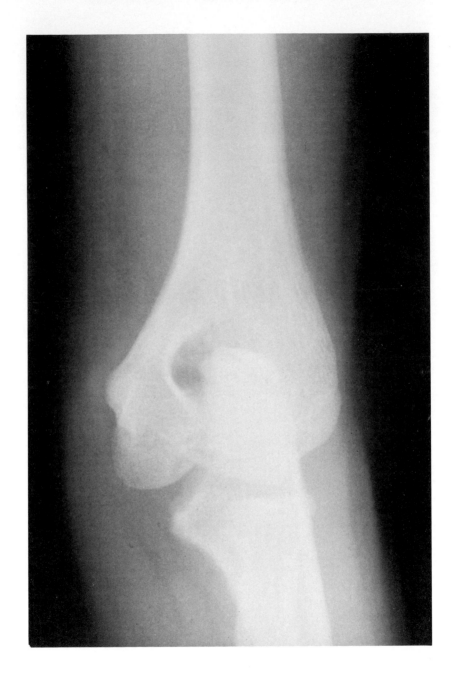

Figure 9

Anteroposterior
oblique radiograph of elbow region
with forearm semipronated
(female aged 11 years).

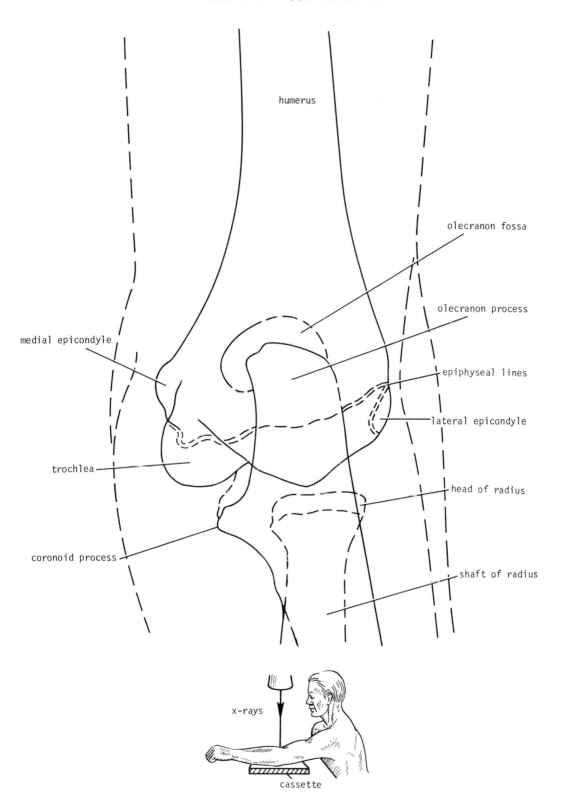

humerus

olecranon fossa

olecranon process

medial epicondyle

epiphyseal lines

lateral epicondyle

trochlea

head of radius

coronoid process

shaft of radius

x-rays

cassette

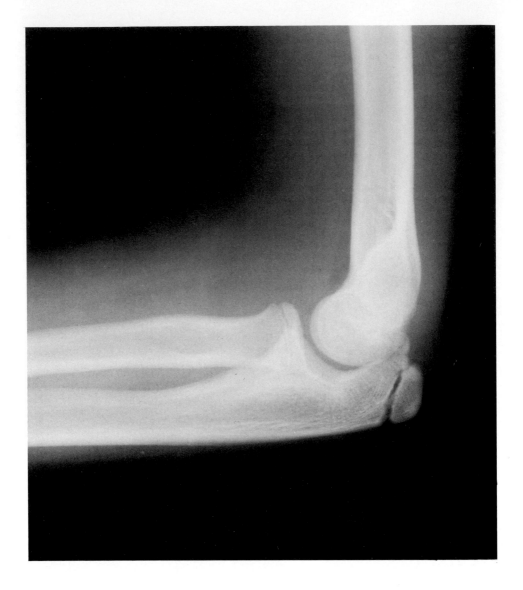

Figure 10

Lateral radiograph of elbow region
(female aged 11 years).

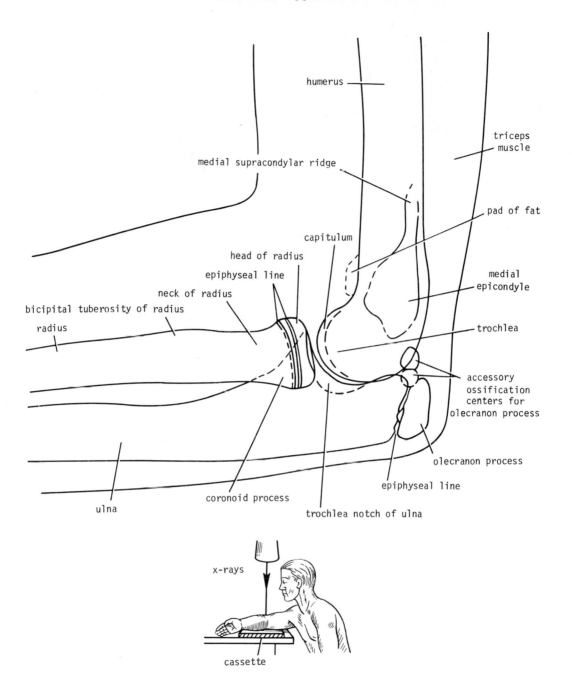

humerus

triceps muscle

medial supracondylar ridge

pad of fat

capitulum

head of radius

epiphyseal line

medial epicondyle

neck of radius

bicipital tuberosity of radius

radius

trochlea

accessory ossification centers for olecranon process

olecranon process

epiphyseal line

coronoid process

ulna

trochlea notch of ulna

x-rays

cassette

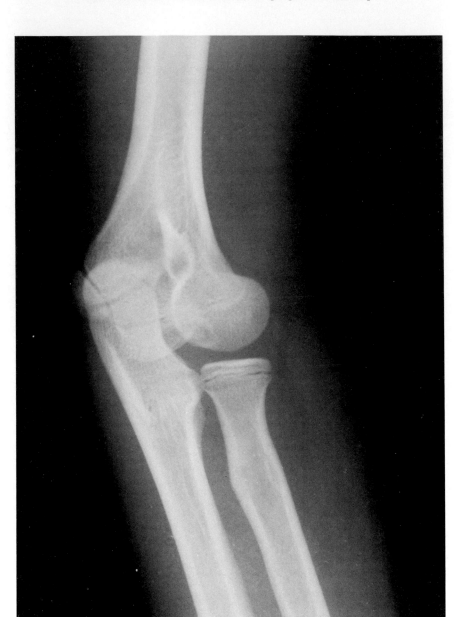

Figure 11

Oblique radiograph of elbow region
(female aged 11 years).

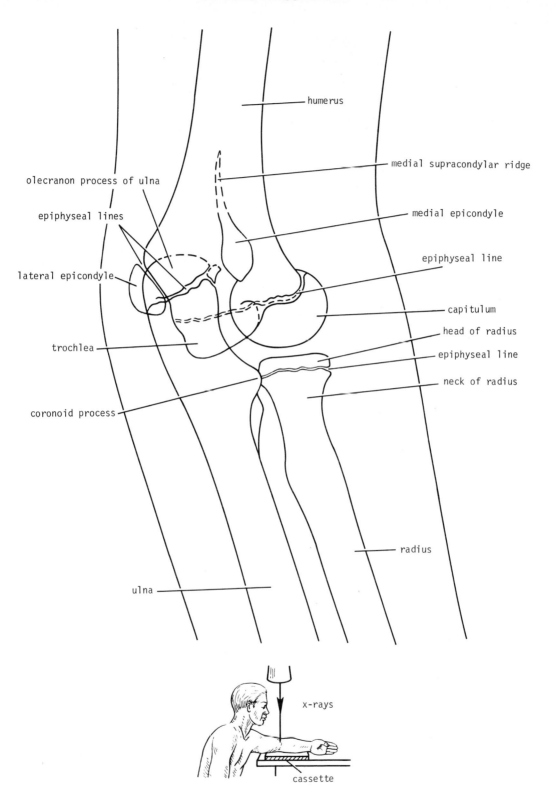

humerus

medial supracondylar ridge

olecranon process of ulna

medial epicondyle

epiphyseal lines

epiphyseal line

lateral epicondyle

capitulum

head of radius

epiphyseal line

trochlea

neck of radius

coronoid process

radius

ulna

x-rays

cassette

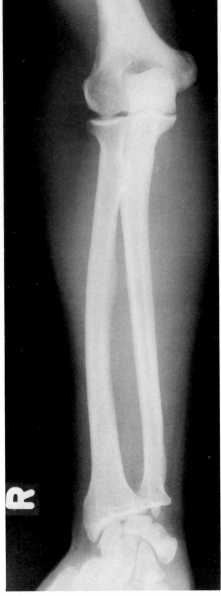

Figure 12

Anteroposterior radiograph of forearm
(male aged 65 years).

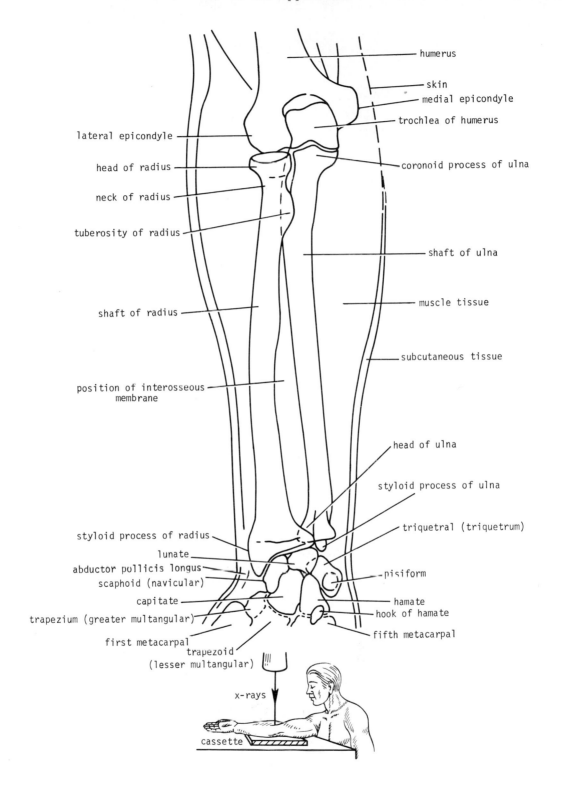

humerus

skin

medial epicondyle

trochlea of humerus

lateral epicondyle

head of radius

coronoid process of ulna

neck of radius

tuberosity of radius

shaft of ulna

muscle tissue

shaft of radius

subcutaneous tissue

position of interosseous
membrane

head of ulna

styloid process of ulna

triquetral (triquetrum)

styloid process of radius

lunate

abductor pollicis longus

scaphoid (navicular)

capitate

trapezium (greater multangular)

first metacarpal

trapezoid
(lesser multangular)

pisiform

hamate

hook of hamate

fifth metacarpal

x-rays

cassette

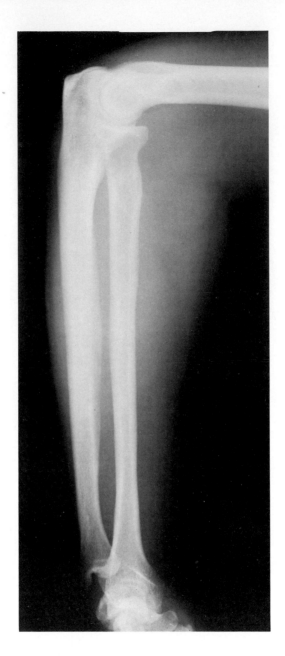

Figure 13

Lateral radiograph of forearm
(male aged 65 years).

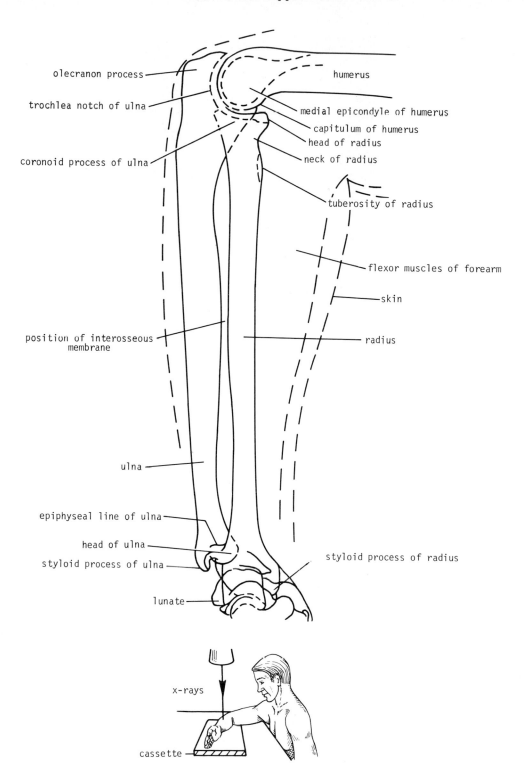

olecranon process

trochlea notch of ulna

coronoid process of ulna

humerus

medial epicondyle of humerus

capitulum of humerus

head of radius

neck of radius

tuberosity of radius

flexor muscles of forearm

skin

position of interosseous membrane

radius

ulna

epiphyseal line of ulna

head of ulna

styloid process of ulna

styloid process of radius

lunate

x-rays

cassette

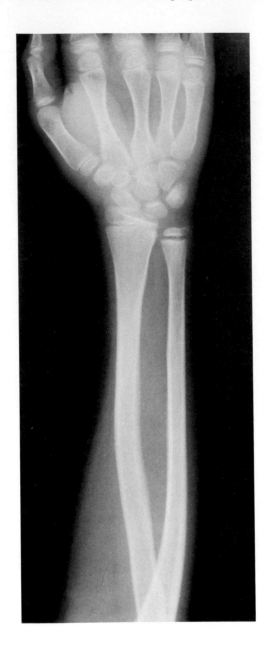

Figure 14

Posteroanterior
radiograph of pronated forearm
(male aged 10 years).

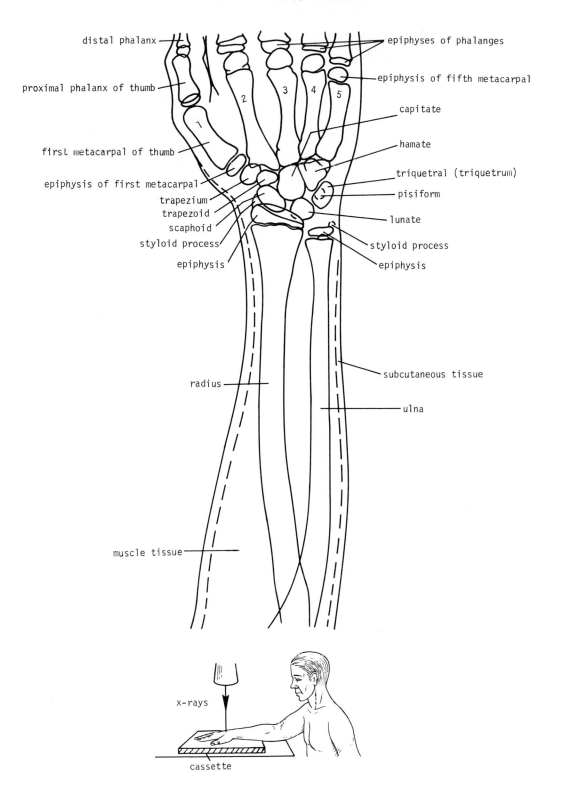

distal phalanx

epiphyses of phalanges

proximal phalanx of thumb

epiphysis of fifth metacarpal

capitate

first metacarpal of thumb

hamate

epiphysis of first metacarpal

triquetral (triquetrum)

trapezium

pisiform

trapezoid

lunate

scaphoid

styloid process

styloid process

epiphysis

epiphysis

subcutaneous tissue

radius

ulna

muscle tissue

x-rays

cassette

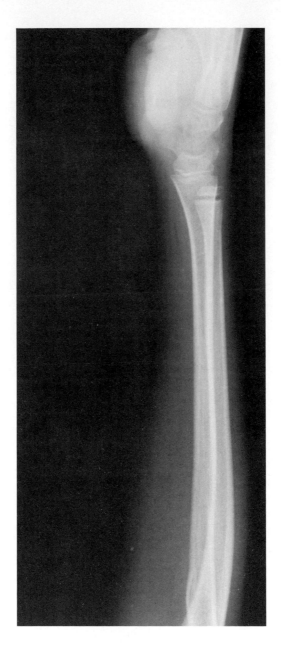

Figure 15

Lateral radiograph of forearm
(male aged 10 years).

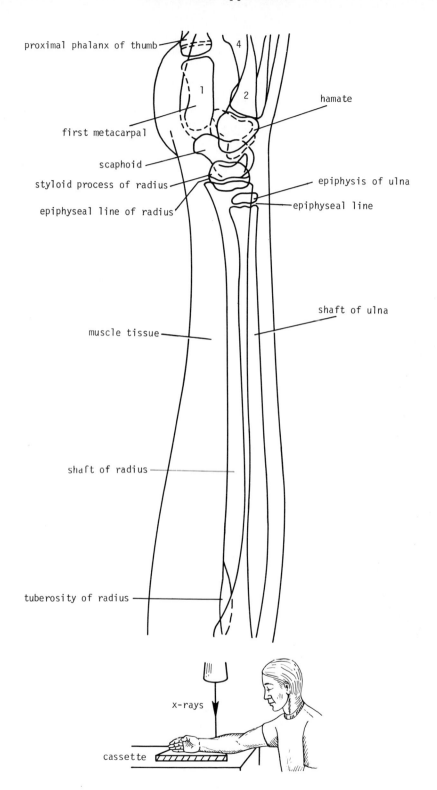

proximal phalanx of thumb

4

hamate

1

2

first metacarpal

scaphoid

styloid process of radius

epiphysis of ulna

epiphyseal line of radius

epiphyseal line

shaft of ulna

muscle tissue

shaft of radius

tuberosity of radius

x-rays

cassette

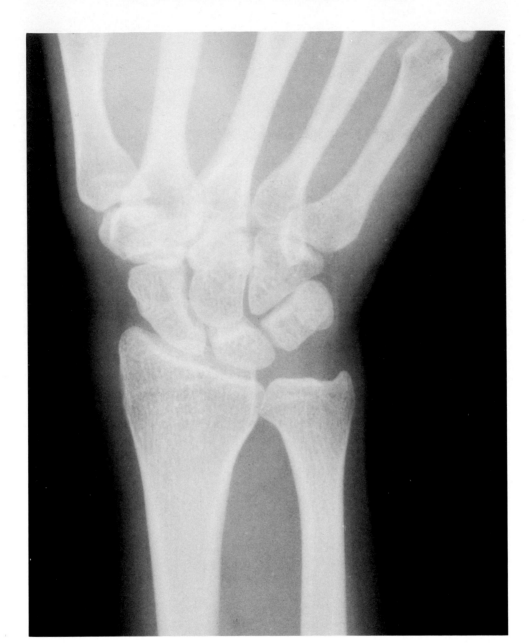

Figure 16

Posteroanterior radiograph of
the wrist with forearm pronated
(male aged 24 years).

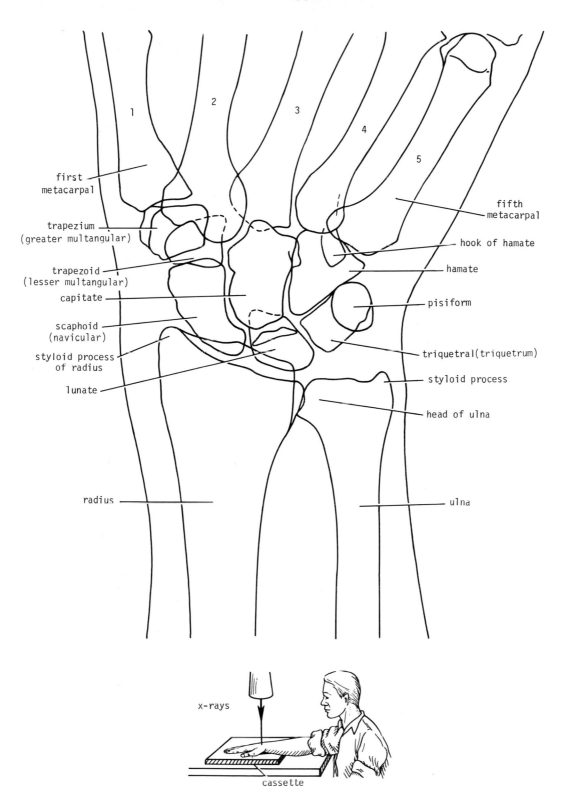

1

2

3

4

5

first
metacarpal

fifth
metacarpal

trapezium
(greater multangular)

hook of hamate

trapezoid
(lesser multangular)

hamate

capitate

pisiform

scaphoid
(navicular)

styloid process
of radius

triquetral (triquetrum)

styloid process

lunate

head of ulna

radius

ulna

x-rays

cassette

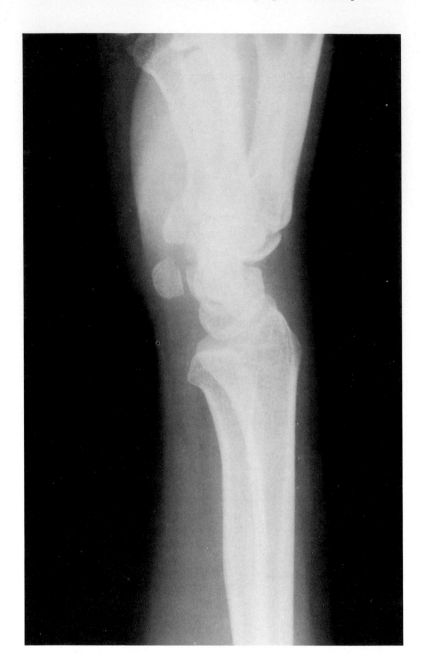

Figure 17

Lateral radiograph of the wrist
(male aged 24 years).

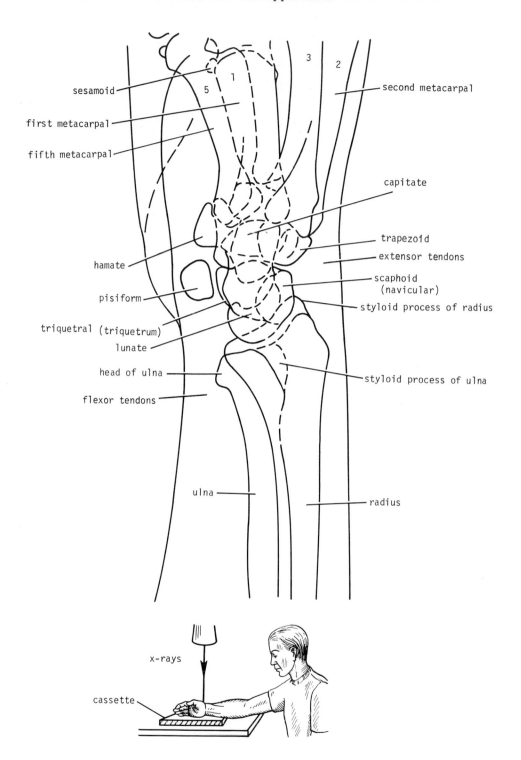

sesamoid

first metacarpal

fifth metacarpal

second metacarpal

capitate

trapezoid

extensor tendons

hamate

scaphoid
(navicular)

pisiform

styloid process of radius

triquetral (triquetrum)

lunate

head of ulna

styloid process of ulna

flexor tendons

ulna

radius

x-rays

cassette

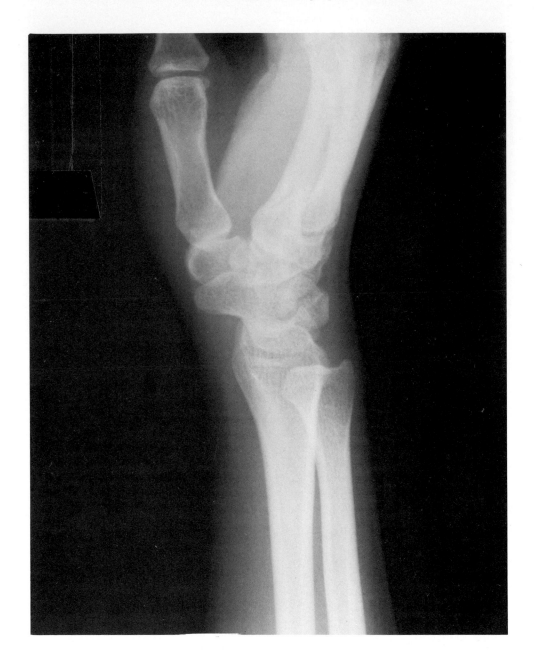

Figure 18

Oblique radiograph of the wrist
(male aged 24 years).

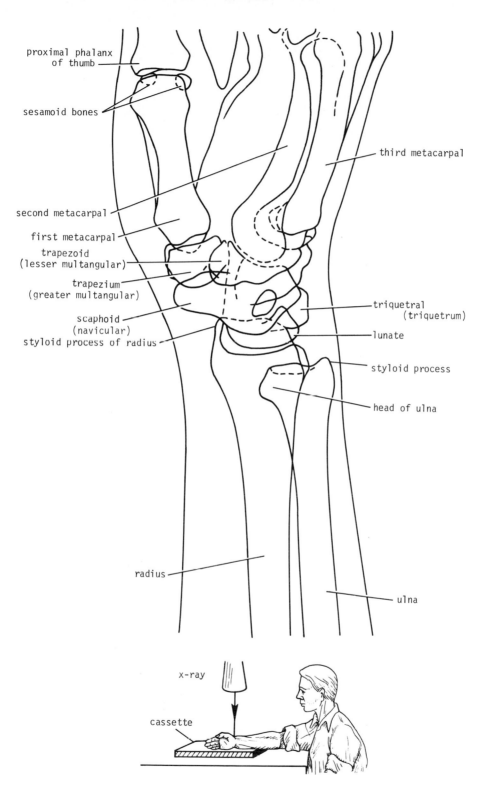

proximal phalanx
of thumb

sesamoid bones

third metacarpal

second metacarpal

first metacarpal

trapezoid
(lesser multangular)

trapezium
(greater multangular)

triquetral
(triquetrum)

scaphoid
(navicular)

lunate

styloid process of radius

styloid process

head of ulna

radius

ulna

x-ray

cassette

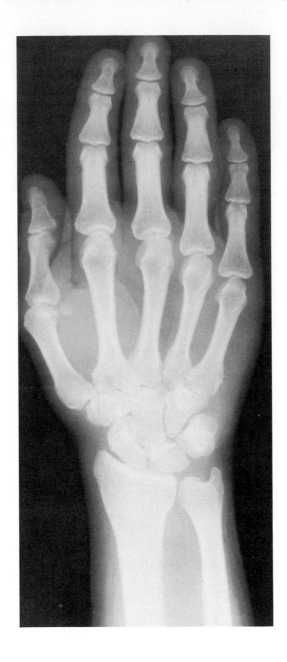

Figure 19

Posteroanterior radiograph of the hand
(male aged 28 years).

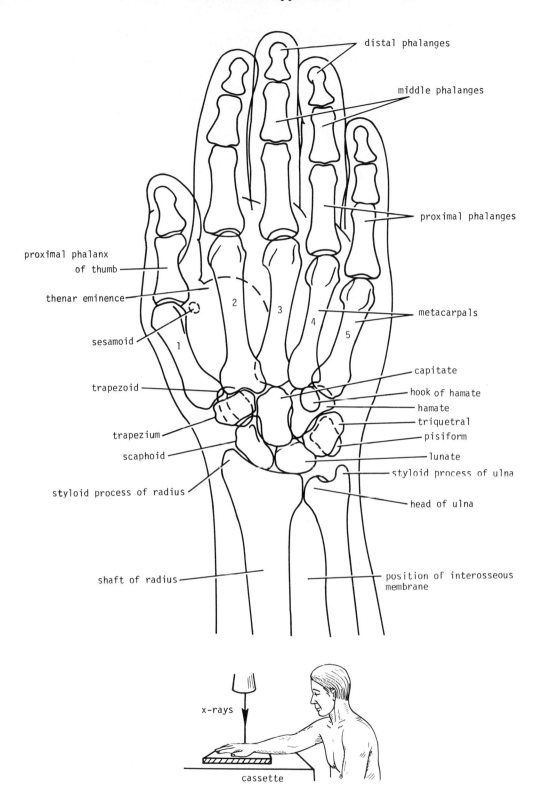

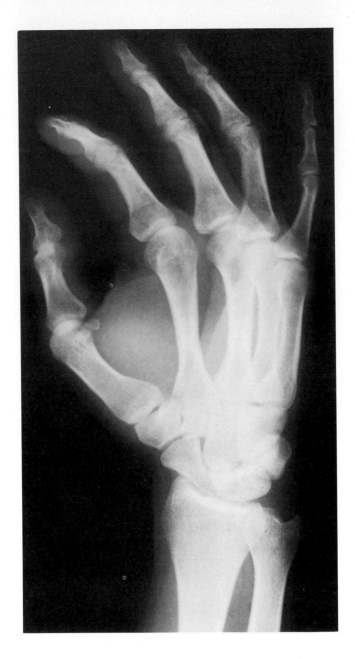

Figure 20

Oblique radiograph of the hand
(male aged 27 years).

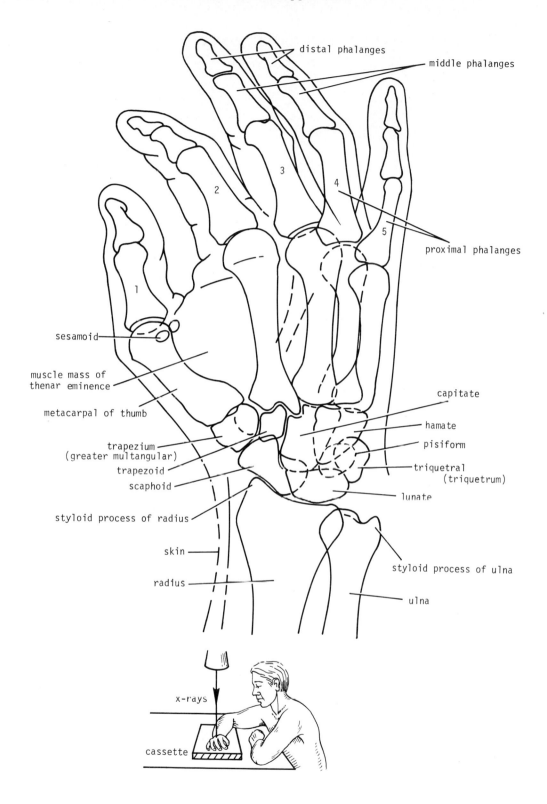

distal phalanges

middle phalanges

proximal phalanges

sesamoid

muscle mass of
thenar eminence

metacarpal of thumb

trapezium
(greater multangular)

trapezoid

scaphoid

styloid process of radius

skin

radius

capitate

hamate

pisiform

triquetral
(triquetrum)

lunate

styloid process of ulna

ulna

x-rays

cassette

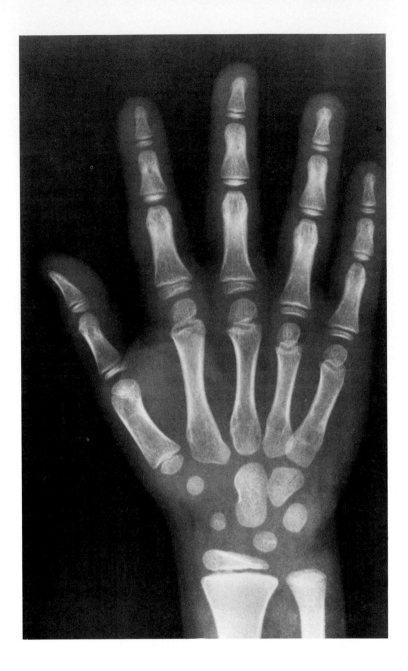

Figure 21

Posteroanterior radiograph of the hand
(male aged 8 years).

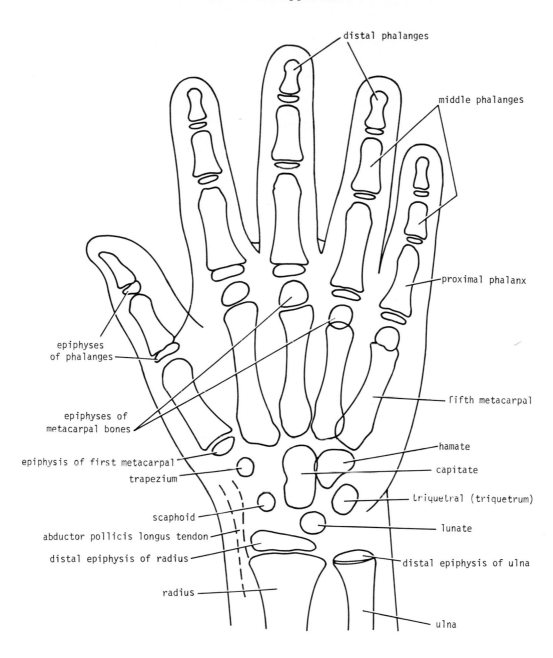

distal phalanges

middle phalanges

proximal phalanx

epiphyses
of phalanges

epiphyses of
metacarpal bones

fifth metacarpal

epiphysis of first metacarpal

trapezium

hamate

capitate

triquetral (triquetrum)

scaphoid

abductor pollicis longus tendon

distal epiphysis of radius

lunate

distal epiphysis of ulna

radius

ulna

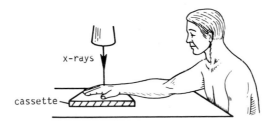

x-rays

cassette

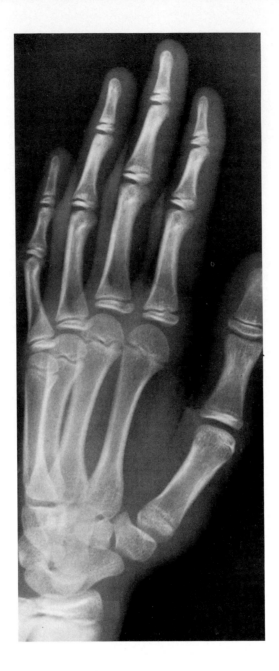

Figure 22

Oblique radiograph of the hand
(male aged 13 years).

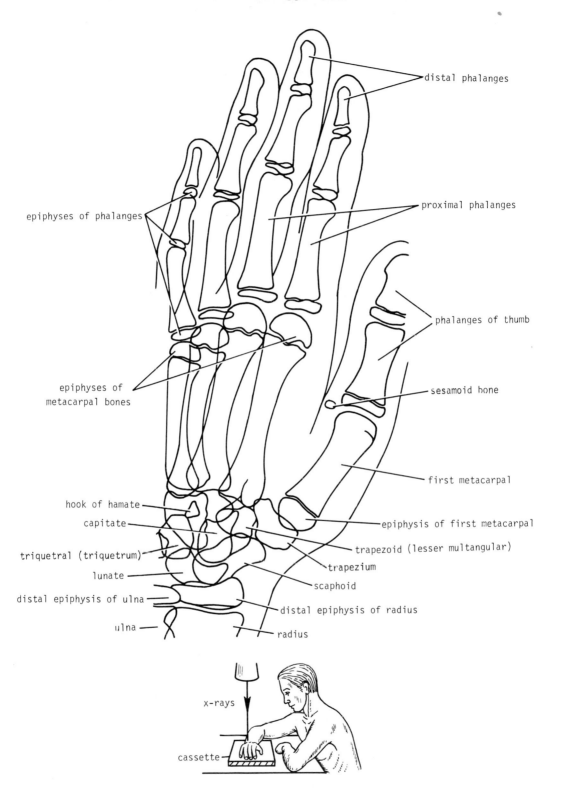

distal phalanges

proximal phalanges

epiphyses of phalanges

phalanges of thumb

epiphyses of
metacarpal bones

sesamoid hone

first metacarpal

hook of hamate

epiphysis of first metacarpal

capitate

trapezoid (lesser multangular)

triquetral (triquetrum)

trapezium

lunate

scaphoid

distal epiphysis of ulna

distal epiphysis of radius

ulna

radius

x-rays

cassette

3

THE THORAX

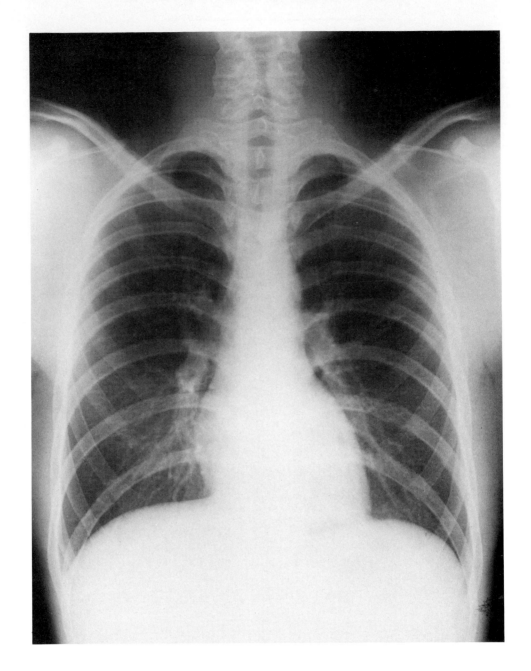

Figure 1

Posteroanterior radiograph of thorax
(male aged 20 years).

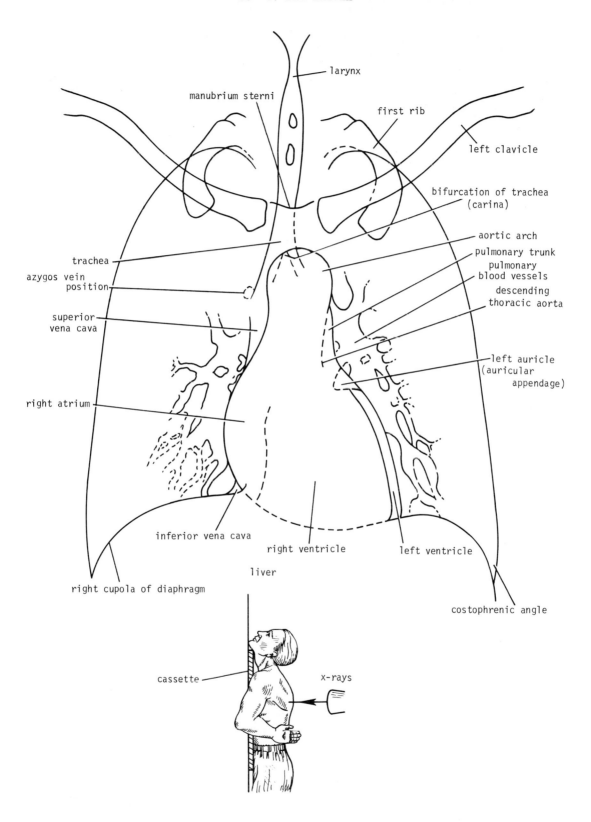

larynx

manubrium sterni

first rib

left clavicle

bifurcation of trachea
(carina)

aortic arch

pulmonary trunk

pulmonary
blood vessels

descending
thoracic aorta

trachea

azygos vein
position

superior
vena cava

left auricle
(auricular
appendage)

right atrium

inferior vena cava

right ventricle

left ventricle

liver

right cupola of diaphragm

costophrenic angle

cassette

x-rays

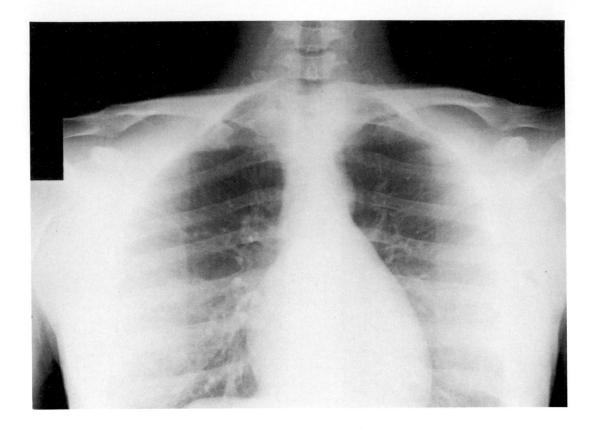

Figure 2

Apical lordotic radiograph of thorax
(female aged 30 years).

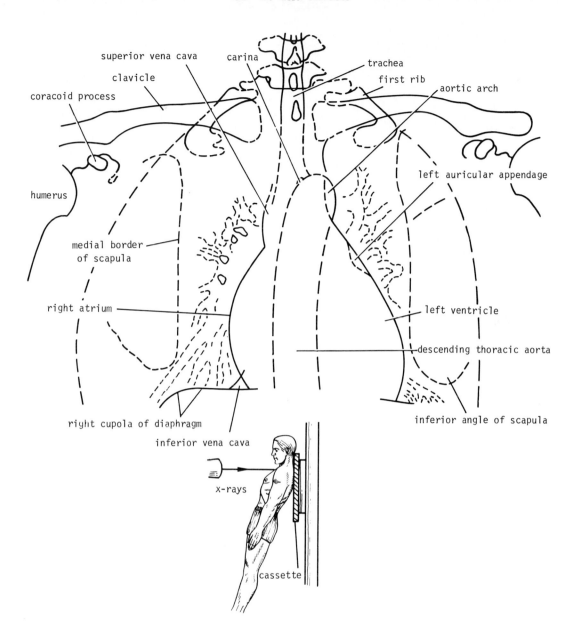

coracoid process

clavicle

superior vena cava

carina

trachea

first rib

aortic arch

humerus

left auricular appendage

medial border
of scapula

right atrium

left ventricle

descending thoracic aorta

inferior angle of scapula

right cupola of diaphragm

inferior vena cava

x-rays

cassette

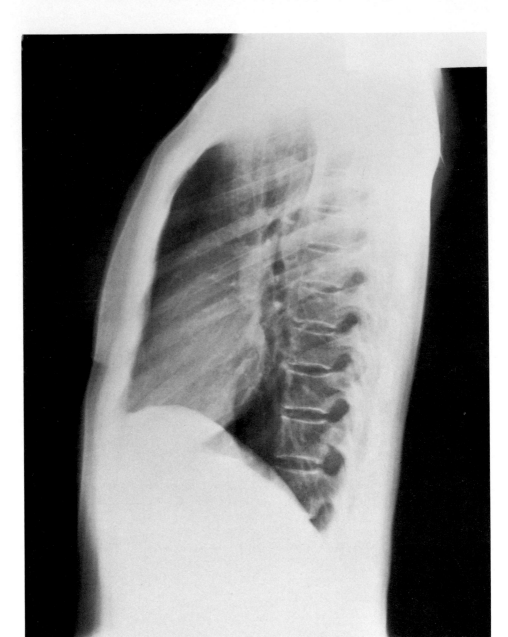

Figure 3

Left lateral radiograph of thorax
(female aged 30 years).

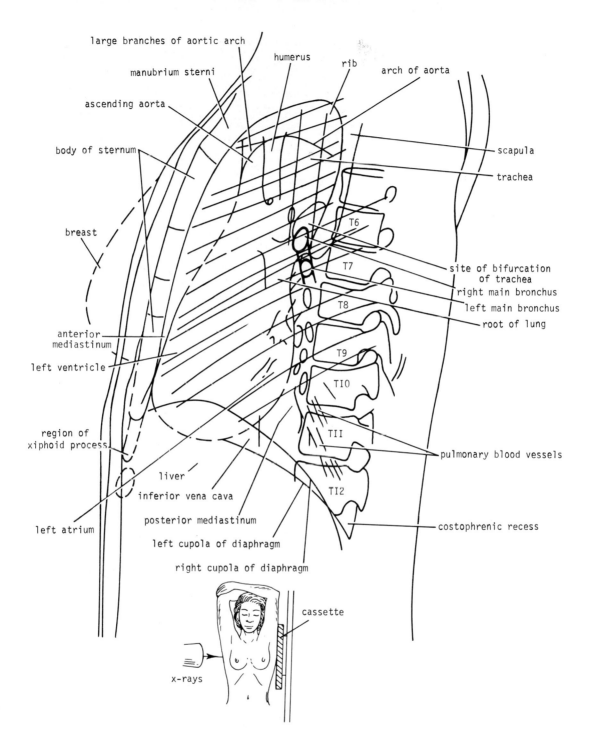

large branches of aortic arch

manubrium sterni

humerus

rib

arch of aorta

ascending aorta

body of sternum

scapula

trachea

breast

T6

T7

site of bifurcation
of trachea

right main bronchus

left main bronchus

T8

root of lung

anterior
mediastinum

T9

left ventricle

T10

region of
xiphoid process

T11

pulmonary blood vessels

liver

T12

inferior vena cava

left atrium

posterior mediastinum

costophrenic recess

left cupola of diaphragm

right cupola of diaphragm

cassette

x-rays

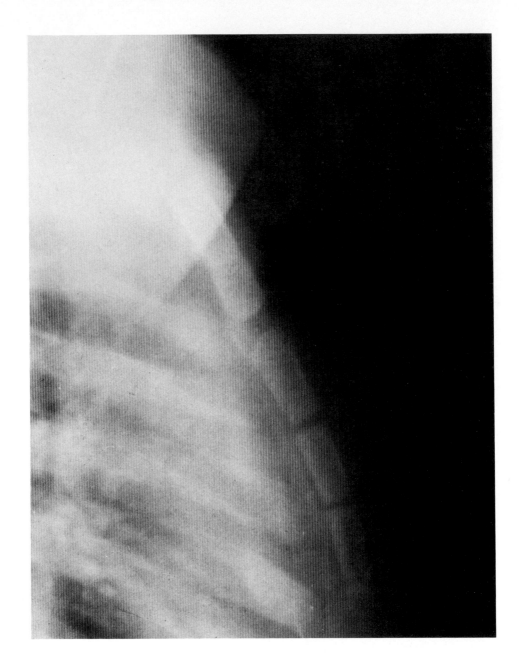

Figure 4

Right lateral radiograph of sternum
(male aged 8 years).

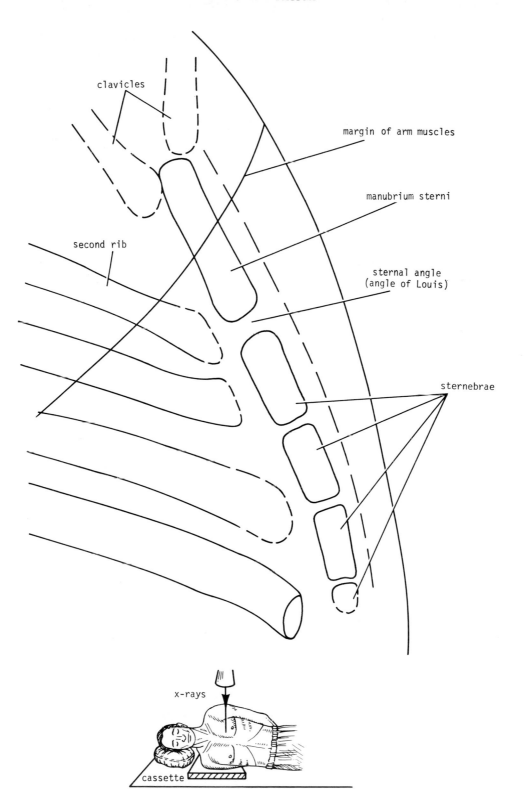

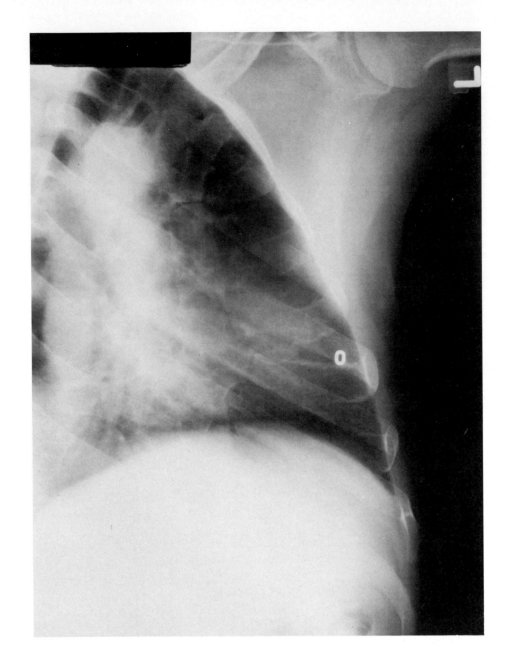

Figure 5

Right oblique radiograph of sternum
and sternoclavicular joints
(male aged 59 years).

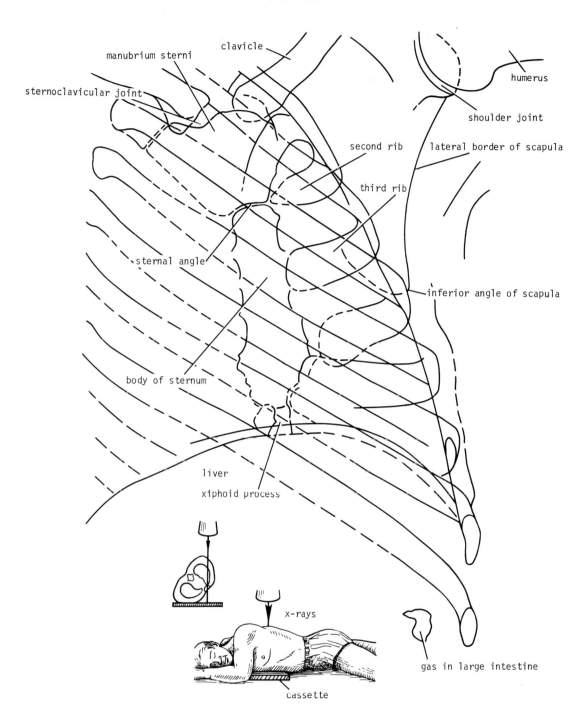

manubrium sterni

clavicle

humerus

sternoclavicular joint

shoulder joint

second rib

lateral border of scapula

third rib

inferior angle of scapula

sternal angle

body of sternum

liver

xiphoid process

x-rays

gas in large intestine

cassette

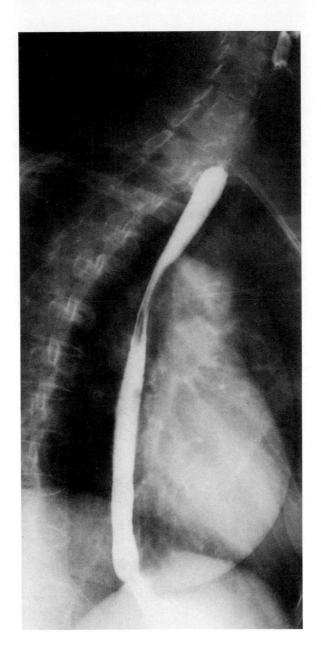

Figure 6

Right oblique radiograph of thorax
following a barium swallow
(female aged 62 years).

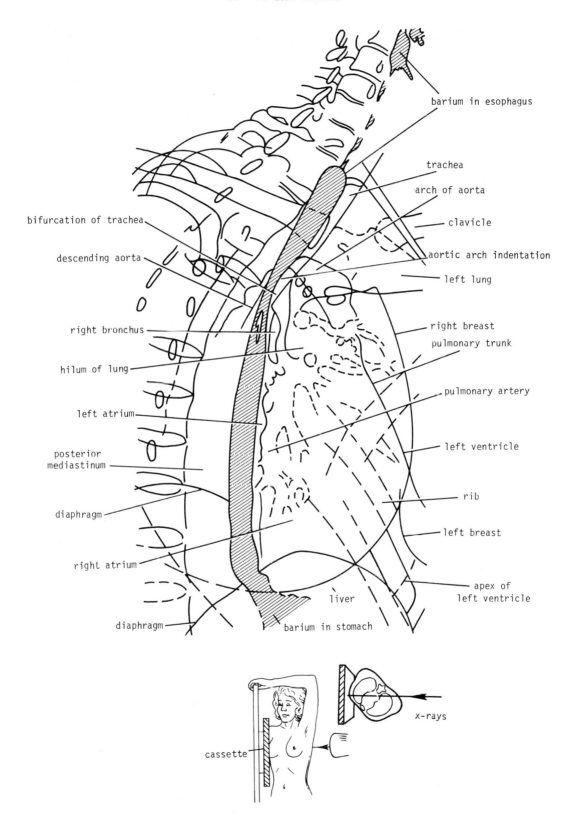

barium in esophagus

trachea

arch of aorta

clavicle

aortic arch indentation

bifurcation of trachea

left lung

descending aorta

right breast

pulmonary trunk

right bronchus

pulmonary artery

hilum of lung

left atrium

left ventricle

posterior mediastinum

rib

diaphragm

left breast

right atrium

apex of
left ventricle

diaphragm

liver

barium in stomach

x-rays

cassette

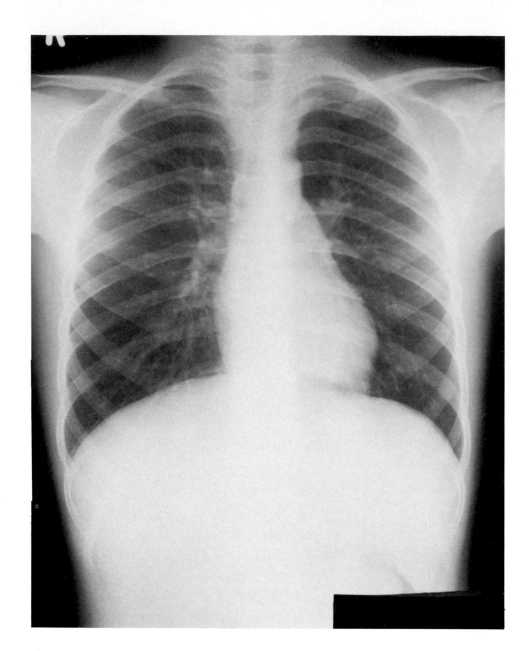

Figure 7

Posteroanterior radiograph of thorax
(male aged 9½ years).

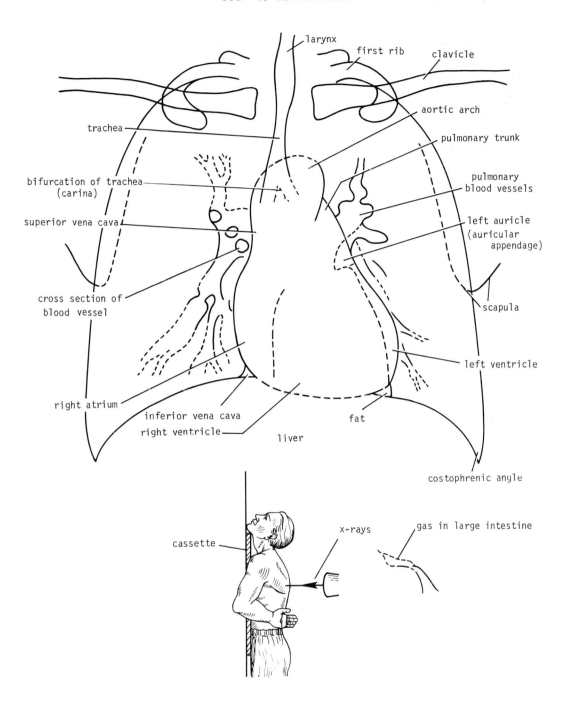

larynx

first rib

clavicle

aortic arch

trachea

pulmonary trunk

pulmonary
blood vessels

bifurcation of trachea
(carina)

superior vena cava

left auricle
(auricular
appendage)

cross section of
blood vessel

scapula

left ventricle

right atrium

inferior vena cava

right ventricle

fat

liver

costophrenic angle

cassette

x-rays

gas in large intestine

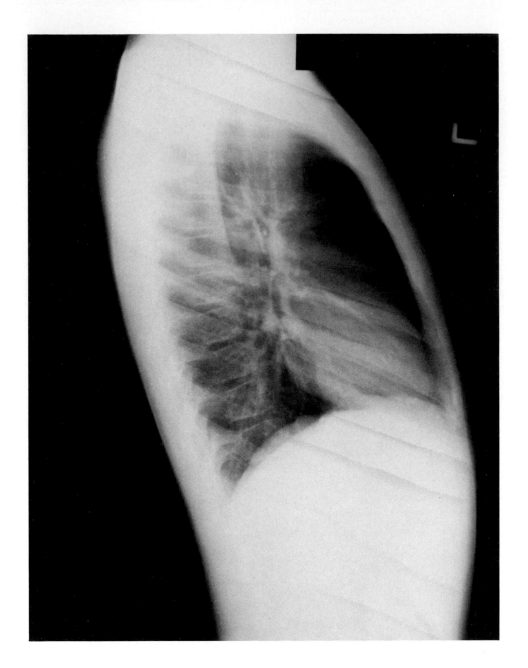

Figure 8

Left lateral radiograph of thorax
(male aged 9½ years).

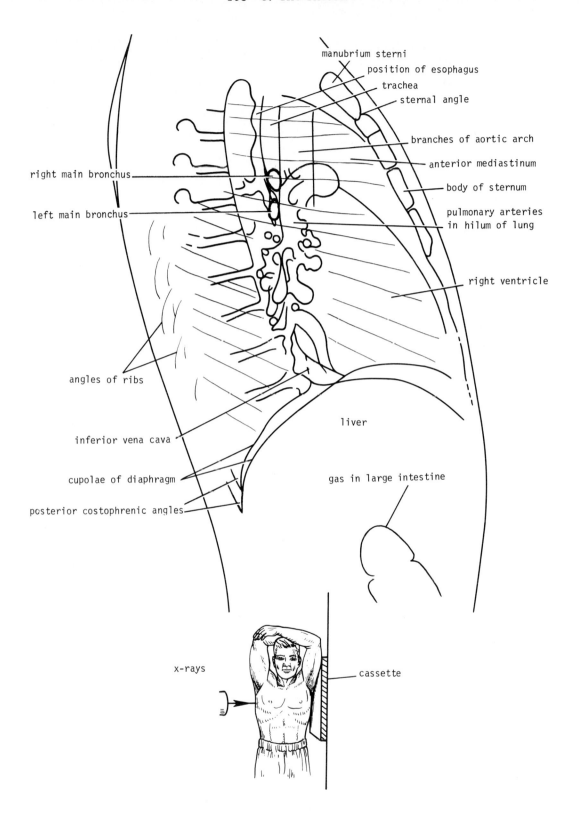

manubrium sterni

position of esophagus

trachea

sternal angle

branches of aortic arch

anterior mediastinum

body of sternum

pulmonary arteries
in hilum of lung

right ventricle

right main bronchus

left main bronchus

angles of ribs

inferior vena cava

cupolae of diaphragm

posterior costophrenic angles

liver

gas in large intestine

x-rays

cassette

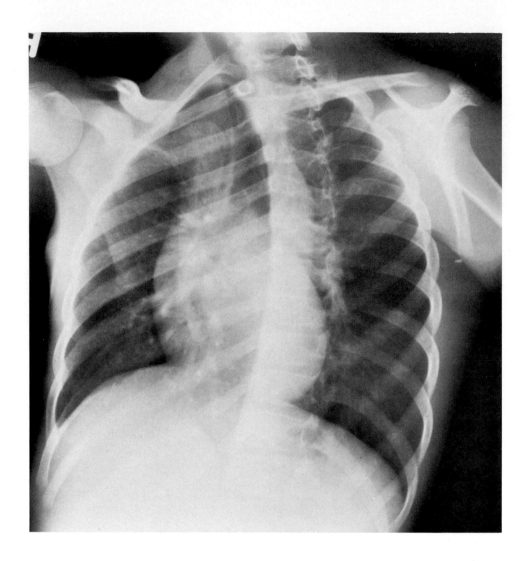

Figure 9

Left anterior
oblique radiograph of thorax
(female aged 10 years).

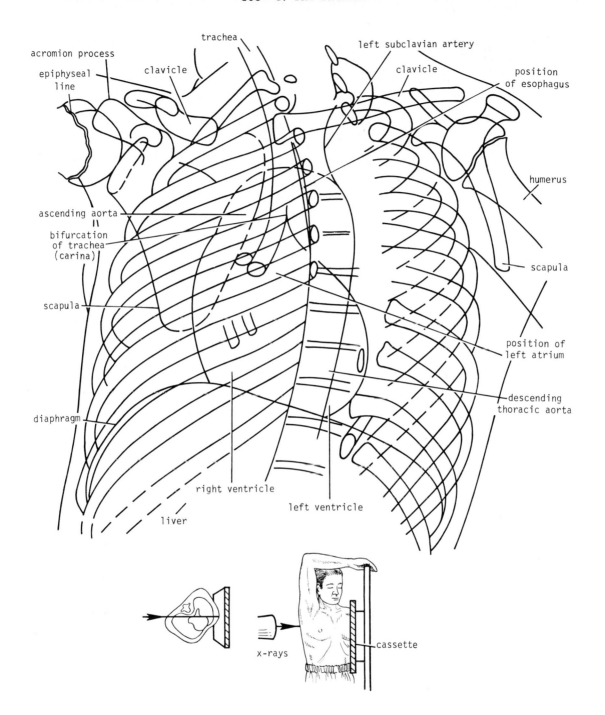

acromion process
epiphyseal line
clavicle
trachea
left subclavian artery
clavicle
position of esophagus
humerus
ascending aorta
bifurcation of trachea (carina)
scapula
scapula
position of left atrium
descending thoracic aorta
diaphragm
right ventricle
left ventricle
liver
x-rays
cassette

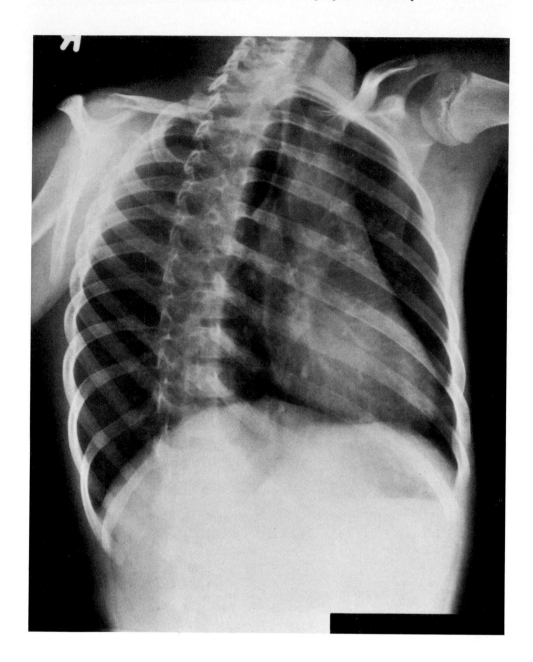

Figure 10

Right anterior
oblique radiograph of thorax
(male aged 10 years).

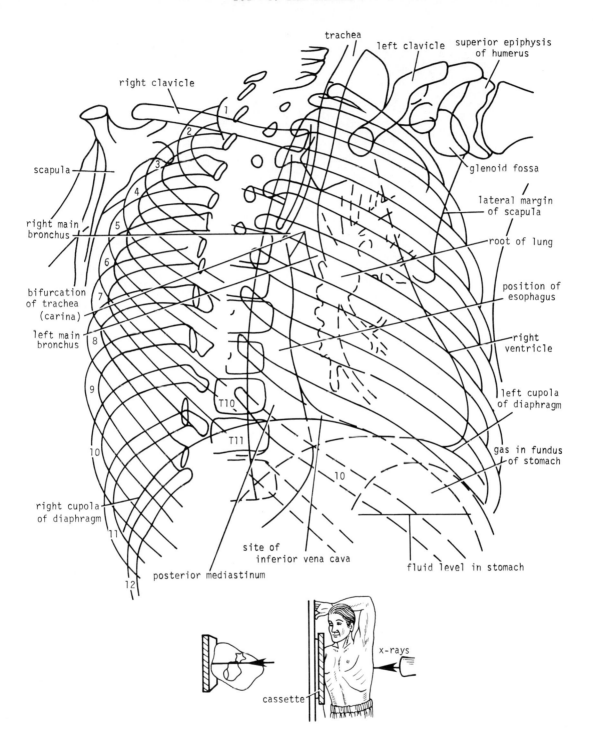

trachea

left clavicle

superior epiphysis of humerus

right clavicle

scapula

1

2

3

4

5

6

7

8

9

T10

T11

10

11

12

glenoid fossa

lateral margin of scapula

root of lung

position of esophagus

right ventricle

left cupola of diaphragm

gas in fundus of stomach

fluid level in stomach

right main bronchus

bifurcation of trachea (carina)

left main bronchus

right cupola of diaphragm

site of inferior vena cava

posterior mediastinum

x-rays

cassette

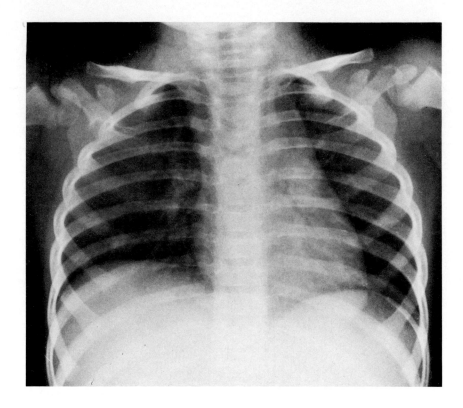

Figure 11

Anteroposterior
supine radiograph of thorax
(female aged 1 year).

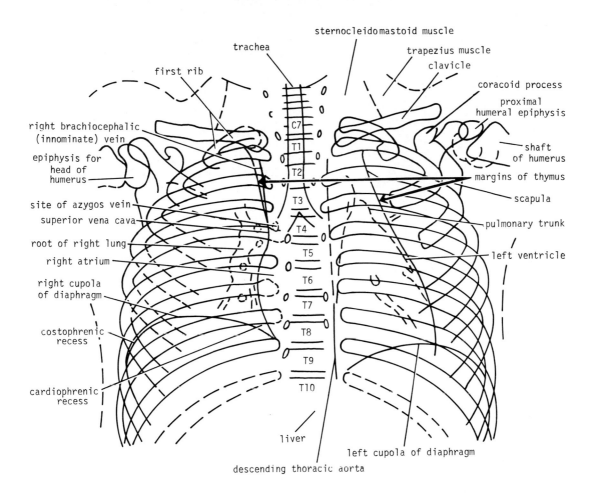

sternocleidomastoid muscle

trachea

first rib

trapezius muscle

clavicle

coracoid process

proximal
humeral epiphysis

right brachiocephalic
(innominate) vein

C7

T1

shaft
of humerus

epiphysis for
head of
humerus

T2

margins of thymus

scapula

site of azygos vein

T3

superior vena cava

T4

pulmonary trunk

root of right lung

T5

right atrium

left ventricle

T6

right cupola
of diaphragm

T7

costophrenic
recess

T8

T9

cardiophrenic
recess

T10

liver

left cupola of diaphragm

descending thoracic aorta

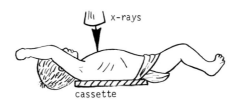

x-rays

cassette

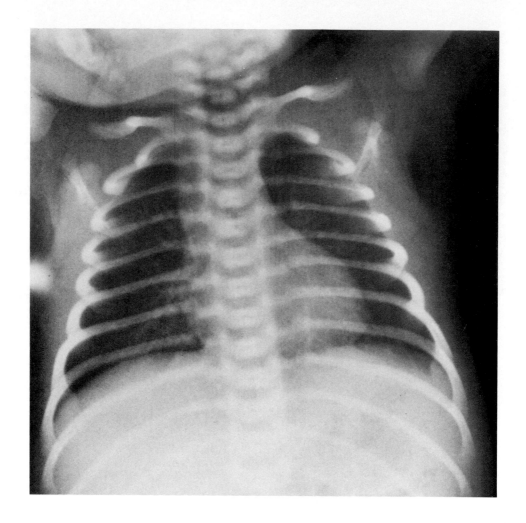

Figure 12

Anteroposterior supine
radiograph of thorax
(male aged 2 days).

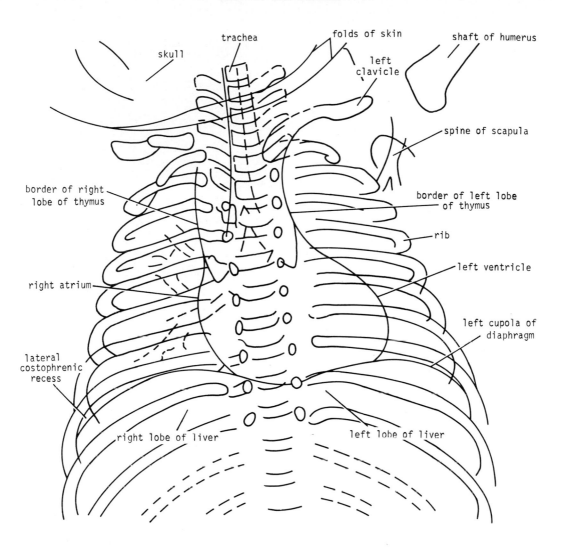

skull

trachea

folds of skin

left
clavicle

shaft of humerus

spine of scapula

border of right
lobe of thymus

border of left lobe
of thymus

rib

right atrium

left ventricle

lateral
costophrenic
recess

left cupola of
diaphragm

right lobe of liver

left lobe of liver

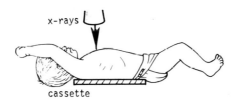

x-rays

cassette

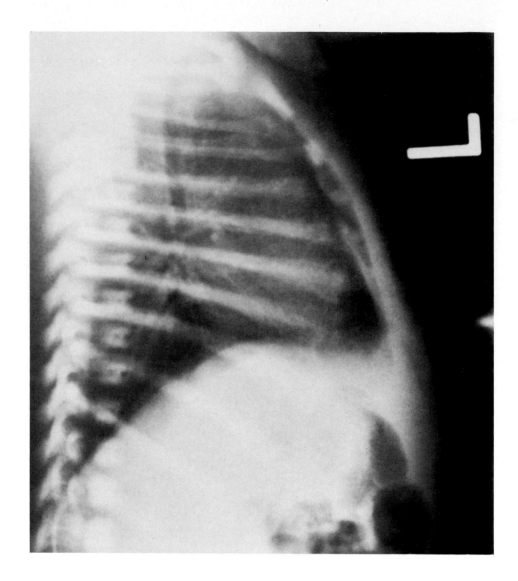

Figure 13

Left lateral radiograph of thorax
(male aged 2 days).

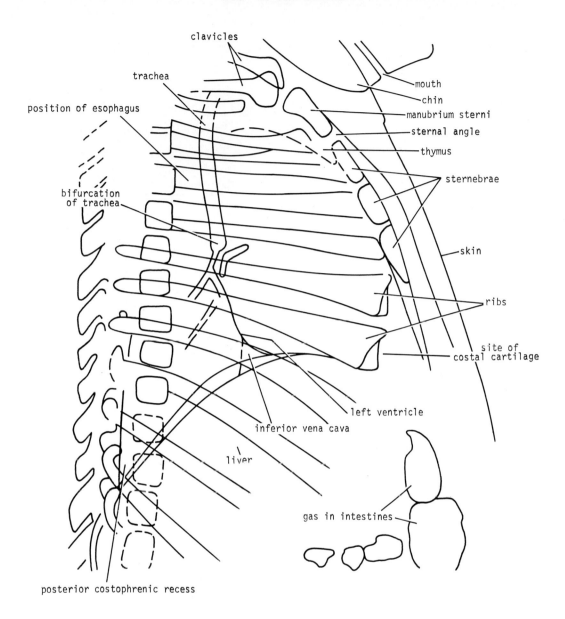

clavicles

trachea

position of esophagus

bifurcation
of trachea

mouth
chin
manubrium sterni
sternal angle
thymus

sternebrae

skin

ribs

site of
costal cartilage

left ventricle

inferior vena cava

liver

gas in intestines

posterior costophrenic recess

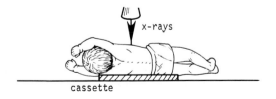

x-rays

cassette

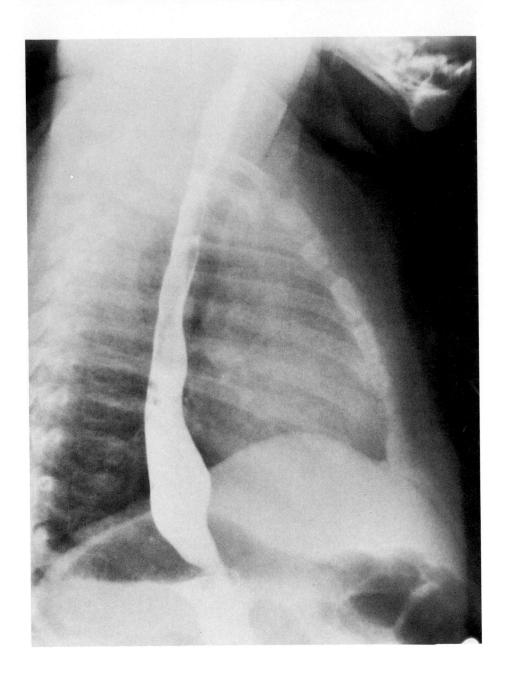

Figure 14

Left lateral radiograph of thorax
following a barium swallow
(female aged 4 months).

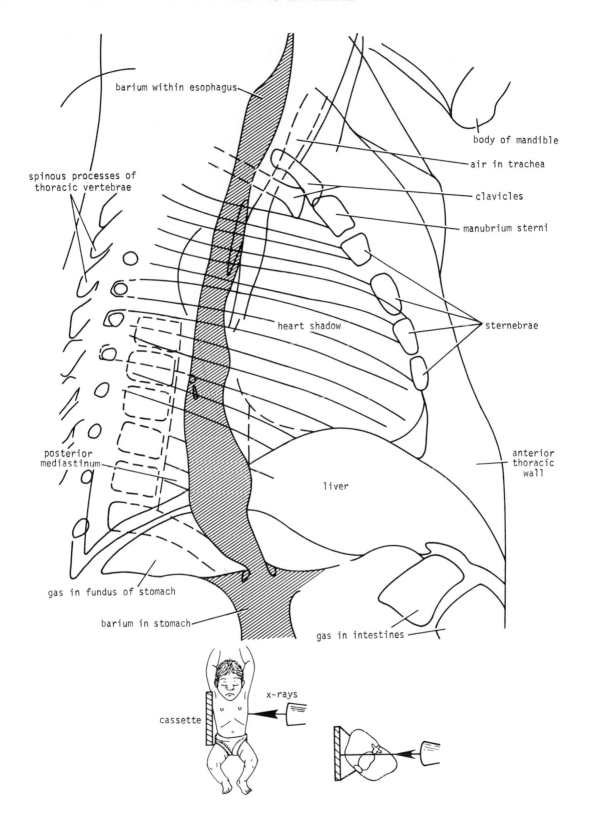

barium within esophagus

body of mandible

air in trachea

clavicles

manubrium sterni

spinous processes of thoracic vertebrae

heart shadow

sternebrae

posterior mediastinum

liver

anterior thoracic wall

gas in fundus of stomach

barium in stomach

gas in intestines

cassette

x-rays

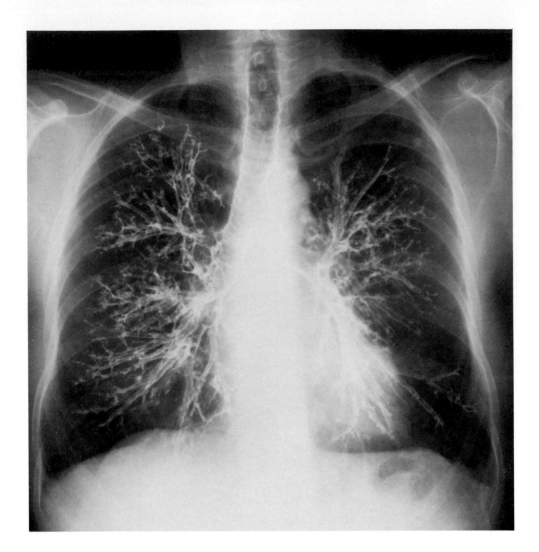

Figure 15

Posteroanterior bronchogram of thorax
(male aged 45 years).

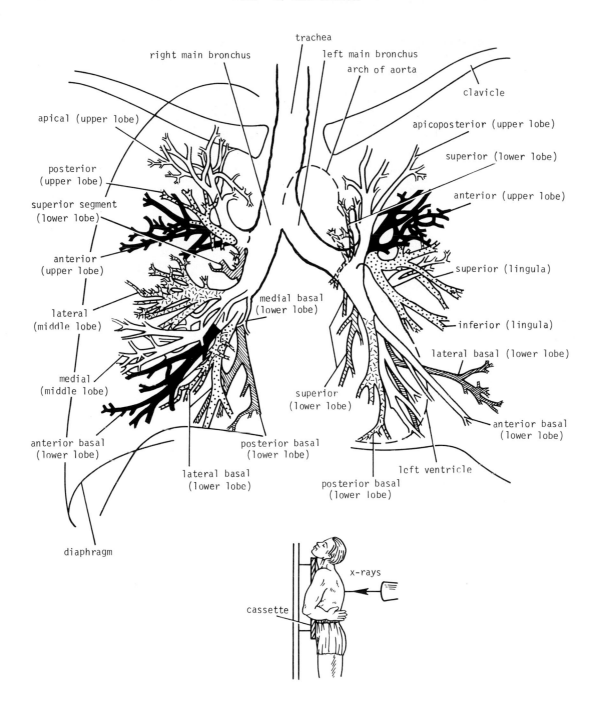

trachea

right main bronchus

left main bronchus

arch of aorta

clavicle

apical (upper lobe)

apicoposterior (upper lobe)

superior (lower lobe)

posterior (upper lobe)

anterior (upper lobe)

superior segment (lower lobe)

superior (lingula)

anterior (upper lobe)

medial basal (lower lobe)

inferior (lingula)

lateral (middle lobe)

lateral basal (lower lobe)

medial (middle lobe)

superior (lower lobe)

anterior basal (lower lobe)

anterior basal (lower lobe)

posterior basal (lower lobe)

left ventricle

lateral basal (lower lobe)

posterior basal (lower lobe)

diaphragm

x-rays

cassette

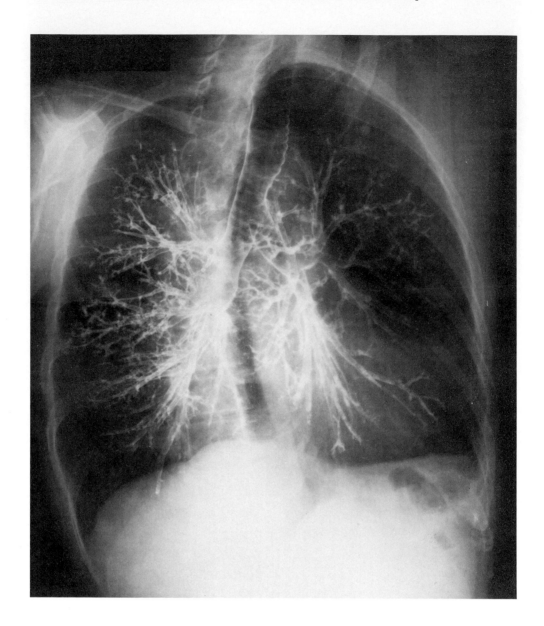

Figure 16

Right anterior
oblique bronchogram of thorax
(male aged 45 years).

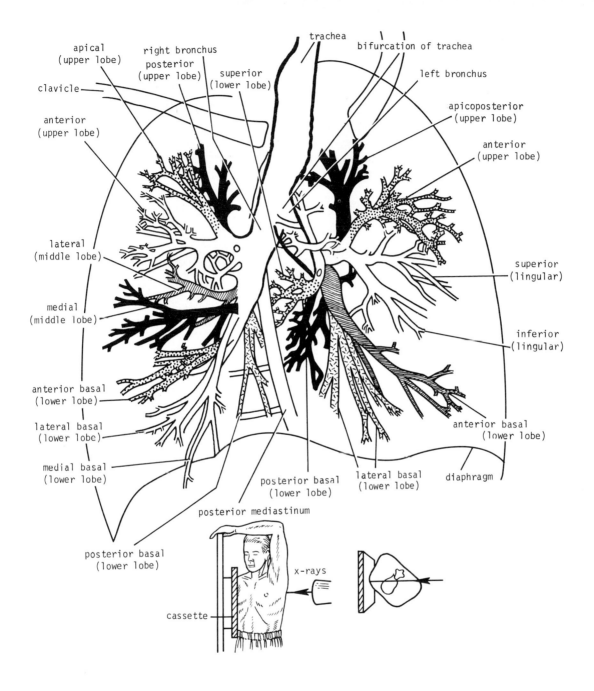

apical
(upper lobe)

right bronchus
posterior
(upper lobe)

trachea

bifurcation of trachea

left bronchus

superior
(lower lobe)

clavicle

apicoposterior
(upper lobe)

anterior
(upper lobe)

anterior
(upper lobe)

lateral
(middle lobe)

superior
(lingular)

medial
(middle lobe)

inferior
(lingular)

anterior basal
(lower lobe)

lateral basal
(lower lobe)

anterior basal
(lower lobe)

medial basal
(lower lobe)

posterior basal
(lower lobe)

lateral basal
(lower lobe)

diaphragm

posterior mediastinum

posterior basal
(lower lobe)

x-rays

cassette

THE ABDOMEN

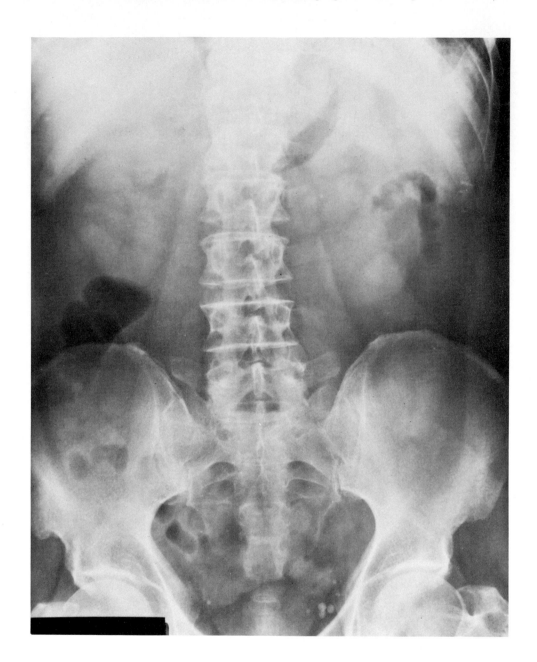

Figure 1

Anteroposterior
radiograph of the abdomen
(male aged 62 years).

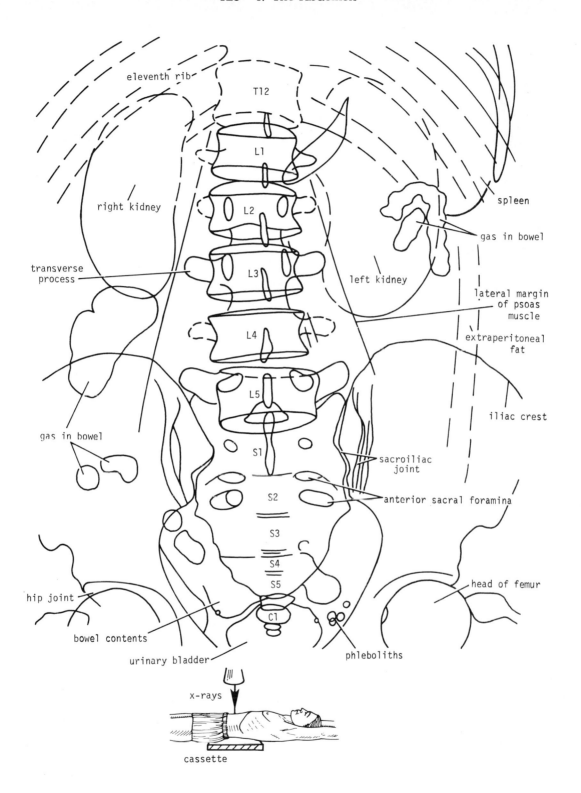

eleventh rib

T12

L1

right kidney

L2

spleen

gas in bowel

transverse
process

L3

left kidney

lateral margin
of psoas
muscle

L4

extraperitoneal
fat

L5

iliac crest

gas in bowel

S1

sacroiliac
joint

S2

anterior sacral foramina

S3

S4

S5

head of femur

hip joint

C1

bowel contents

phleboliths

urinary bladder

x-rays

cassette

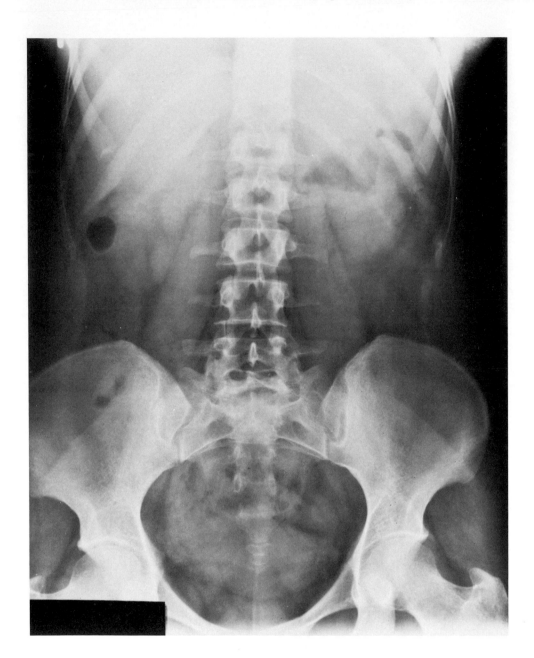

Figure 2

Anteroposterior
radiograph of the abdomen
(female aged 26 years).

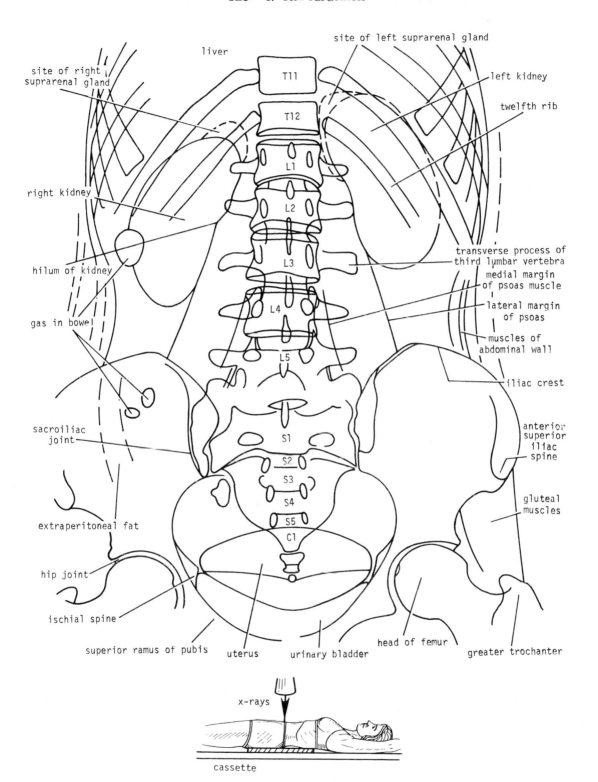

site of left suprarenal gland

liver

site of right suprarenal gland

left kidney

twelfth rib

T11

T12

L1

right kidney

L2

L3

transverse process of third lumbar vertebra

medial margin of psoas muscle

hilum of kidney

L4

lateral margin of psoas

muscles of abdominal wall

gas in bowel

L5

iliac crest

sacroiliac joint

S1

anterior superior iliac spine

S2

S3

S4

gluteal muscles

S5

extraperitoneal fat

C1

hip joint

ischial spine

superior ramus of pubis   uterus   urinary bladder   head of femur   greater trochanter

x-rays

cassette

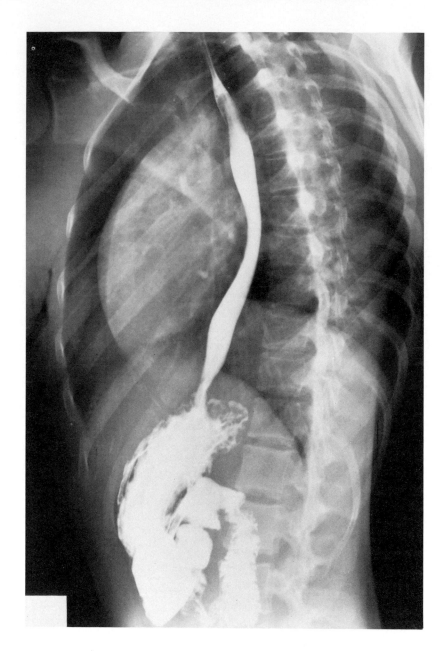

Figure 3

Oblique radiograph
of thorax and abdomen
following a barium swallow
(female aged 30 years).

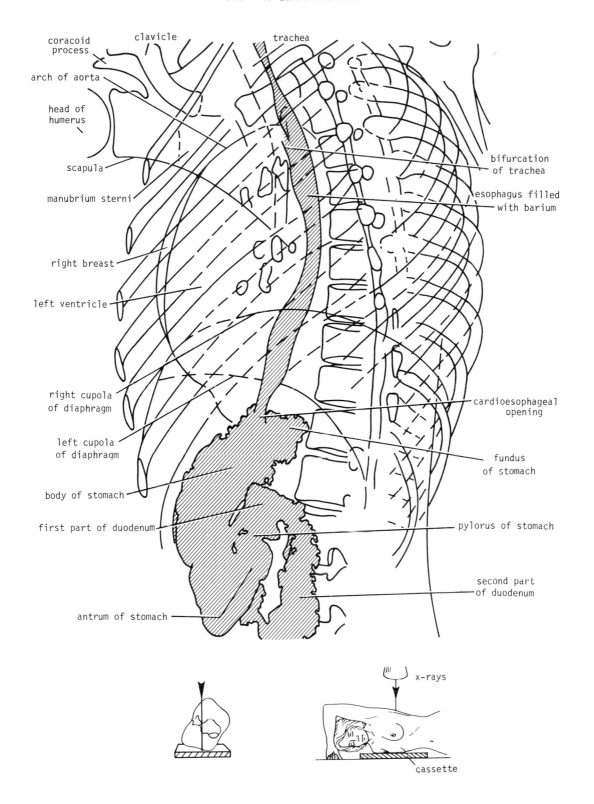

coracoid process

clavicle

trachea

arch of aorta

head of humerus

scapula

bifurcation of trachea

manubrium sterni

esophagus filled with barium

right breast

left ventricle

right cupola of diaphragm

cardioesophageal opening

left cupola of diaphragm

fundus of stomach

body of stomach

first part of duodenum

pylorus of stomach

second part of duodenum

antrum of stomach

x-rays

cassette

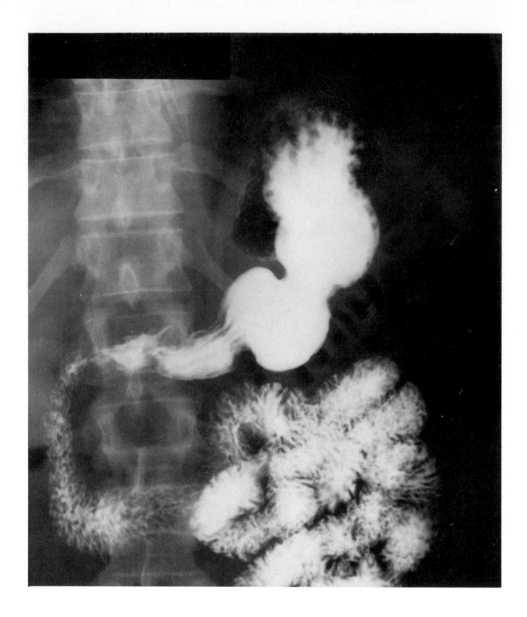

Figure 4

Posteroanterior radiograph of the
stomach, duodenum, and jejunum
following a barium meal
(male aged 38 years).

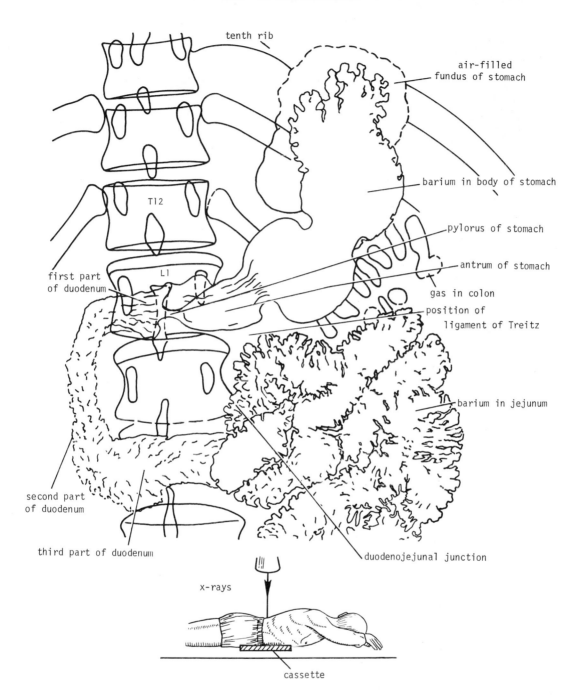

tenth rib

air-filled
fundus of stomach

barium in body of stomach

pylorus of stomach

antrum of stomach

gas in colon

first part
of duodenum

position of
ligament of Treitz

barium in jejunum

second part
of duodenum

third part of duodenum

duodenojejunal junction

T12

L1

x-rays

cassette

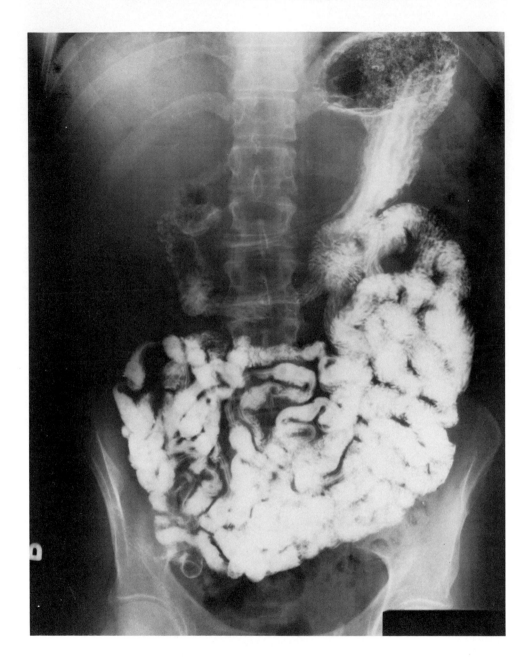

Figure 5

Anteroposterior
radiograph of the stomach,
duodenum, jejunum, and ileum 2 hours
after ingesting a barium meal
(male aged 44 years).

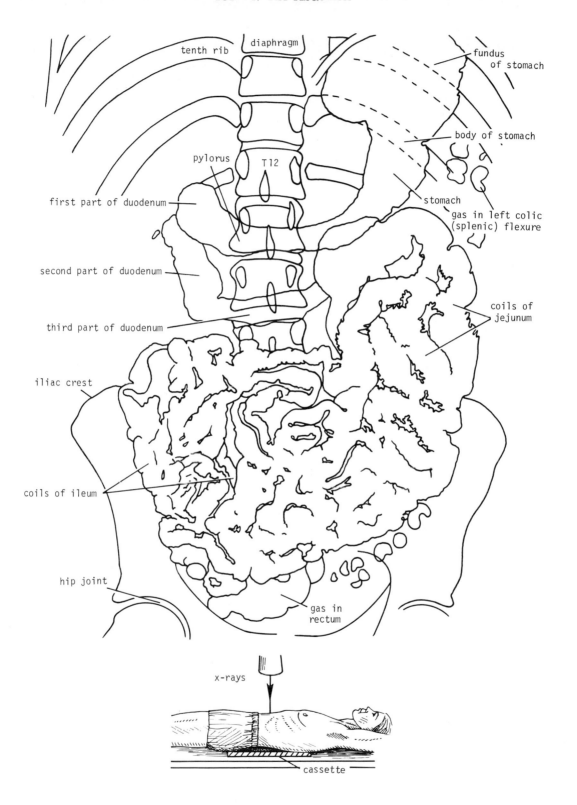

tenth rib
diaphragm
fundus of stomach
body of stomach
pylorus
T 12
first part of duodenum
stomach
gas in left colic (splenic) flexure
second part of duodenum
coils of jejunum
third part of duodenum
iliac crest
coils of ileum
hip joint
gas in rectum
x-rays
cassette

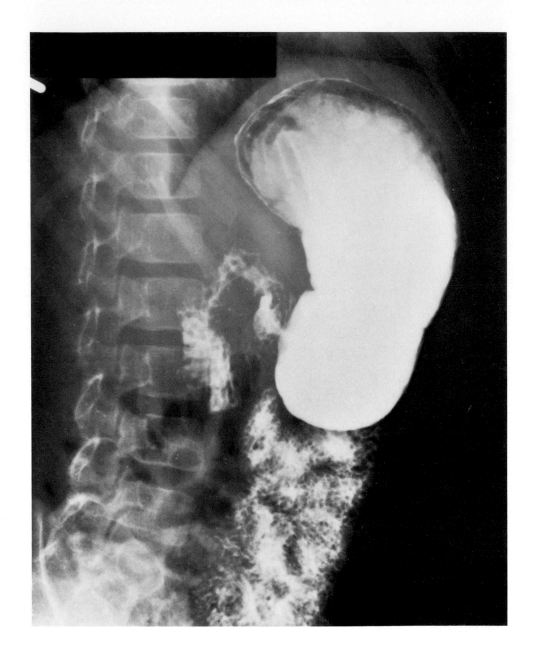

Figure 6

Right anterior oblique
radiograph of the stomach, duodenum,
and jejunum following a barium meal
(male aged 7 years).

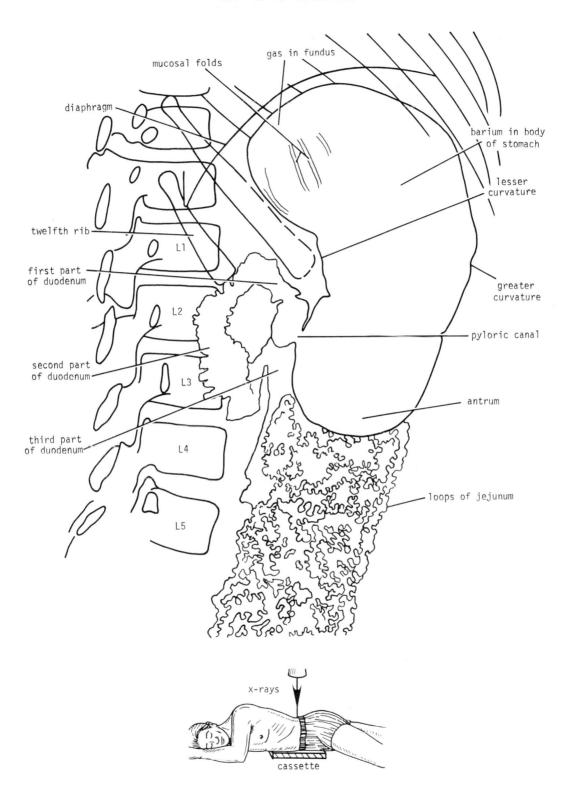

mucosal folds

gas in fundus

diaphragm

barium in body
of stomach

lesser
curvature

twelfth rib

L1

first part
of duodenum

greater
curvature

L2

pyloric canal

second part
of duodenum

L3

antrum

third part
of duodenum

L4

L5

loops of jejunum

x-rays

cassette

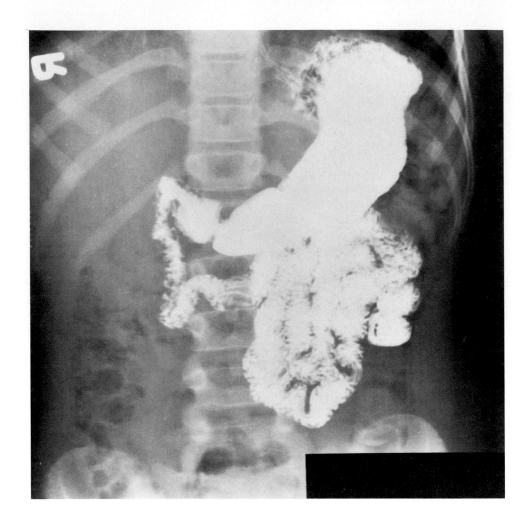

Figure 7

Posteroanterior radiograph of the
stomach, duodenum, and jejunum
following a barium meal
(female aged 6 years).

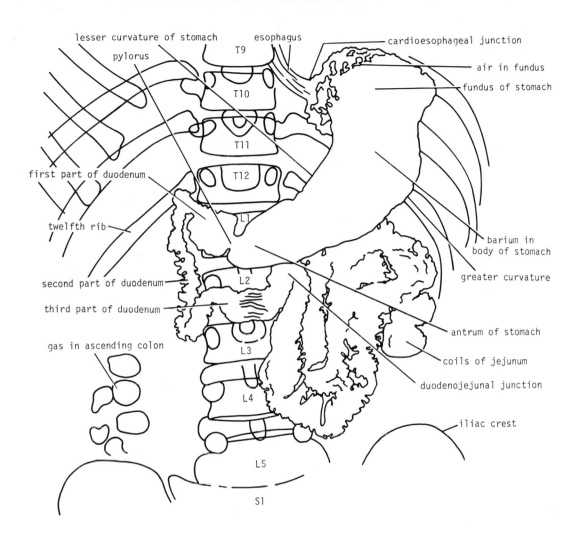

lesser curvature of stomach
esophagus
cardioesophageal junction
pylorus
air in fundus
fundus of stomach
first part of duodenum
twelfth rib
barium in body of stomach
greater curvature
second part of duodenum
third part of duodenum
antrum of stomach
gas in ascending colon
coils of jejunum
duodenojejunal junction
iliac crest

T9
T10
T11
T12
L1
L2
L3
L4
L5
S1

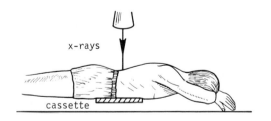

x-rays

cassette

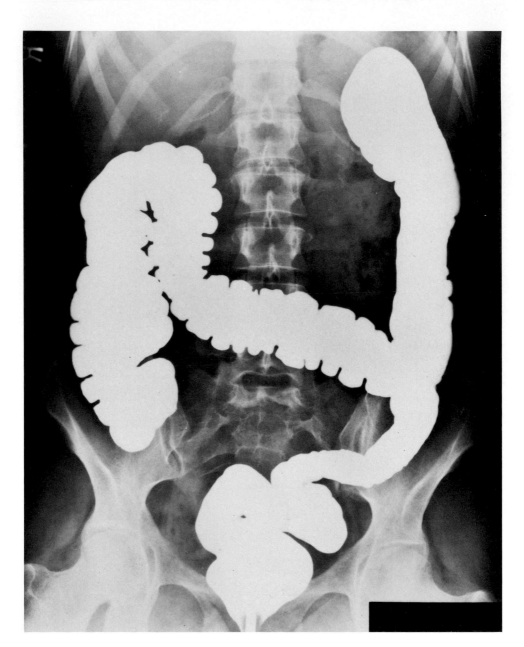

Figure 8

Posteroanterior radiograph of the
colon following a barium enema
(female aged 26 years).

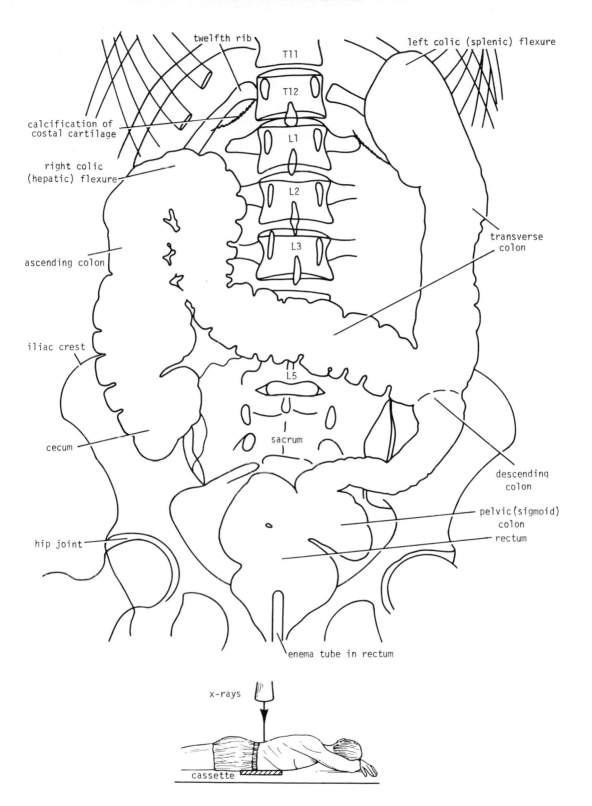

twelfth rib

left colic (splenic) flexure

T11

T12

calcification of
costal cartilage

L1

right colic
(hepatic) flexure

L2

L3

transverse
colon

ascending colon

iliac crest

L5

cecum

sacrum

descending
colon

pelvic (sigmoid)
colon

hip joint

rectum

enema tube in rectum

x-rays

cassette

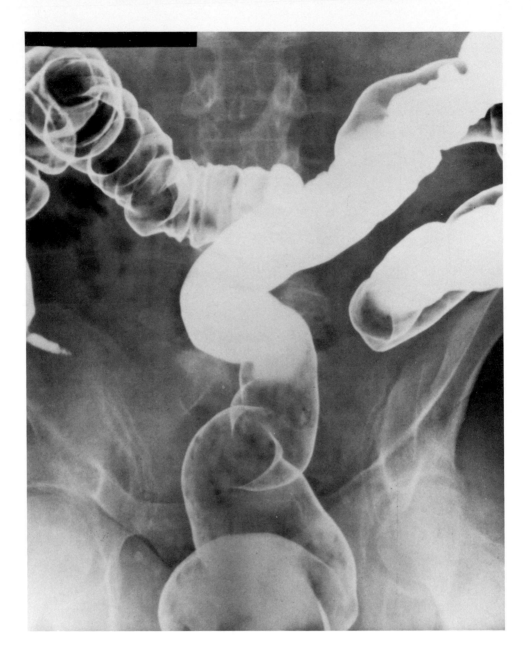

Figure 9

Prone angled radiograph of the pelvic
colon following a barium enema
(female aged 53 years).

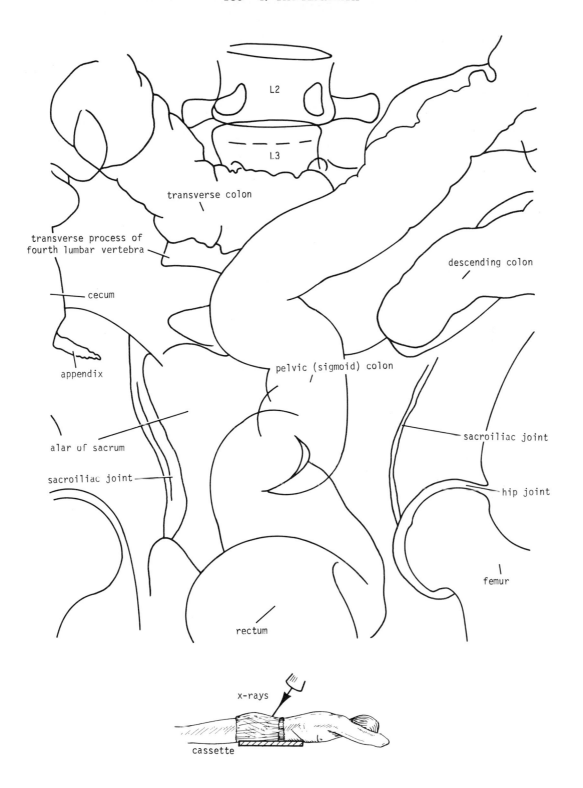

L2

L3

transverse colon

transverse process of
fourth lumbar vertebra

descending colon

cecum

appendix

pelvic (sigmoid) colon

sacroiliac joint

alar of sacrum

sacroiliac joint

hip joint

femur

rectum

x-rays

cassette

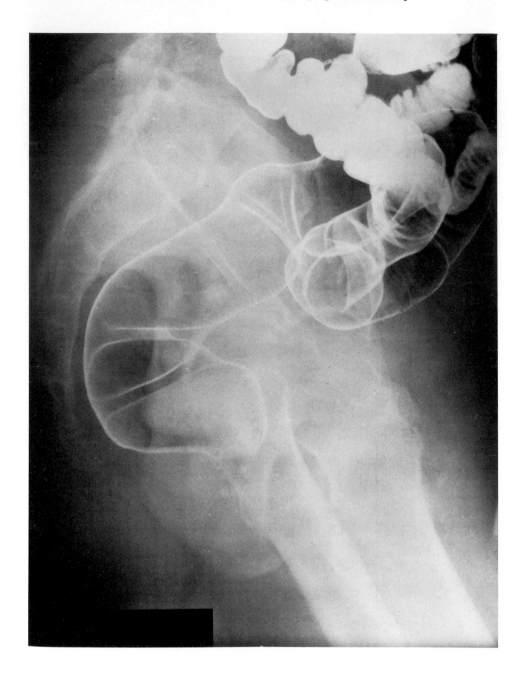

Figure 10

Lateral radiograph of pelvic colon and
rectum following a barium enema
(male aged 48 years).

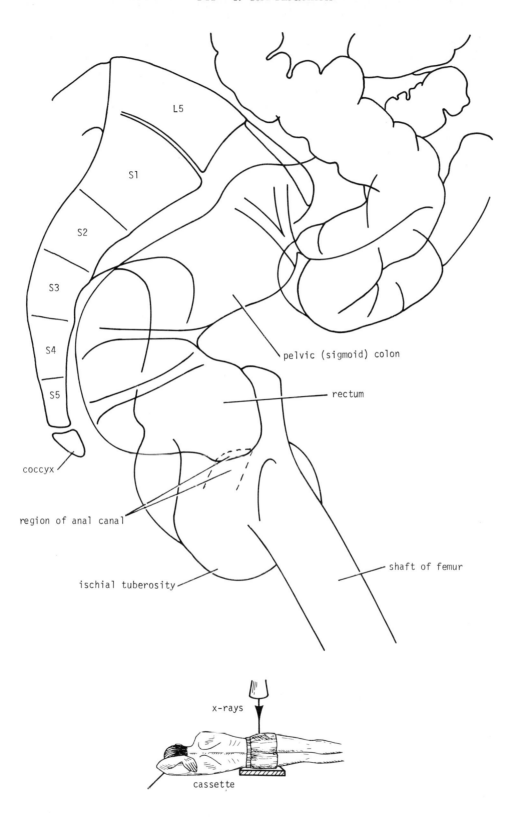

L5

S1

S2

S3

S4

S5

coccyx

region of anal canal

ischial tuberosity

pelvic (sigmoid) colon

rectum

shaft of femur

x-rays

cassette

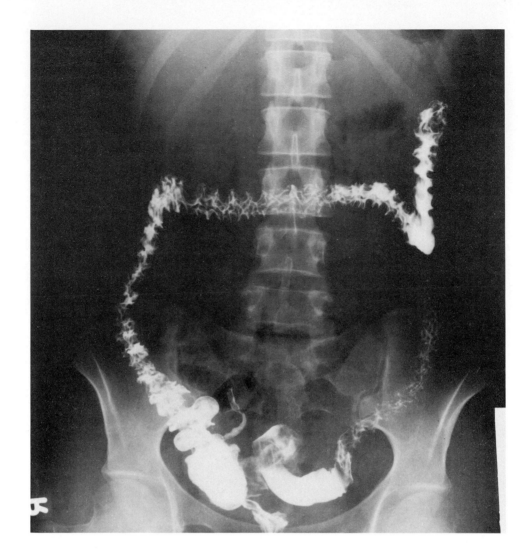

Figure 11

Posteroanterior radiograph of the colon
following evacuation of barium
(female aged 20 years).

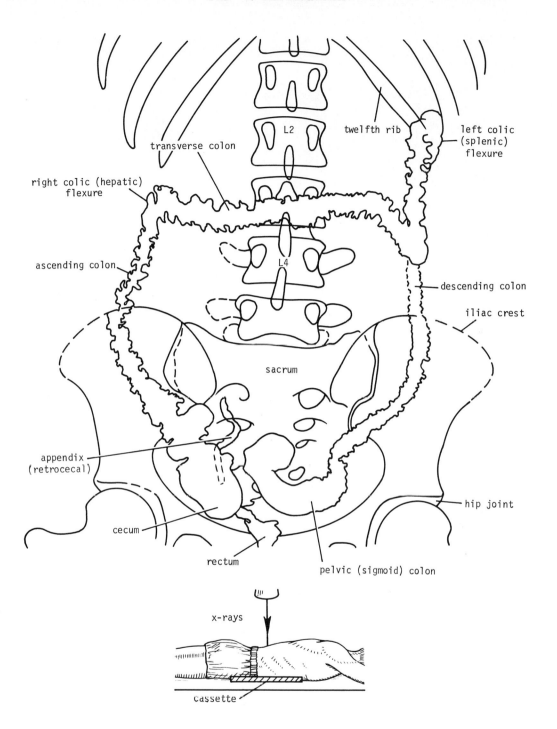

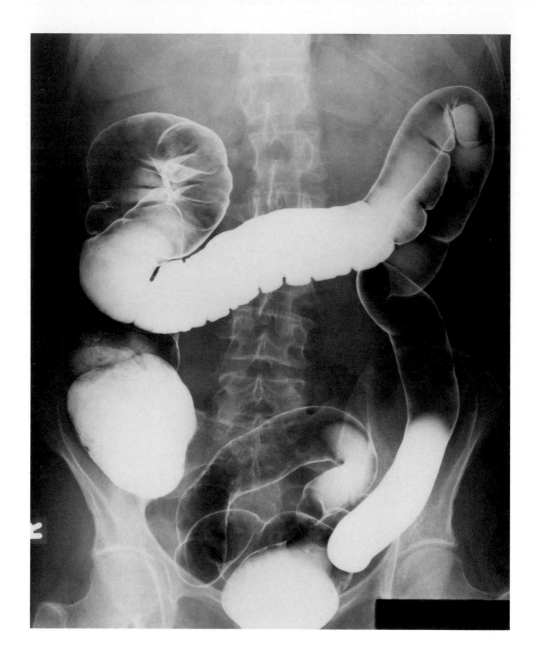

Figure 12

Posteroanterior radiograph of the colon
following an air double-contrast enema
(female aged 55 years).

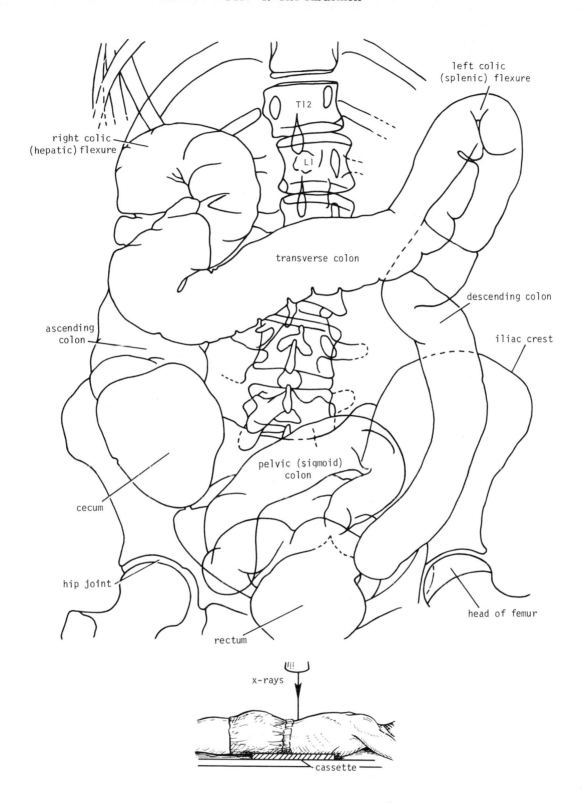

right colic (hepatic) flexure

left colic (splenic) flexure

T12

L1

transverse colon

descending colon

ascending colon

iliac crest

pelvic (sigmoid) colon

cecum

hip joint

head of femur

rectum

x-rays

cassette

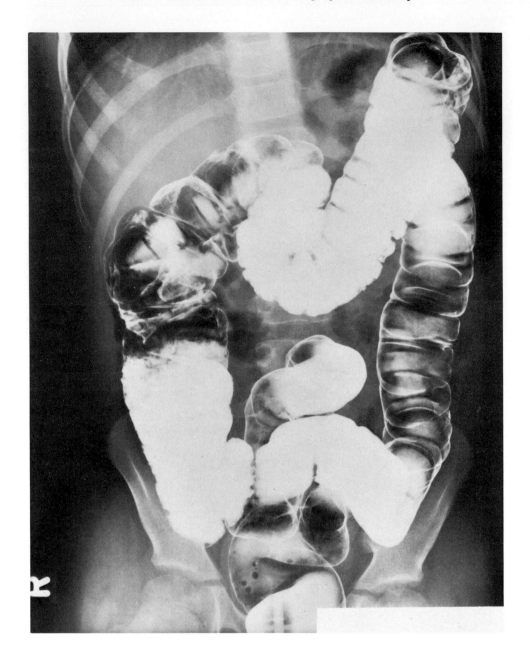

Figure 13

Posteroanterior radiograph of the colon
following a barium enema
(male aged 8 years).

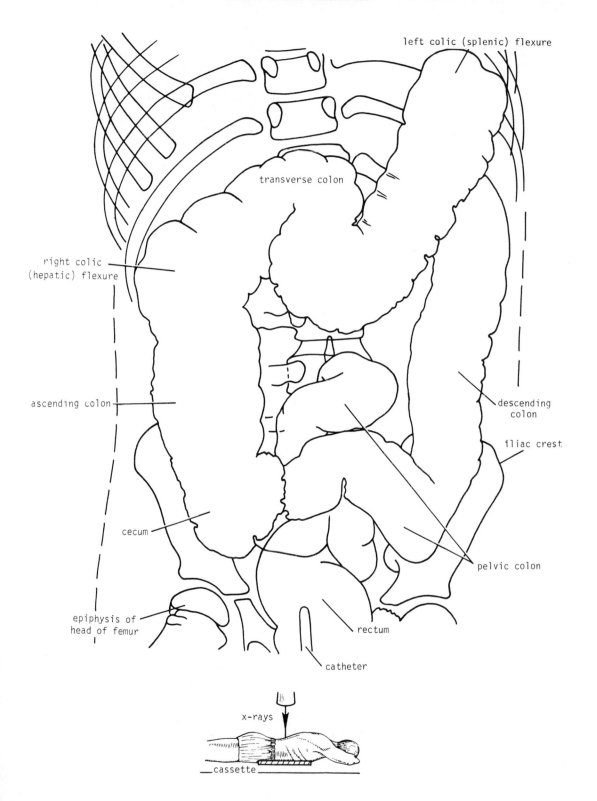

left colic (splenic) flexure

transverse colon

right colic
(hepatic) flexure

ascending colon

descending
colon

iliac crest

cecum

pelvic colon

epiphysis of
head of femur

rectum

pelvic colon

catheter

x-rays

cassette

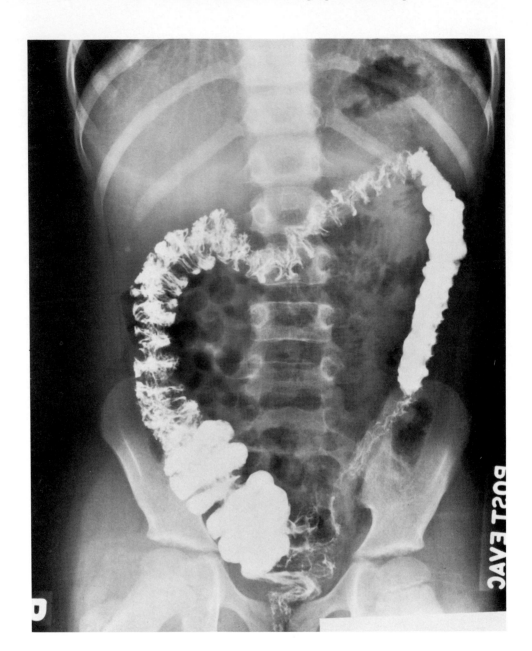

Figure 14

Posteroanterior radiograph of the colon
following evacuation of barium
(male aged 8 years).

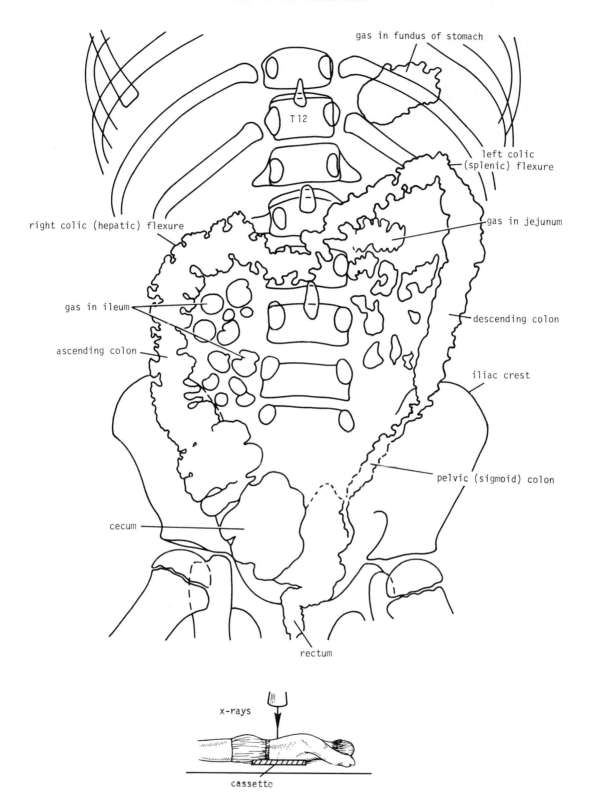

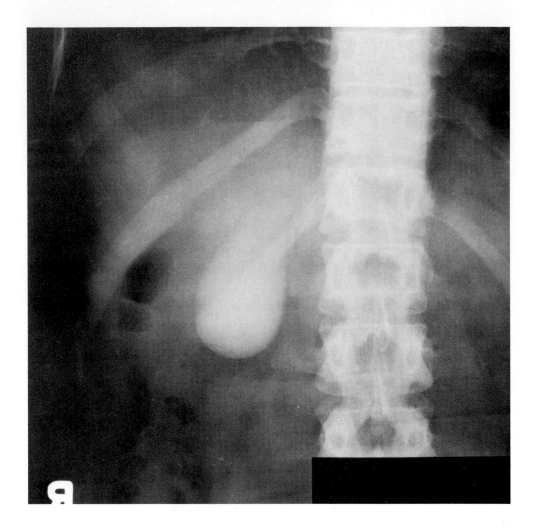

Figure 15

A cholecystogram following
the oral administration of an
iodine-containing compound
(male aged 29 years).

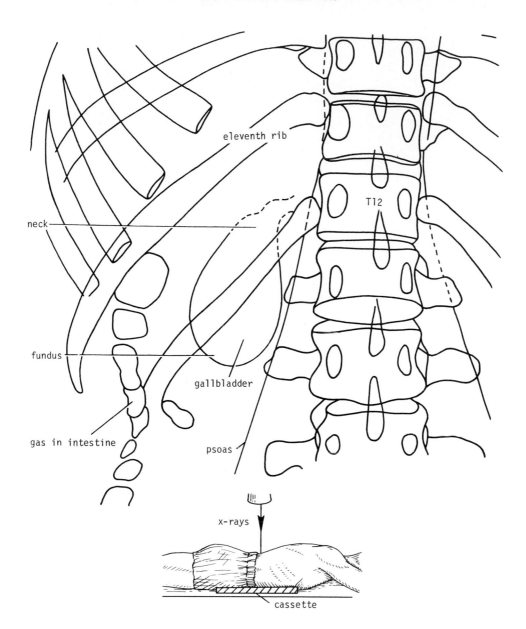

eleventh rib

neck

T12

fundus

gallbladder

gas in intestine

psoas

x-rays

cassette

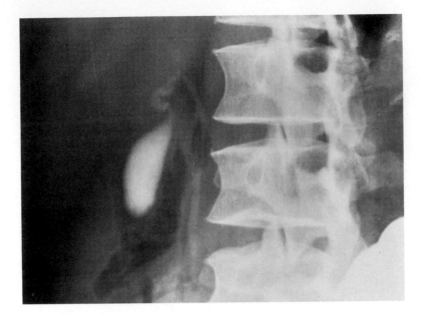

Figure 16

A cholecystogram after the
ingestion of a fatty meal
(female aged 45 years).

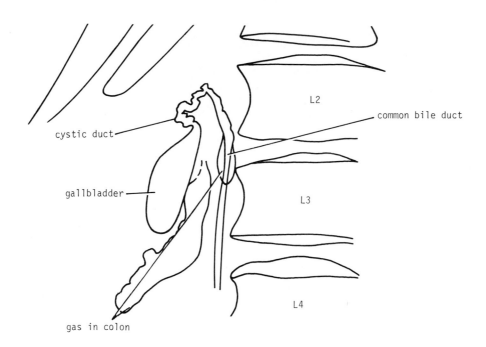

cystic duct

common bile duct

L2

gallbladder

L3

gas in colon

L4

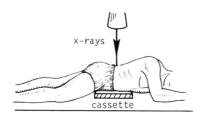

x-rays

cassette

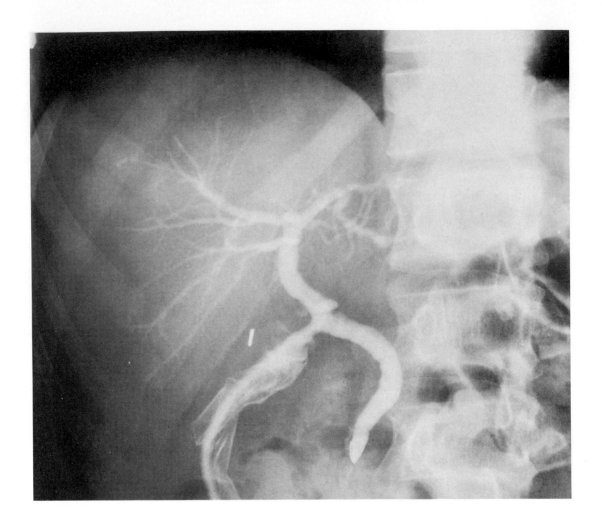

Figure 17

A cholangiogram following the operative
introduction of radiopaque material
into the common bile duct
(male aged 43 years).

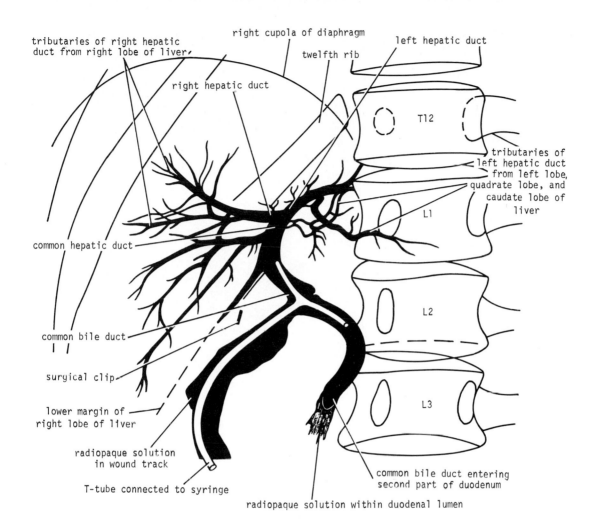

tributaries of right hepatic duct from right lobe of liver

right cupola of diaphragm

left hepatic duct

right hepatic duct

twelfth rib

T12

tributaries of left hepatic duct from left lobe, quadrate lobe, and caudate lobe of liver

L1

common hepatic duct

L2

common bile duct

surgical clip

L3

lower margin of right lobe of liver

radiopaque solution in wound track

common bile duct entering second part of duodenum

T-tube connected to syringe

radiopaque solution within duodenal lumen

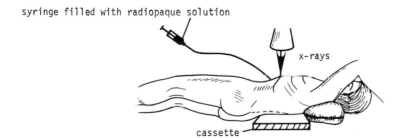

syringe filled with radiopaque solution

x-rays

cassette

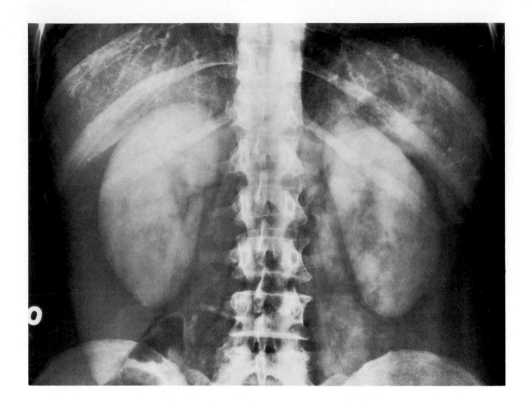

Figure 18

A nephrogram immediately after
the intravenous injection of a
suitable contrast medium
(female aged 61 years).

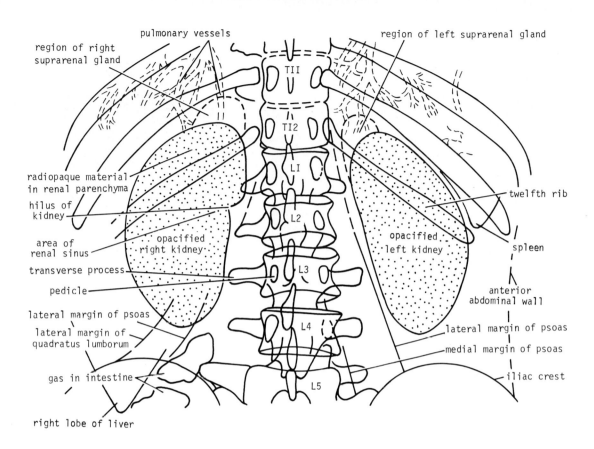

region of right suprarenal gland

pulmonary vessels

region of left suprarenal gland

TII

TI2

LI

radiopaque material in renal parenchyma

hilus of kidney

twelfth rib

L2

area of renal sinus

opacified right kidney

opacified left kidney

spleen

transverse process

L3

pedicle

anterior abdominal wall

lateral margin of psoas

L4

lateral margin of psoas

lateral margin of quadratus lumborum

medial margin of psoas

gas in intestine

L5

iliac crest

right lobe of liver

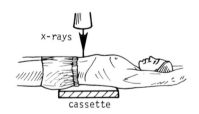

x-rays

cassette

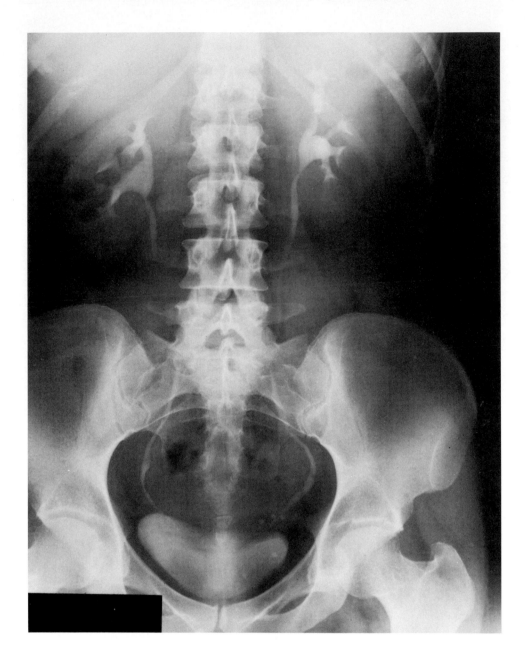

Figure 19

An intravenous pyelogram obtained 30
minutes after the injection of
a suitable contrast medium
(female aged 39 years).

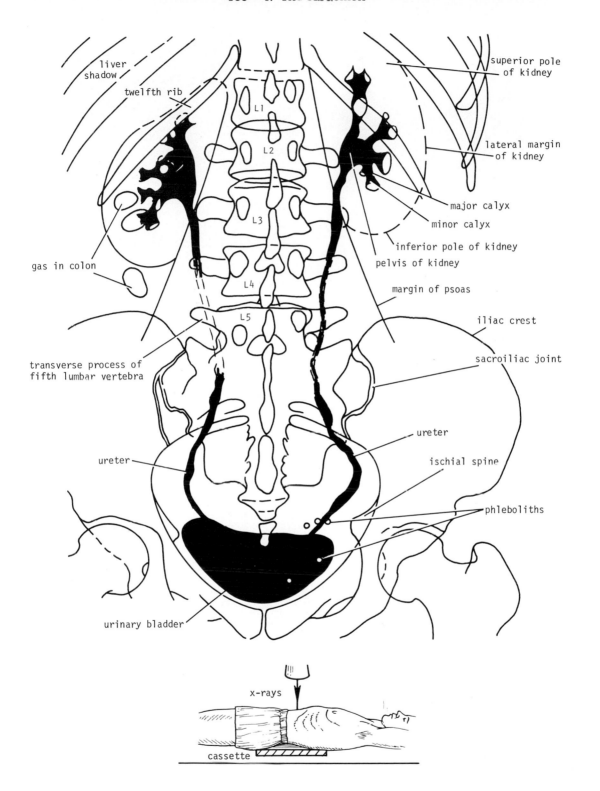

liver shadow

twelfth rib

superior pole of kidney

lateral margin of kidney

L1

L2

major calyx

minor calyx

L3

inferior pole of kidney

pelvis of kidney

gas in colon

margin of psoas

L4

iliac crest

L5

sacroiliac joint

transverse process of fifth lumbar vertebra

ureter

ischial spine

ureter

phleboliths

urinary bladder

x-rays

cassette

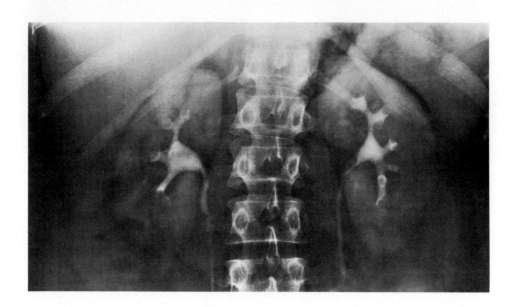

Figure 20

An intravenous pyelogram obtained 5
minutes after the injection of
a suitable contrast medium
(female aged 28 years).

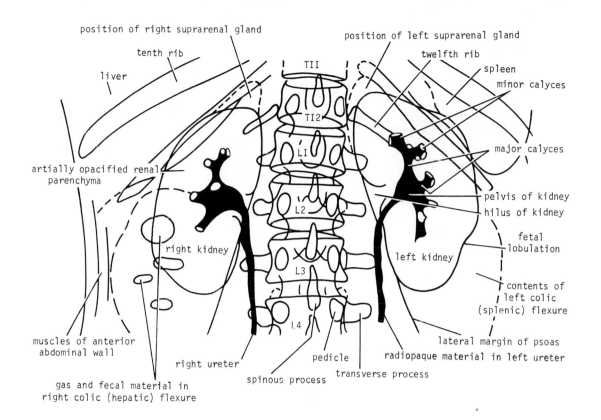

position of right suprarenal gland

tenth rib

liver

TII

position of left suprarenal gland

twelfth rib

spleen

minor calyces

TI2

LI

major calyces

artially opacified renal parenchyma

L2

pelvis of kidney

hilus of kidney

fetal lobulation

right kidney

left kidney

L3

contents of left colic (splenic) flexure

L4

muscles of anterior abdominal wall

right ureter

pedicle

transverse process

lateral margin of psoas

radiopaque material in left ureter

spinous process

gas and fecal material in right colic (hepatic) flexure

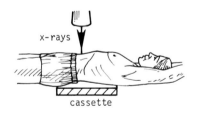

x-rays

cassette

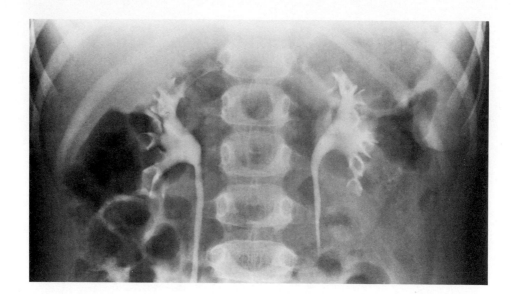

Figure 21

An intravenous pyelogram obtained 15
minutes after the injection of
a suitable contrast medium
(female aged 5 years).

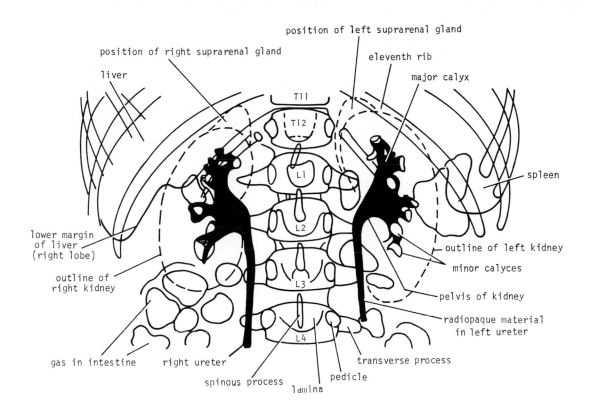

position of left suprarenal gland

position of right suprarenal gland

eleventh rib

liver

major calyx

T11

T12

L1

spleen

L2

lower margin
of liver
(right lobe)

outline of left kidney

minor calyces

outline of
right kidney

L3

pelvis of kidney

radiopaque material
in left ureter

L4

gas in intestine   right ureter

transverse process

spinous process   pedicle

lamina

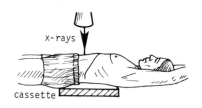

x-rays

cassette

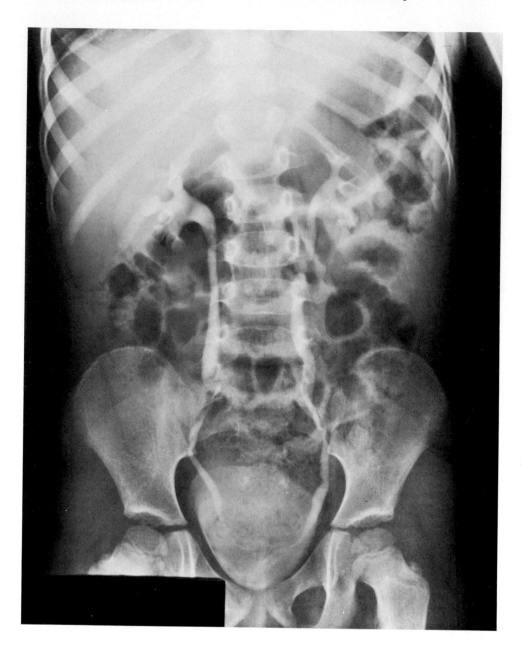

Figure 22

An intravenous pyelogram obtained 20
minutes after the injection of
a suitable contrast medium
(female aged 5 years).

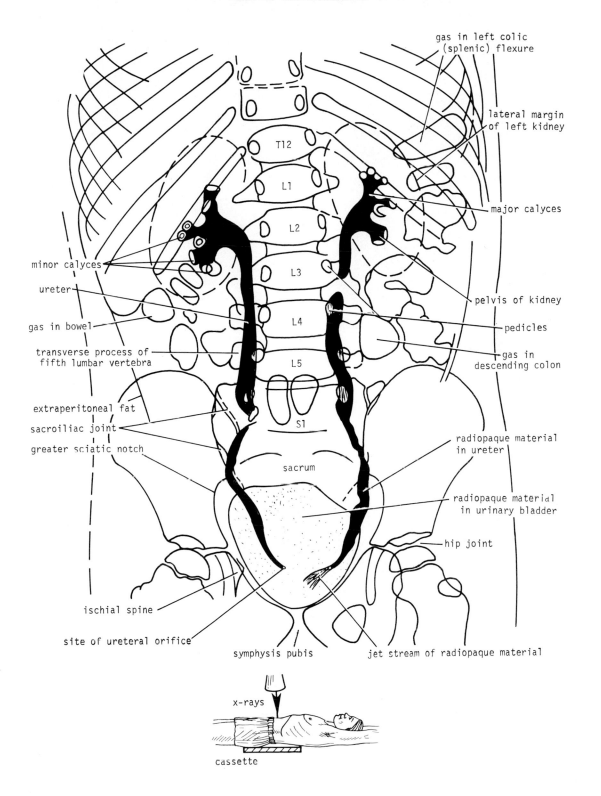

gas in left colic (splenic) flexure

lateral margin of left kidney

major calyces

minor calyces

pelvis of kidney

ureter

gas in bowel

pedicles

transverse process of fifth lumbar vertebra

gas in descending colon

extraperitoneal fat

sacroiliac joint

radiopaque material in ureter

greater sciatic notch

radiopaque material in urinary bladder

hip joint

ischial spine

site of ureteral orifice

symphysis pubis

jet stream of radiopaque material

T12
L1
L2
L3
L4
L5
S1
sacrum

x-rays

cassette

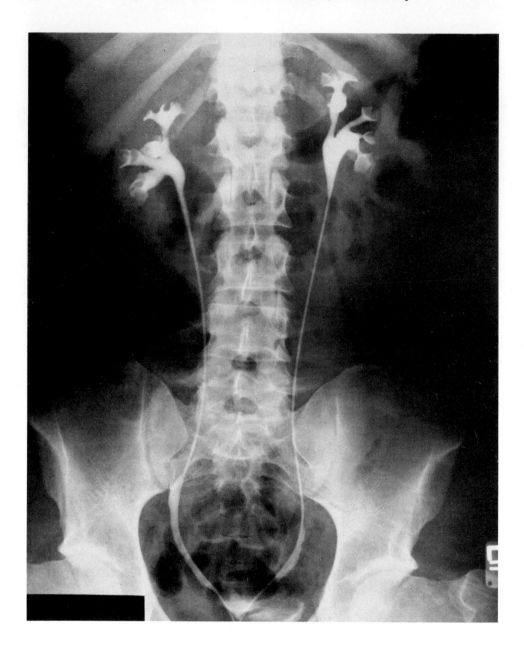

Figure 23

A retrograde pyelogram following
the injection of radiopaque material
into ureteric catheters
(male aged 32 years).

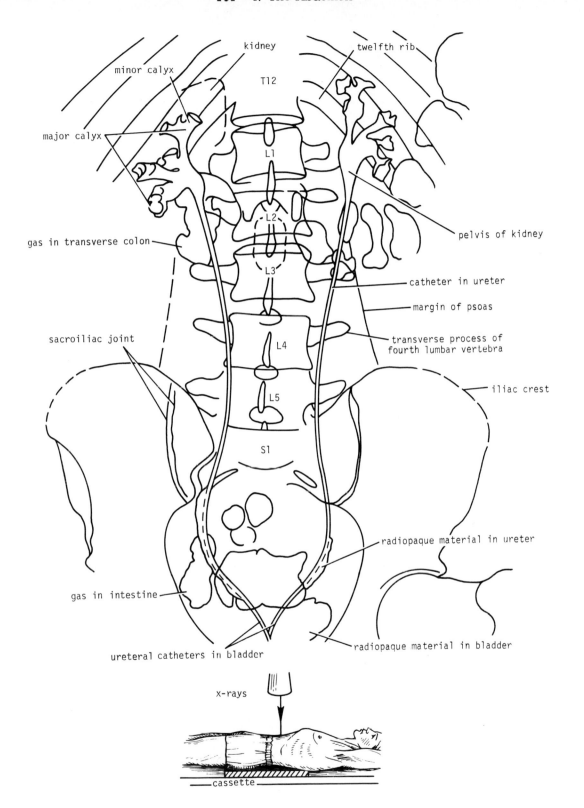

kidney

twelfth rib

minor calyx

T12

major calyx

L1

gas in transverse colon

L2

pelvis of kidney

L3

catheter in ureter

margin of psoas

transverse process of
fourth lumbar vertebra

sacroiliac joint

L4

iliac crest

L5

S1

radiopaque material in ureter

gas in intestine

radiopaque material in bladder

ureteral catheters in bladder

x-rays

cassette

5

THE PELVIS

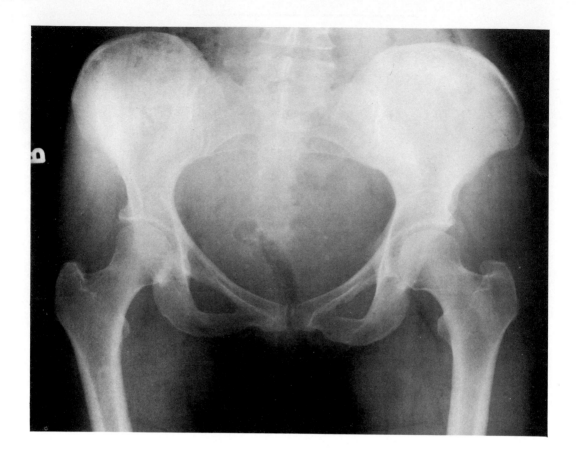

Figure 1

Anteroposterior radiograph of pelvis
(female aged 46 years).

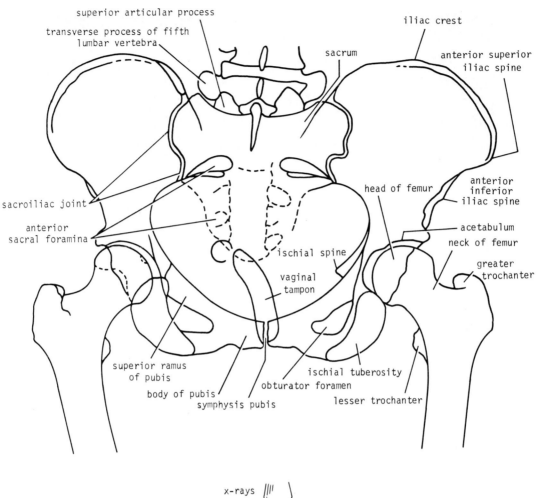

superior articular process

transverse process of fifth
lumbar vertebra

iliac crest

sacrum

anterior superior
iliac spine

sacroiliac joint

anterior
sacral foramina

head of femur

anterior
inferior
iliac spine

acetabulum

neck of femur

greater
trochanter

ischial spine

vaginal
tampon

superior ramus
of pubis

body of pubis

symphysis pubis

obturator foramen

ischial tuberosity

lesser trochanter

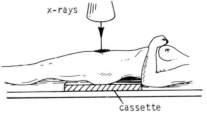

x-rays

cassette

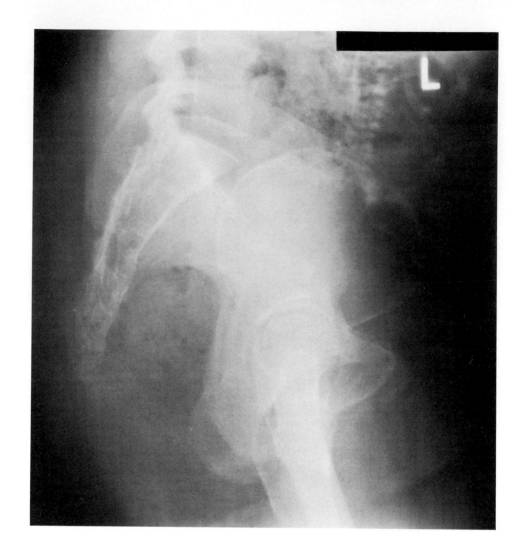

Figure 2

Lateral radiograph of pregnant woman
aged 25 years. The pregnancy
is in the third trimester.

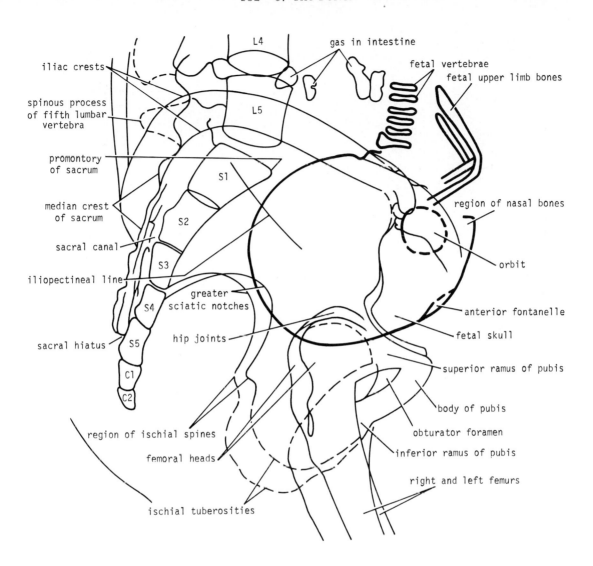

iliac crests

spinous process
of fifth lumbar
vertebra

promontory
of sacrum

median crest
of sacrum

sacral canal

iliopectineal line

sacral hiatus

region of ischial spines

femoral heads

ischial tuberosities

L4

L5

S1

S2

S3

S4

S5

C1

C2

greater
sciatic notches

hip joints

gas in intestine

fetal vertebrae
fetal upper limb bones

region of nasal bones

orbit

anterior fontanelle

fetal skull

superior ramus of pubis

body of pubis

obturator foramen

inferior ramus of pubis

right and left femurs

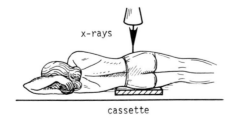

x-rays

cassette

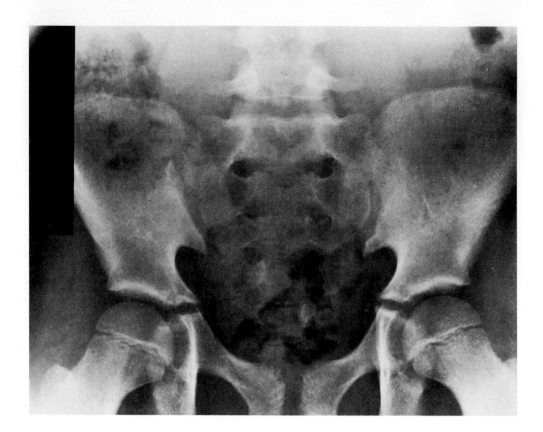

Figure 3

Anteroposterior radiograph of pelvis
(male aged 11 years).

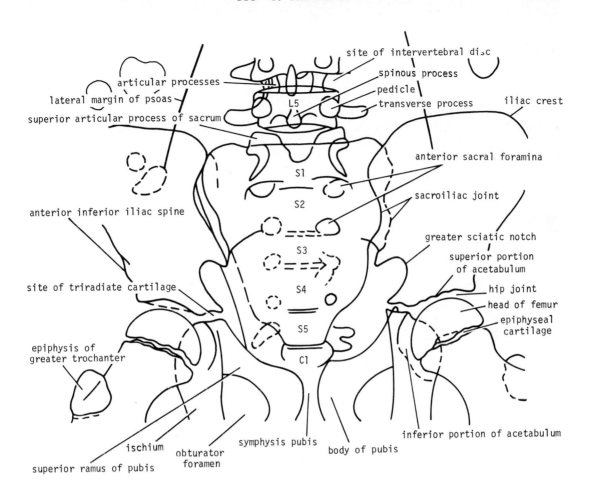

articular processes

lateral margin of psoas

superior articular process of sacrum

site of intervertebral disc

spinous process

pedicle

transverse process

iliac crest

L5

anterior sacral foramina

S1

S2

sacroiliac joint

anterior inferior iliac spine

greater sciatic notch

superior portion of acetabulum

S3

site of triradiate cartilage

hip joint

S4

head of femur

epiphyseal cartilage

S5

epiphysis of greater trochanter

C1

inferior portion of acetabulum

ischium

obturator foramen

symphysis pubis

body of pubis

superior ramus of pubis

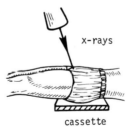

x-rays

cassette

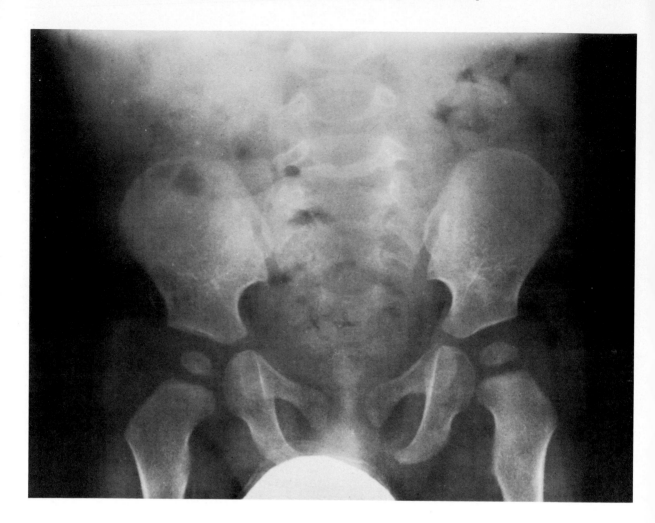

Figure 4

Anteroposterior radiograph of pelvis
(male aged 4 years).

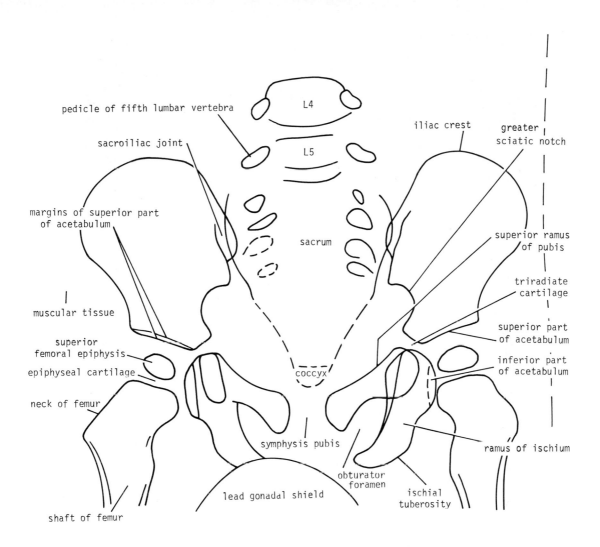

pedicle of fifth lumbar vertebra

sacroiliac joint

margins of superior part
of acetabulum

muscular tissue

superior
femoral epiphysis

epiphyseal cartilage

neck of femur

shaft of femur

L4

L5

sacrum

coccyx

symphysis pubis

lead gonadal shield

iliac crest

greater
sciatic notch

superior ramus
of pubis

triradiate
cartilage

superior part
of acetabulum

inferior part
of acetabulum

ramus of ischium

obturator
foramen

ischial
tuberosity

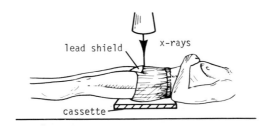

lead shield   x-rays

cassette

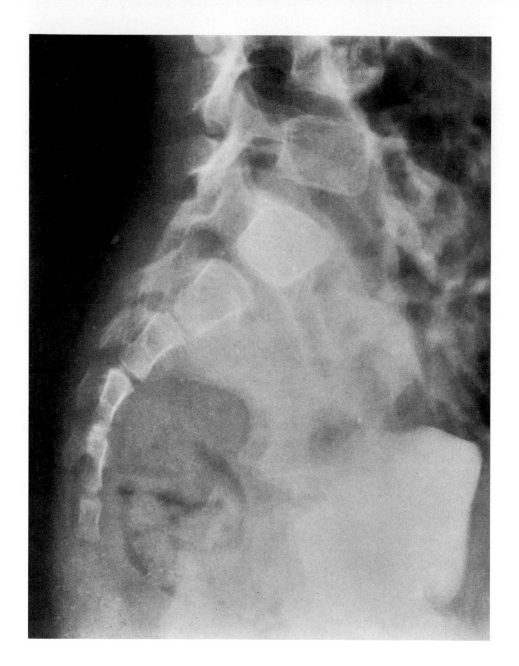

Figure 5

Lateral radiograph of pelvis
(female aged 5 years).

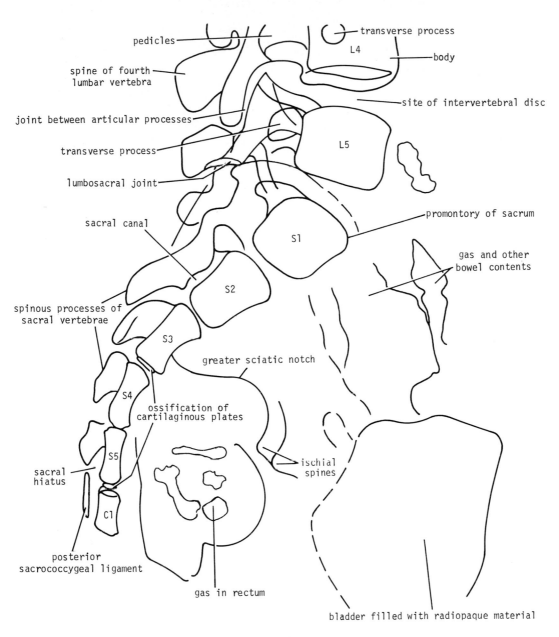

pedicles

transverse process

L4

spine of fourth
lumbar vertebra

body

site of intervertebral disc

joint between articular processes

transverse process

L5

lumbosacral joint

sacral canal

promontory of sacrum

S1

gas and other
bowel contents

spinous processes of
sacral vertebrae

S2

S3

greater sciatic notch

S4

ossification of
cartilaginous plates

S5

ischial
spines

sacral
hiatus

C1

posterior
sacrococcygeal ligament

gas in rectum

bladder filled with radiopaque material

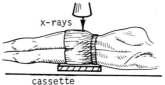

x-rays

cassette

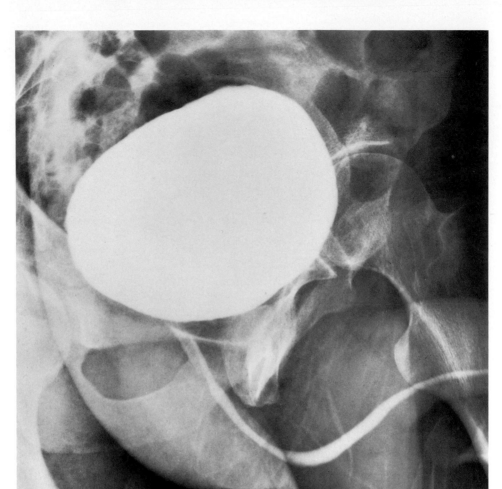

Figure 6

Cystourethrogram following the
intravenous injection of contrast medium
(male aged 28 years).

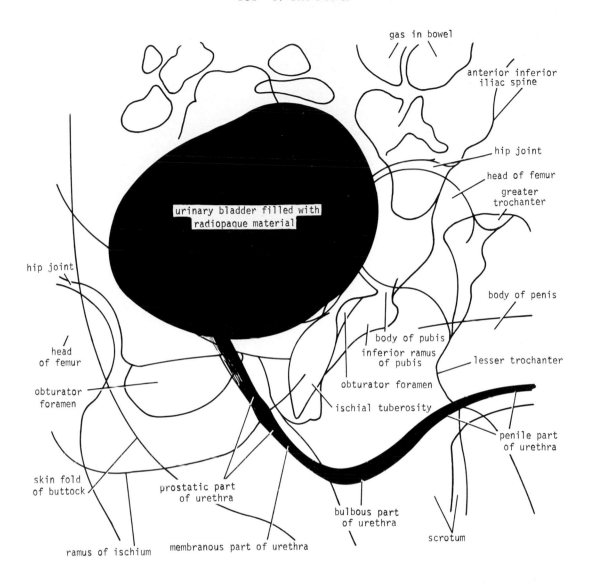

gas in bowel

anterior inferior iliac spine

hip joint

head of femur

greater trochanter

urinary bladder filled with radiopaque material

body of penis

hip joint

body of pubis

inferior ramus of pubis

lesser trochanter

head of femur

obturator foramen

obturator foramen

ischial tuberosity

penile part of urethra

skin fold of buttock

prostatic part of urethra

bulbous part of urethra

membranous part of urethra

scrotum

ramus of ischium

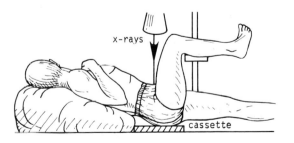

x-rays

cassette

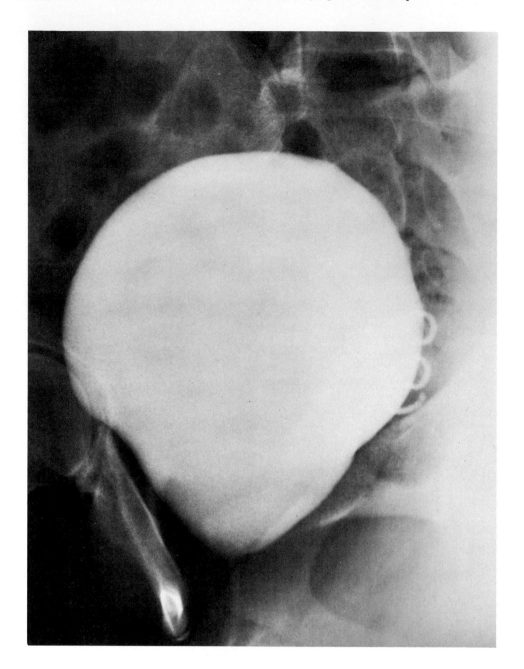

Figure 7

Voiding cystourethrogram
following the intravenous
injection of contrast medium
(female aged 19 years).

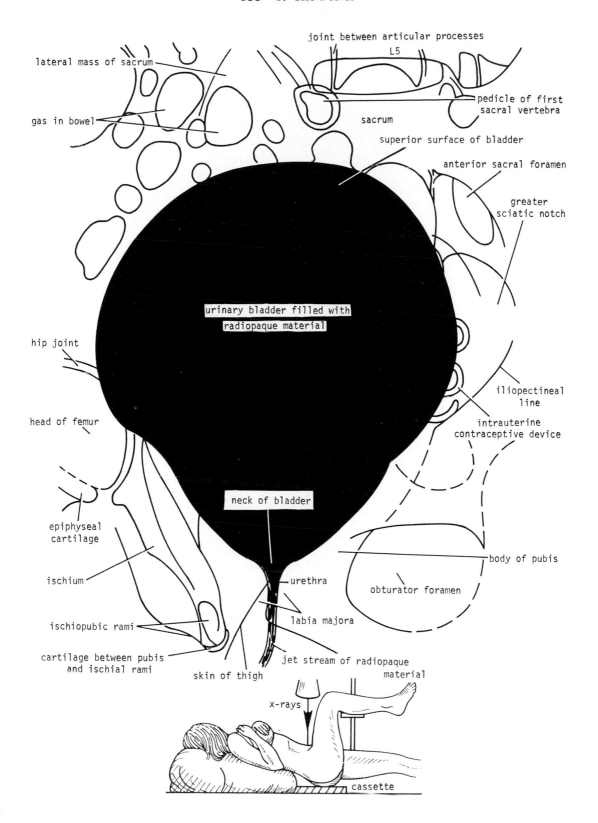

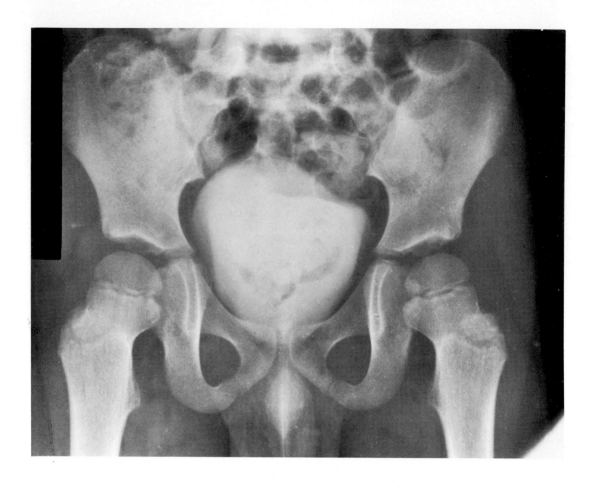

Figure 8

Anteroposterior cystogram
following the intravenous
injection of contrast medium
(male aged 5 years).

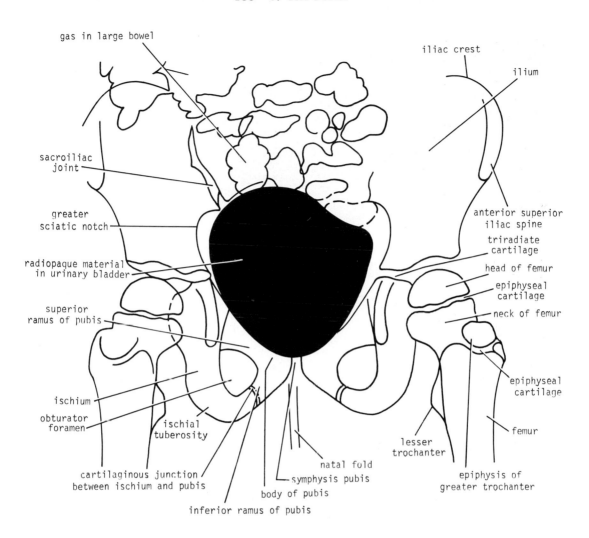

gas in large bowel

iliac crest

ilium

sacroiliac joint

anterior superior iliac spine

greater sciatic notch

triradiate cartilage

radiopaque material in urinary bladder

head of femur

epiphyseal cartilage

neck of femur

superior ramus of pubis

epiphyseal cartilage

ischium

femur

obturator foramen

ischial tuberosity

lesser trochanter

cartilaginous junction between ischium and pubis

natal fold

symphysis pubis

epiphysis of greater trochanter

body of pubis

inferior ramus of pubis

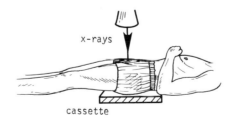

x-rays

cassette

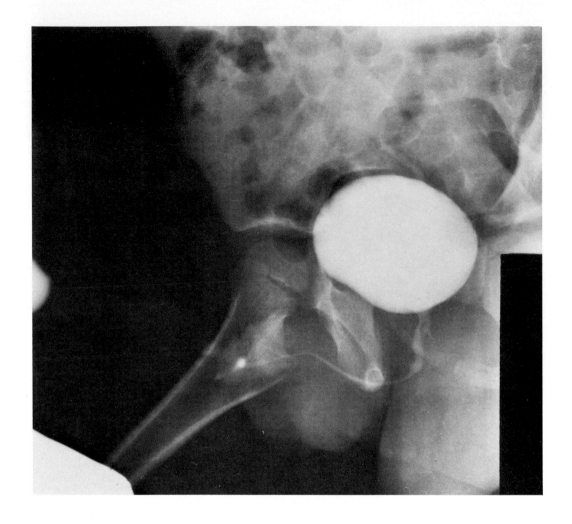

Figure 9

Lateral voiding cystourethrogram
following the intravenous
injection of contrast medium
(male aged 5 years).

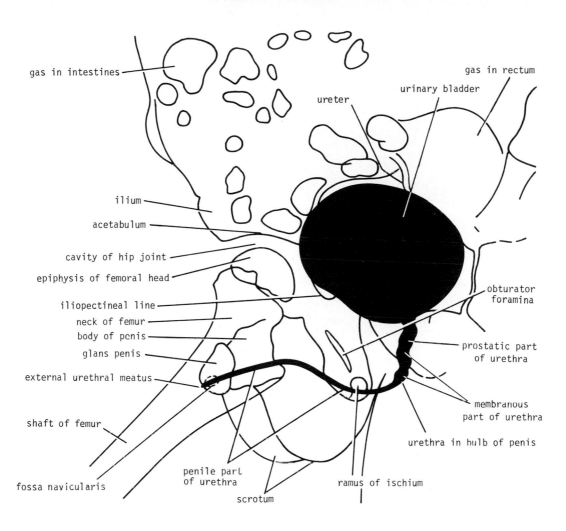

gas in intestines

gas in rectum

ureter

urinary bladder

ilium

acetabulum

cavity of hip joint

epiphysis of femoral head

obturator
foramina

iliopectineal line

neck of femur

body of penis

glans penis

prostatic part
of urethra

external urethral meatus

shaft of femur

membranous
part of urethra

urethra in bulb of penis

fossa navicularis

penile part
of urethra

ramus of ischium

scrotum

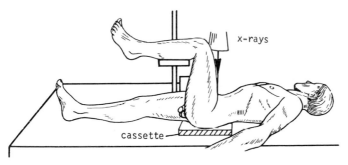

x-rays

cassette

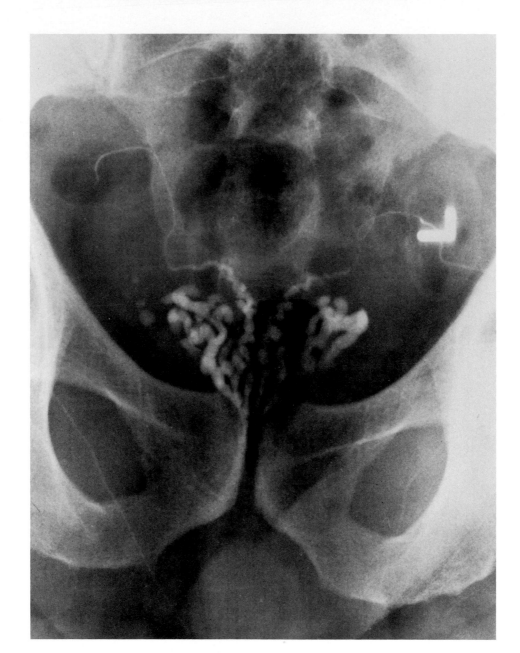

Figure 10

Seminal vesiculogram following the
injection of radiopaque material into
the lumen of the vas deferens
(male aged 40 years).

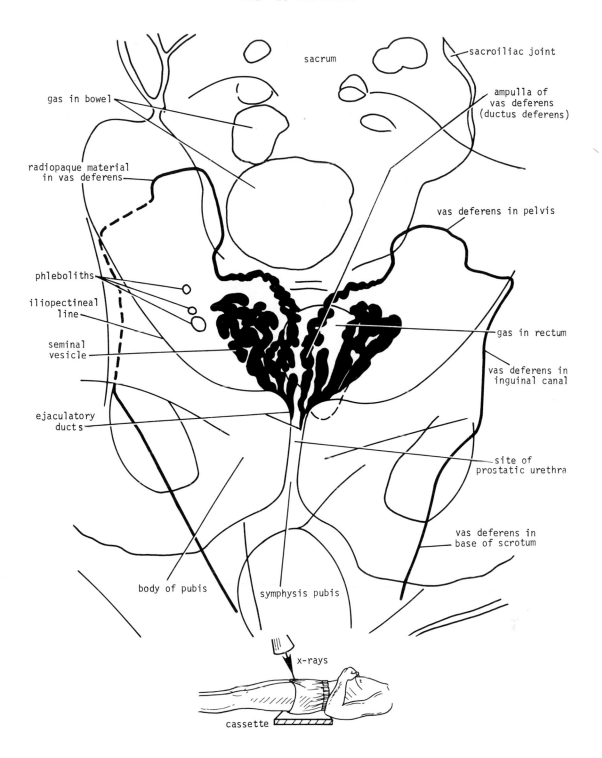

sacrum

sacroiliac joint

gas in bowel

ampulla of
vas deferens
(ductus deferens)

radiopaque material
in vas deferens

vas deferens in pelvis

phleboliths

iliopectineal
line

gas in rectum

seminal
vesicle

vas deferens in
inguinal canal

ejaculatory
ducts

site of
prostatic urethra

vas deferens in
base of scrotum

body of pubis

symphysis pubis

x-rays

cassette

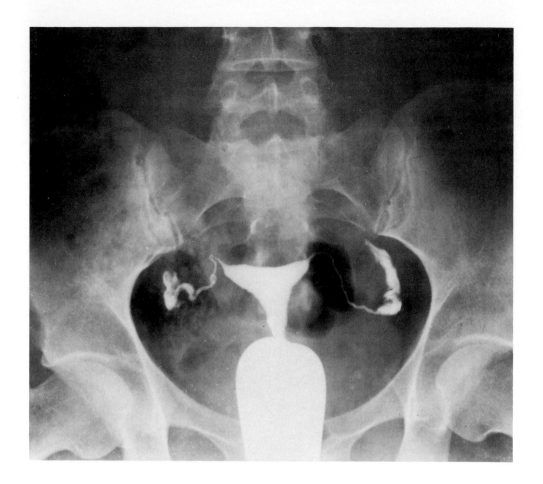

Figure 11

Hysterosalpingogram following the
injection of radiopaque material
into the canal of the cervix
(female aged 25 years).

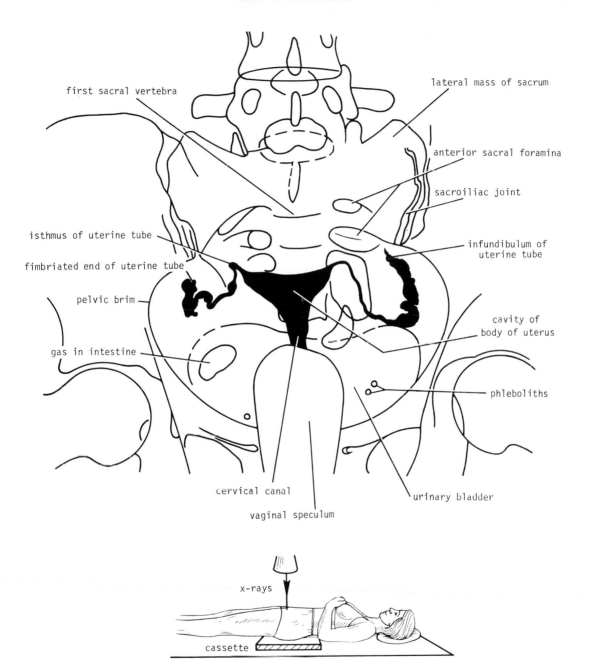

first sacral vertebra

lateral mass of sacrum

anterior sacral foramina

sacroiliac joint

isthmus of uterine tube

infundibulum of uterine tube

fimbriated end of uterine tube

pelvic brim

cavity of body of uterus

gas in intestine

phleboliths

cervical canal

urinary bladder

vaginal speculum

x-rays

cassette

6

THE LOWER LIMB

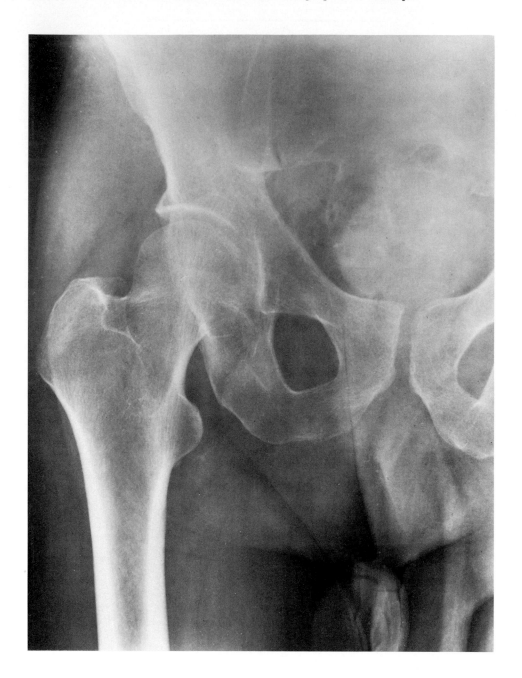

Figure 1

Anteroposterior radiograph of hip joint
(male aged 49 years).

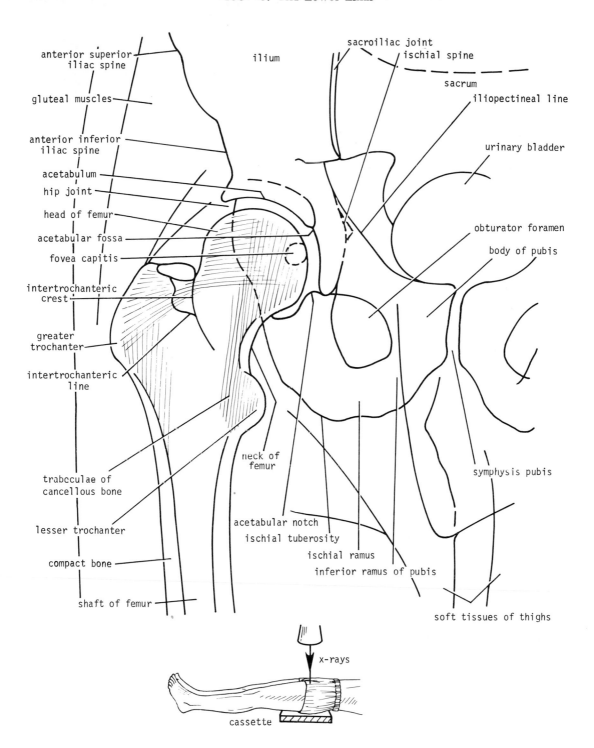

anterior superior
iliac spine

ilium

sacroiliac joint

ischial spine

sacrum

iliopectineal line

gluteal muscles

anterior inferior
iliac spine

urinary bladder

acetabulum

hip joint

head of femur

acetabular fossa

fovea capitis

obturator foramen

body of pubis

intertrochanteric
crest

greater
trochanter

intertrochanteric
line

trabeculae of
cancellous bone

neck of
femur

symphysis pubis

lesser trochanter

compact bone

acetabular notch

ischial tuberosity

ischial ramus

inferior ramus of pubis

soft tissues of thighs

shaft of femur

x-rays

cassette

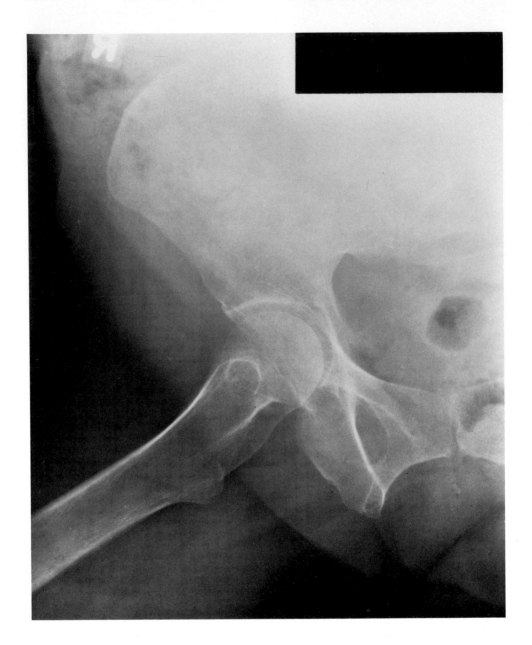

Figure 2

Lateral radiograph of hip joint
(female aged 54 years).

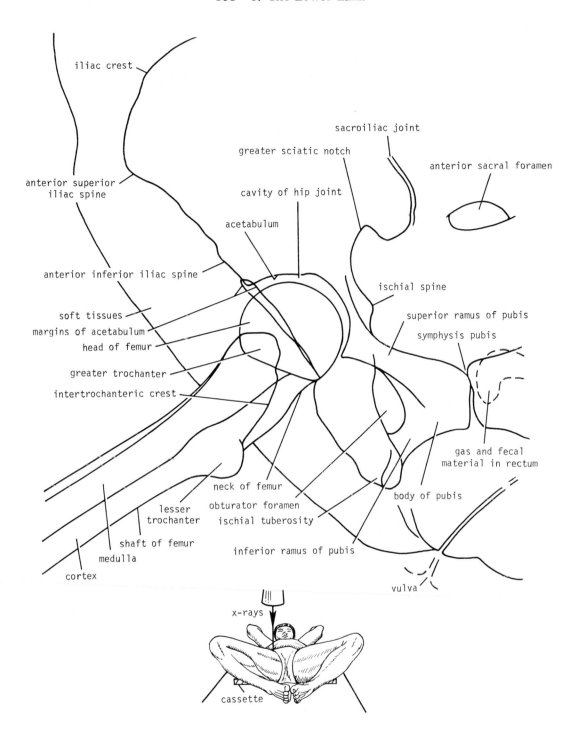

iliac crest

sacroiliac joint

greater sciatic notch

anterior sacral foramen

anterior superior
iliac spine

cavity of hip joint

acetabulum

anterior inferior iliac spine

ischial spine

superior ramus of pubis

soft tissues
margins of acetabulum
head of femur

symphysis pubis

greater trochanter

intertrochanteric crest

gas and fecal
material in rectum

neck of femur

lesser
trochanter

obturator foramen
ischial tuberosity

body of pubis

shaft of femur

medulla

inferior ramus of pubis

cortex

vulva

x-rays

cassette

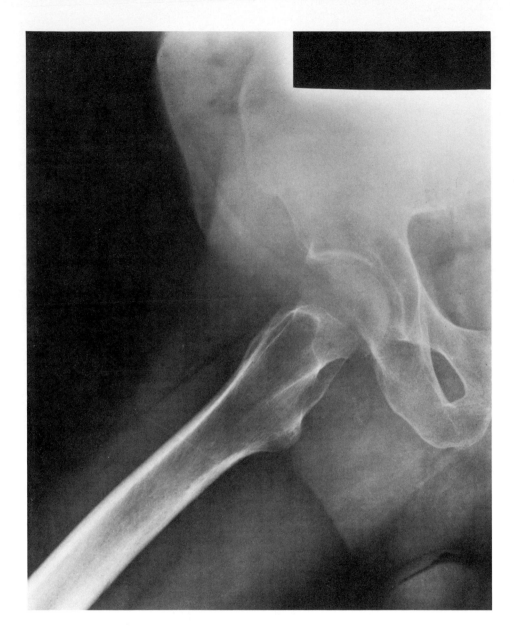

Figure 3

Lateral radiograph of hip joint
(male aged 49 years).

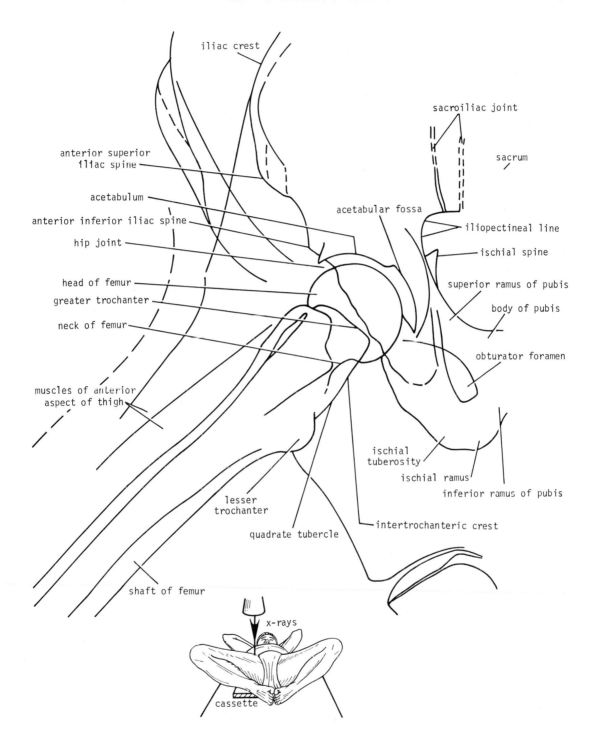

iliac crest

sacroiliac joint

sacrum

anterior superior
iliac spine

acetabulum

anterior inferior iliac spine

hip joint

acetabular fossa

iliopectineal line

ischial spine

superior ramus of pubis

body of pubis

head of femur

greater trochanter

neck of femur

obturator foramen

muscles of anterior
aspect of thigh

ischial
tuberosity

ischial ramus

inferior ramus of pubis

lesser
trochanter

quadrate tubercle

intertrochanteric crest

shaft of femur

x-rays

cassette

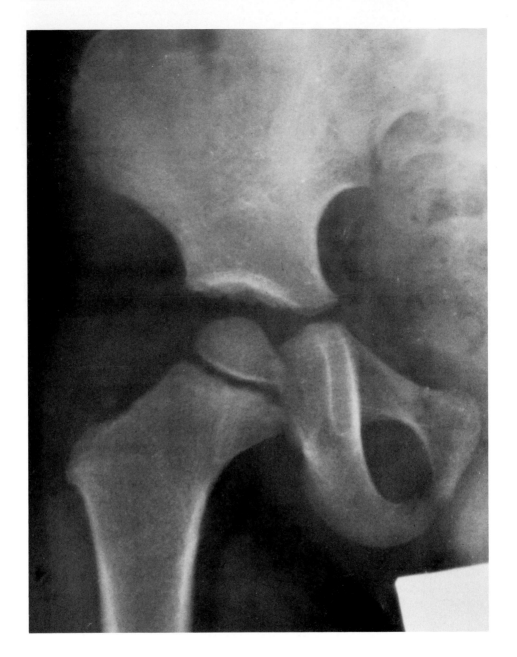

Figure 4

Anteroposterior radiograph of hip joint
(male aged 3 years).

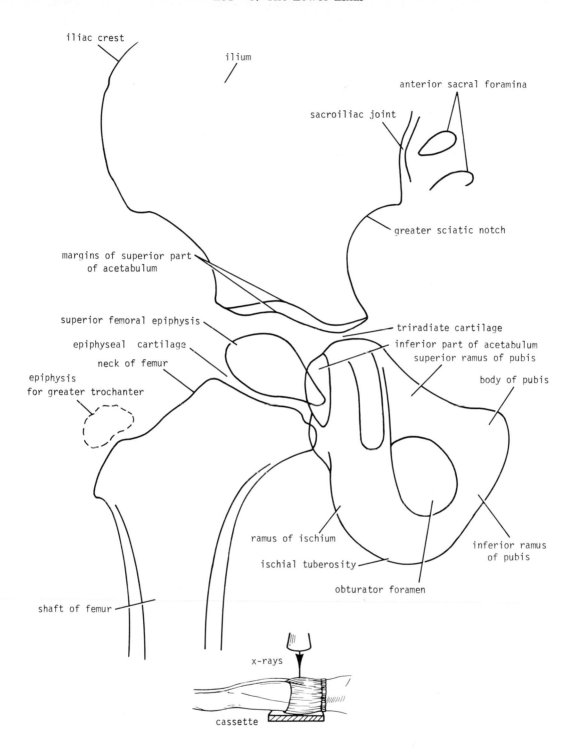

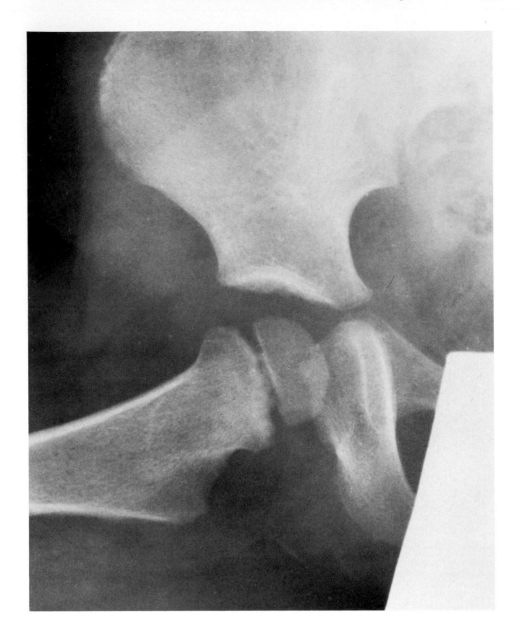

Figure 5

Lateral radiograph of hip joint
(male aged 8 years).

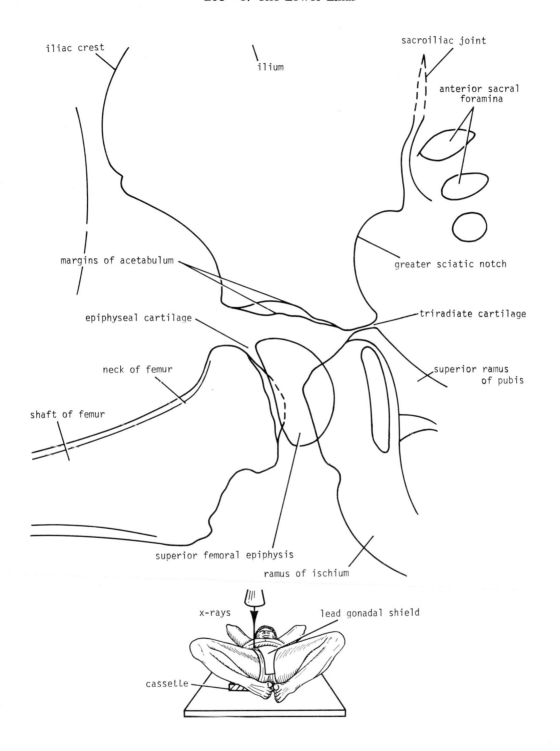

iliac crest

ilium

sacroiliac joint

anterior sacral
foramina

margins of acetabulum

greater sciatic notch

epiphyseal cartilage

triradiate cartilage

neck of femur

superior ramus
of pubis

shaft of femur

superior femoral epiphysis

ramus of ischium

x-rays

lead gonadal shield

cassette

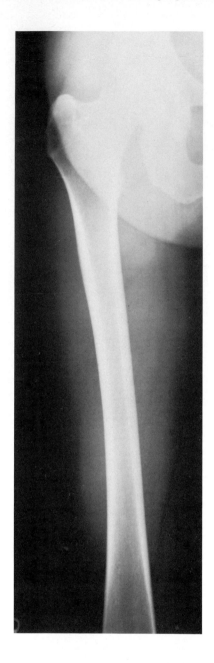

Figure 6

Anteroposterior radiograph of thigh
(female aged 32 years).

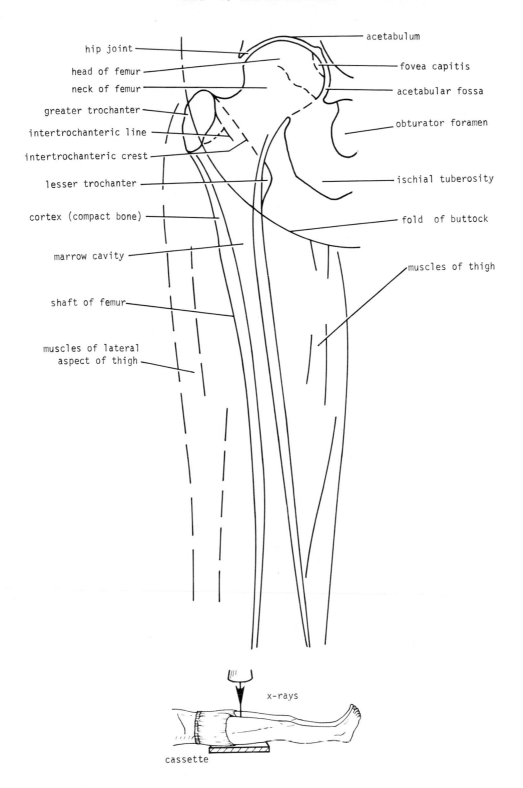

hip joint

head of femur

neck of femur

greater trochanter

intertrochanteric line

intertrochanteric crest

lesser trochanter

cortex (compact bone)

marrow cavity

shaft of femur

muscles of lateral
aspect of thigh

acetabulum

fovea capitis

acetabular fossa

obturator foramen

ischial tuberosity

fold of buttock

muscles of thigh

x-rays

cassette

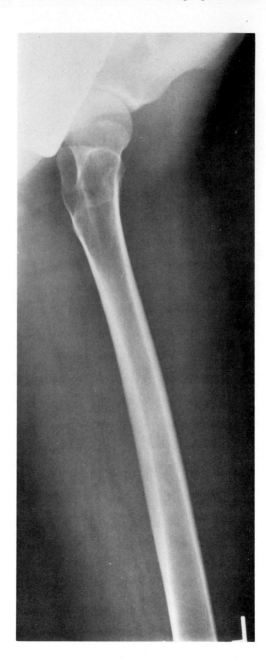

Figure 7

Lateral radiograph of thigh
(female aged 32 years).

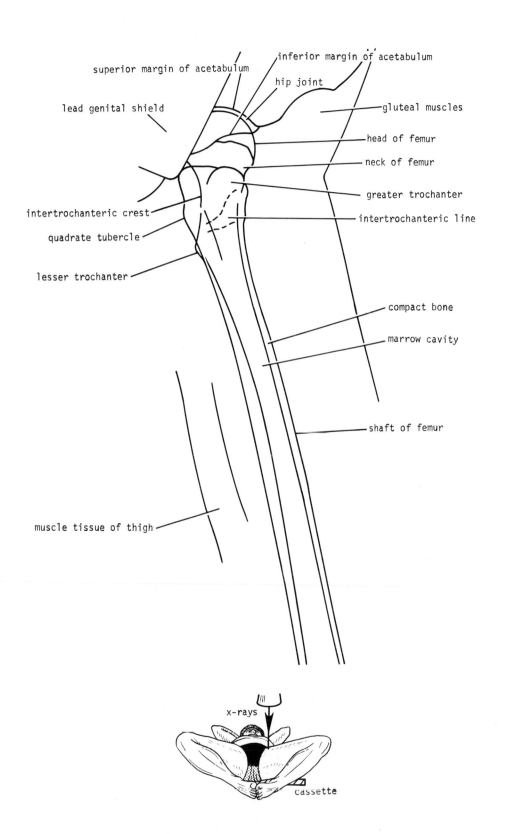

superior margin of acetabulum

inferior margin of acetabulum

hip joint

lead genital shield

gluteal muscles

head of femur

neck of femur

greater trochanter

intertrochanteric crest

intertrochanteric line

quadrate tubercle

lesser trochanter

compact bone

marrow cavity

shaft of femur

muscle tissue of thigh

x-rays

cassette

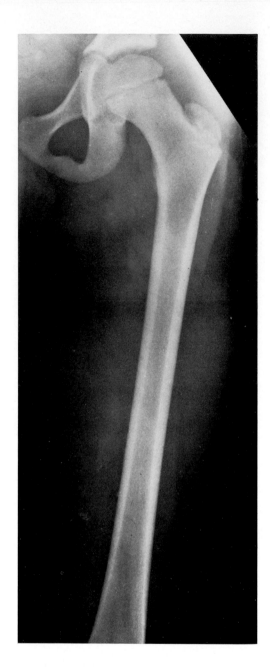

Figure 8

Anteroposterior radiograph of thigh
(male aged 8 years).

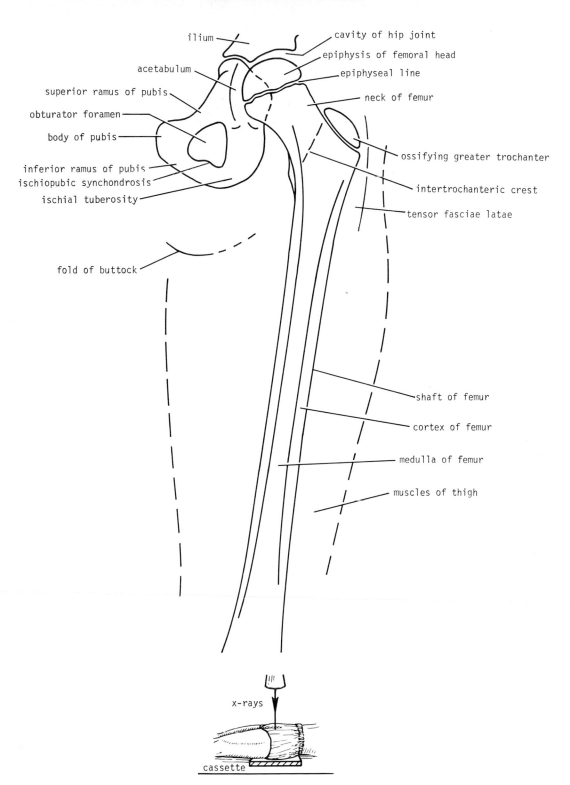

ilium

cavity of hip joint

epiphysis of femoral head

acetabulum

epiphyseal line

superior ramus of pubis

neck of femur

obturator foramen

body of pubis

ossifying greater trochanter

inferior ramus of pubis

intertrochanteric crest

ischiopubic synchondrosis

ischial tuberosity

tensor fasciae latae

fold of buttock

shaft of femur

cortex of femur

medulla of femur

muscles of thigh

x-rays

cassette

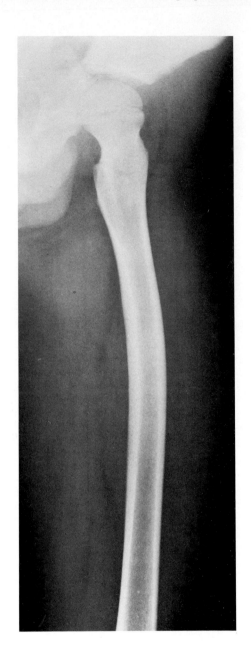

Figure 9

Lateral radiograph of thigh
(male aged 8 years).

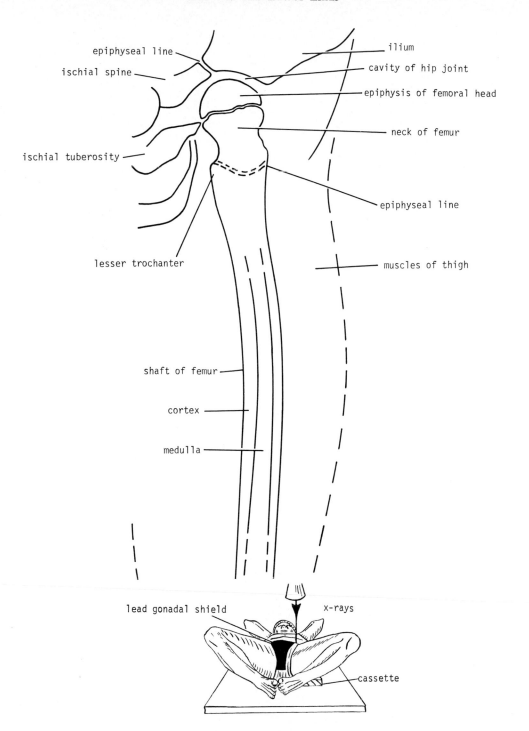

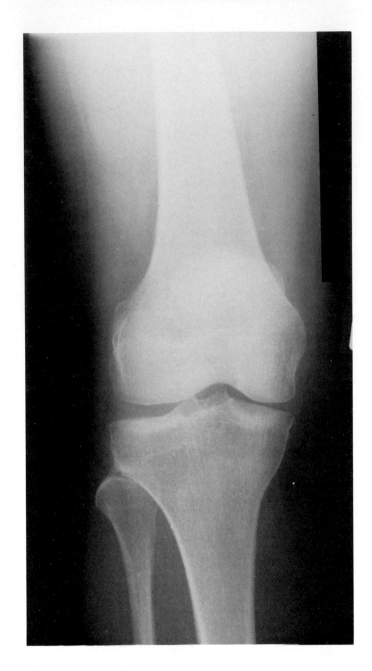

Figure 10

Anteroposterior radiograph of knee joint
(female aged 46 years).

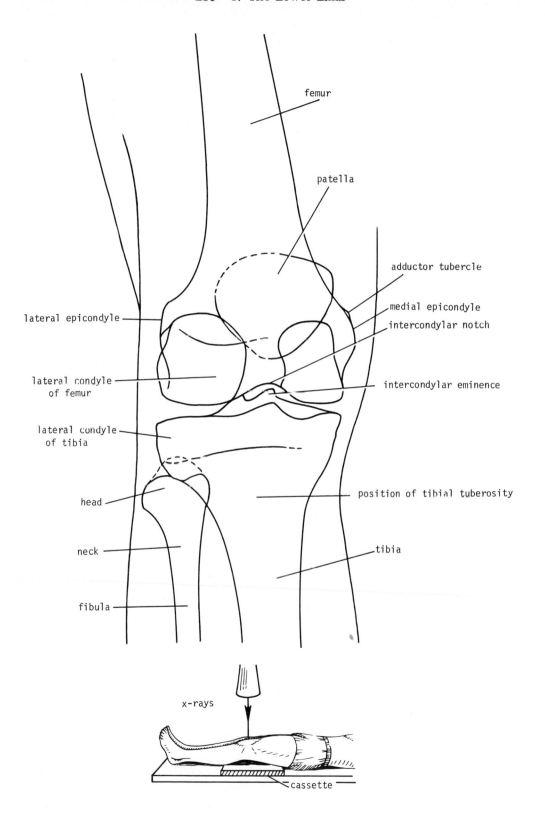

femur

patella

adductor tubercle

lateral epicondyle

medial epicondyle

intercondylar notch

lateral condyle
of femur

intercondylar eminence

lateral condyle
of tibia

position of tibial tuberosity

head

neck

tibia

fibula

x-rays

cassette

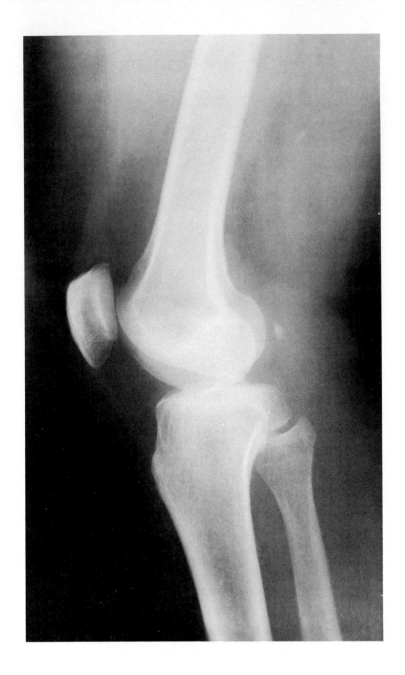

Figure 11

Lateral radiograph of knee joint
(female aged 46 years).

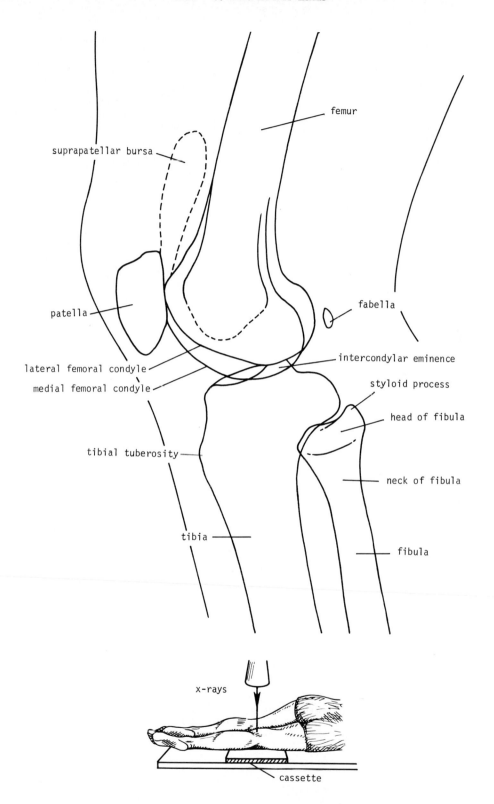

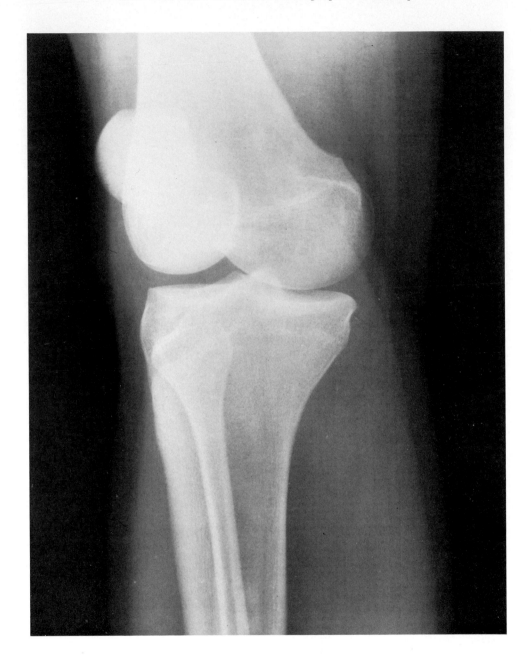

Figure 12

Anteroposterior oblique
radiograph of knee joint
(male aged 22 years).

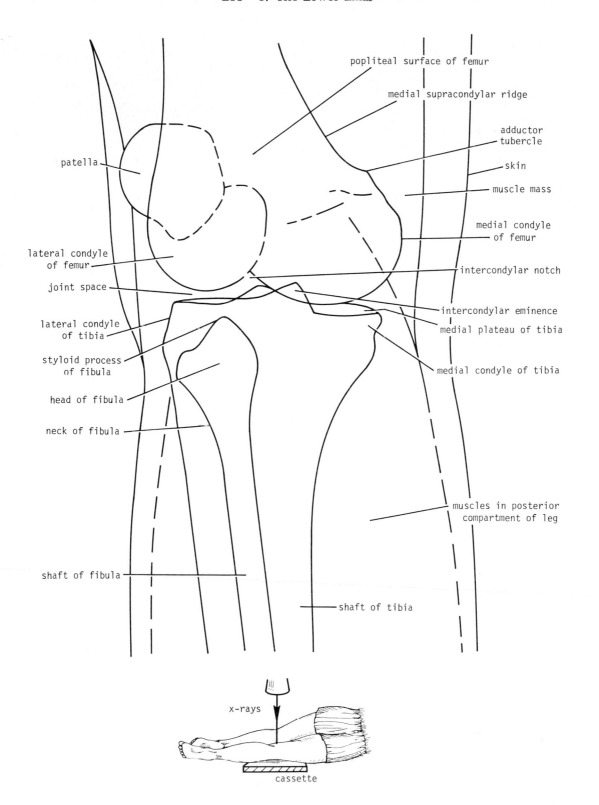

popliteal surface of femur

medial supracondylar ridge

adductor tubercle

skin

muscle mass

medial condyle of femur

intercondylar notch

intercondylar eminence

medial plateau of tibia

medial condyle of tibia

muscles in posterior compartment of leg

shaft of tibia

patella

lateral condyle of femur

joint space

lateral condyle of tibia

styloid process of fibula

head of fibula

neck of fibula

shaft of fibula

x-rays

cassette

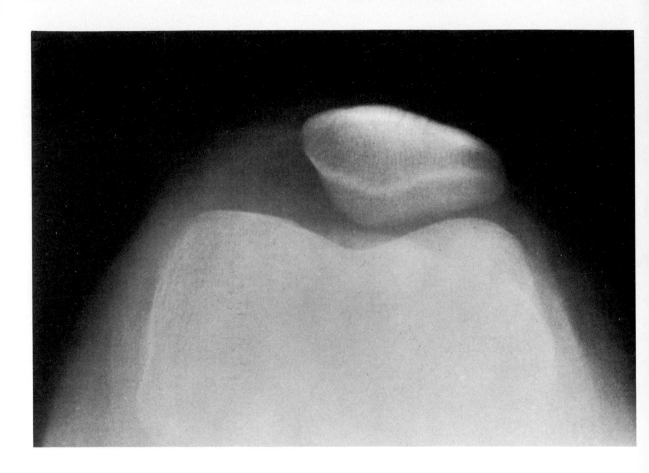

Figure 13

Tangential view of patella
(female aged 19 years).

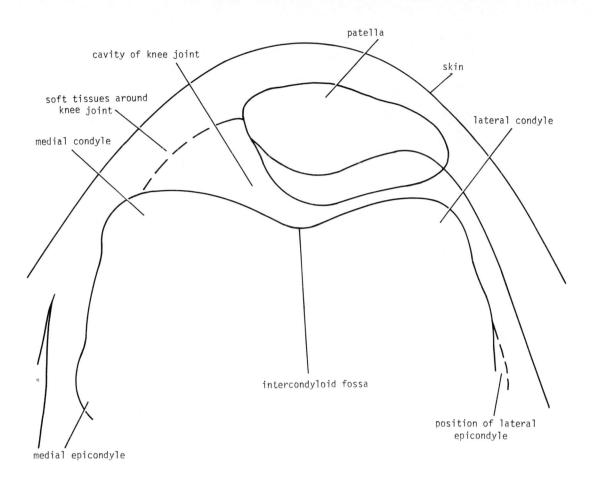

cavity of knee joint

soft tissues around
knee joint

medial condyle

patella

skin

lateral condyle

intercondyloid fossa

position of lateral
epicondyle

medial epicondyle

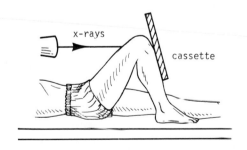

x-rays

cassette

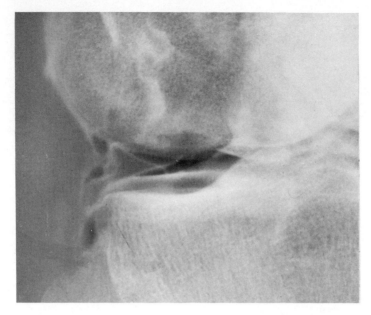

A

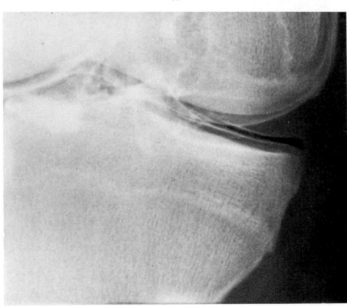

B

Figure 14

Pneumoarthrography of the knee
(A. male aged 17 years;
B. male aged 32 years).

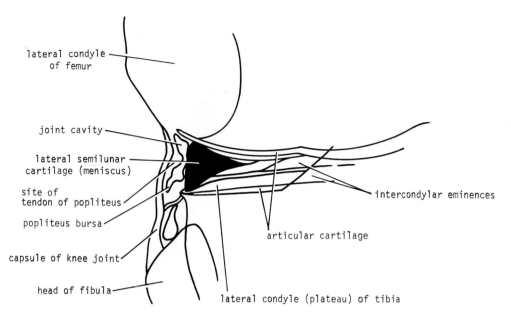

lateral condyle
of femur

joint cavity

lateral semilunar
cartilage (meniscus)

site of
tendon of popliteus

popliteus bursa

capsule of knee joint

head of fibula

intercondylar eminences

articular cartilage

lateral condyle (plateau) of tibia

A

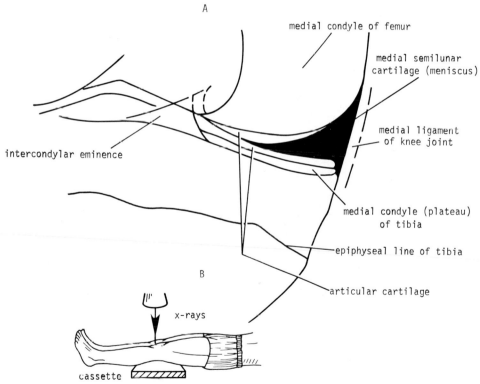

medial condyle of femur

medial semilunar
cartilage (meniscus)

medial ligament
of knee joint

intercondylar eminence

medial condyle (plateau)
of tibia

epiphyseal line of tibia

B

articular cartilage

x-rays

cassette

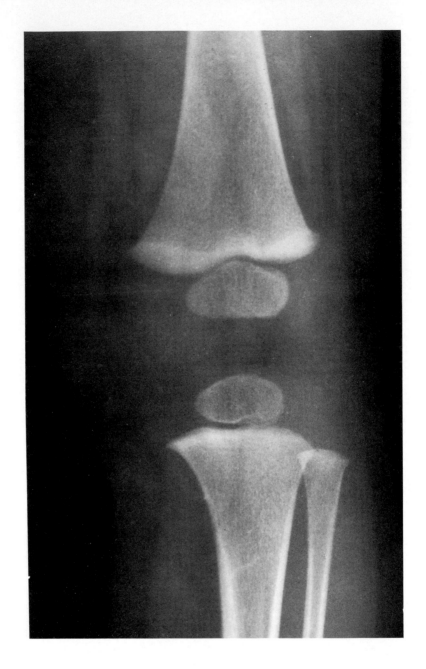

Figure 15

Anteroposterior radiograph of knee joint
(female aged 1 year).

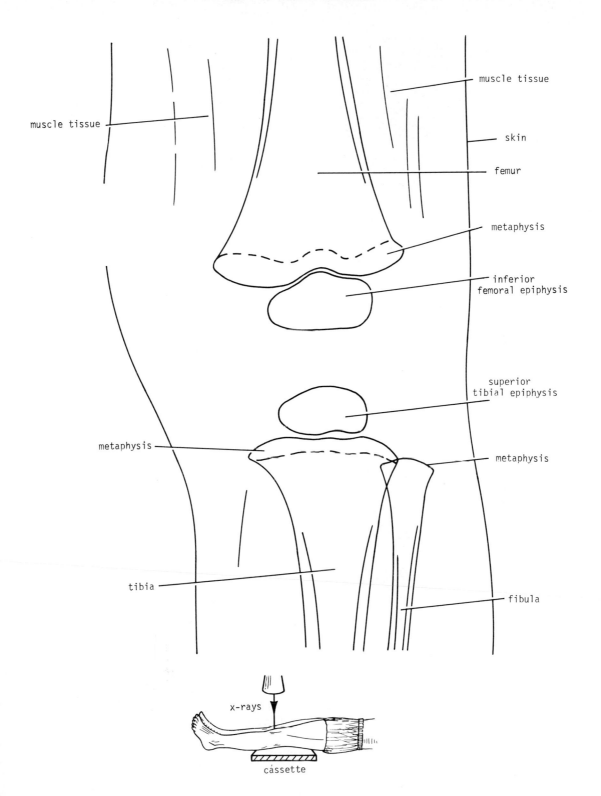

muscle tissue

muscle tissue

skin

femur

metaphysis

inferior
femoral epiphysis

superior
tibial epiphysis

metaphysis

metaphysis

tibia

fibula

x-rays

cassette

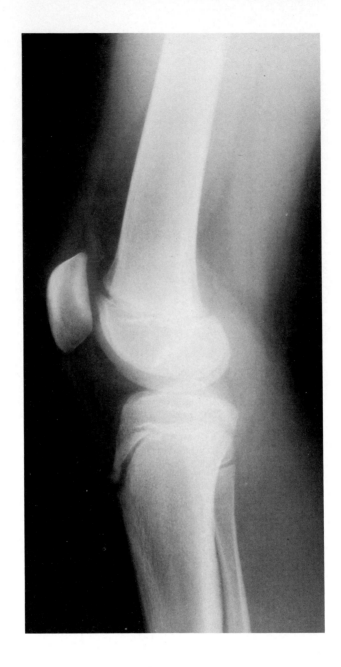

Figure 16

Lateral radiograph of knee joint
(female aged 12 years).

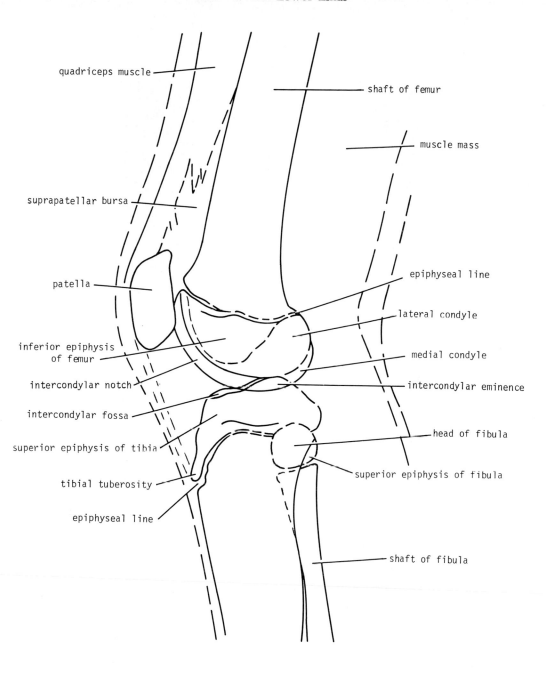

quadriceps muscle

shaft of femur

muscle mass

suprapatellar bursa

patella

epiphyseal line

lateral condyle

inferior epiphysis
of femur

medial condyle

intercondylar notch

intercondylar eminence

intercondylar fossa

head of fibula

superior epiphysis of tibia

superior epiphysis of fibula

tibial tuberosity

epiphyseal line

shaft of fibula

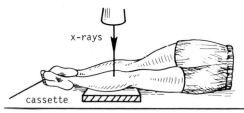

x-rays

cassette

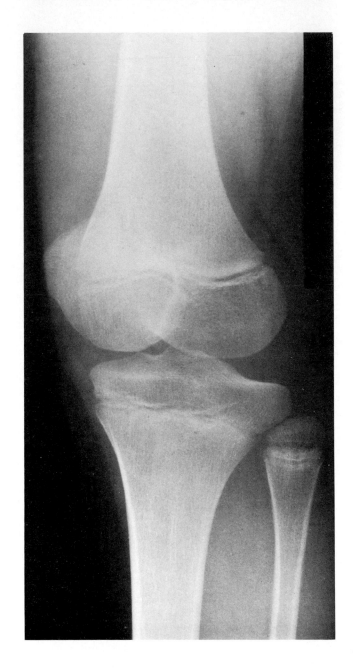

Figure 17

Anteroposterior internal oblique
radiograph of knee joint
(male aged 12 years).

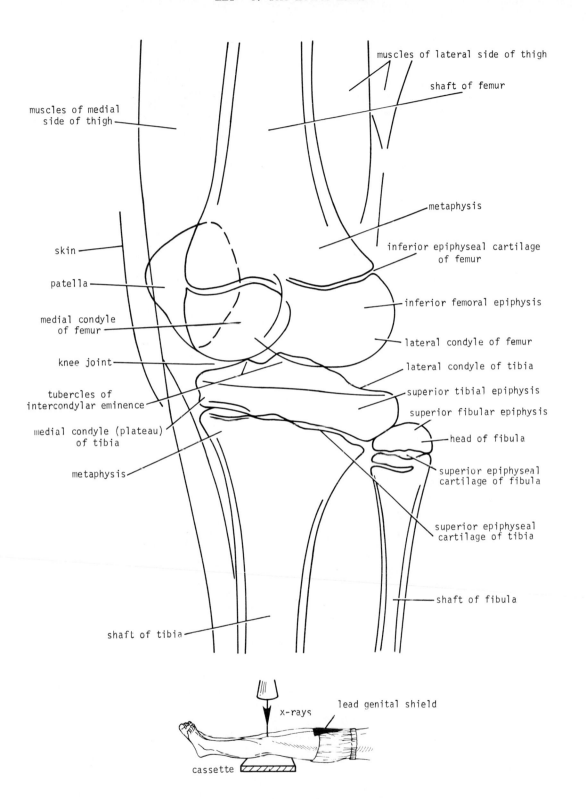

muscles of lateral side of thigh

shaft of femur

muscles of medial side of thigh

metaphysis

inferior epiphyseal cartilage of femur

skin

inferior femoral epiphysis

patella

medial condyle of femur

lateral condyle of femur

knee joint

lateral condyle of tibia

tubercles of intercondylar eminence

superior tibial epiphysis

superior fibular epiphysis

medial condyle (plateau) of tibia

head of fibula

superior epiphyseal cartilage of fibula

metaphysis

superior epiphyseal cartilage of tibia

shaft of fibula

shaft of tibia

lead genital shield

x-rays

cassette

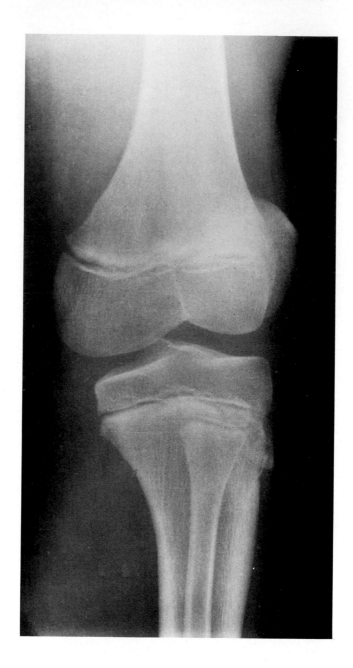

Figure 18

Anteroposterior external oblique
radiograph of knee joint
(male aged 12 years).

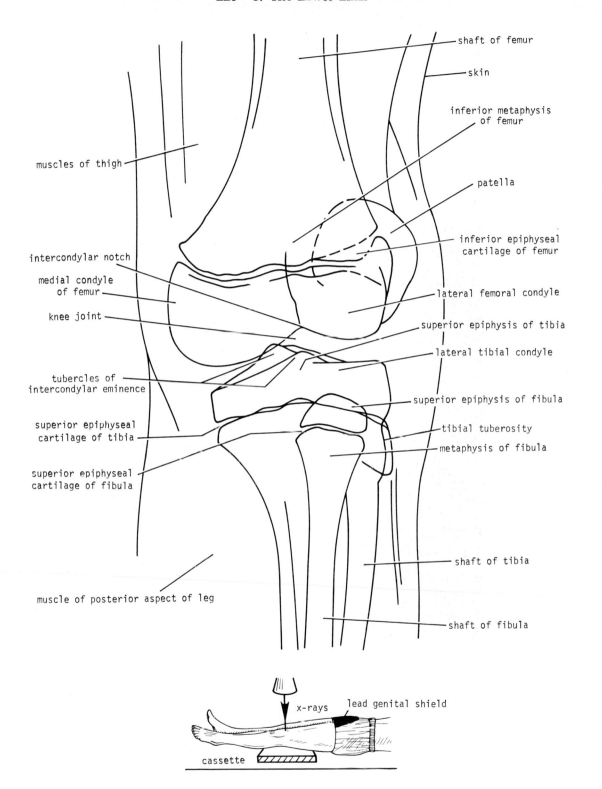

shaft of femur

skin

inferior metaphysis
of femur

patella

muscles of thigh

inferior epiphyseal
cartilage of femur

intercondylar notch

medial condyle
of femur

lateral femoral condyle

knee joint

superior epiphysis of tibia

lateral tibial condyle

tubercles of
intercondylar eminence

superior epiphysis of fibula

superior epiphyseal
cartilage of tibia

tibial tuberosity

metaphysis of fibula

superior epiphyseal
cartilage of fibula

shaft of tibia

muscle of posterior aspect of leg

shaft of fibula

x-rays   lead genital shield

cassette

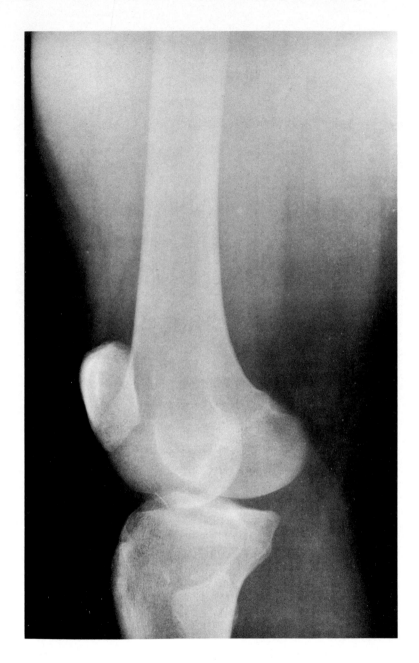

Figure 19

Anteroposterior external oblique
radiograph of knee joint
(male aged 17 years).

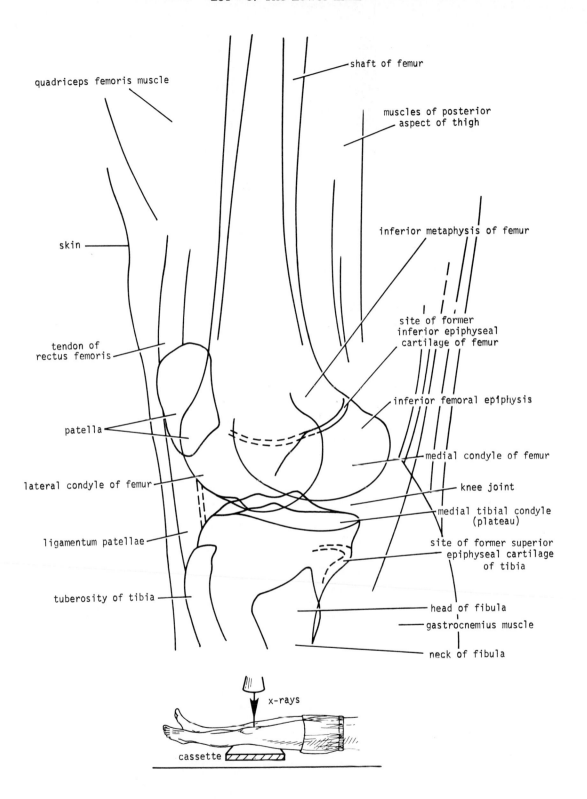

quadriceps femoris muscle

shaft of femur

muscles of posterior
aspect of thigh

skin

inferior metaphysis of femur

tendon of
rectus femoris

site of former
inferior epiphyseal
cartilage of femur

patella

inferior femoral epiphysis

medial condyle of femur

lateral condyle of femur

knee joint

medial tibial condyle
(plateau)

ligamentum patellae

site of former superior
epiphyseal cartilage
of tibia

tuberosity of tibia

head of fibula

gastrocnemius muscle

neck of fibula

x-rays

cassette

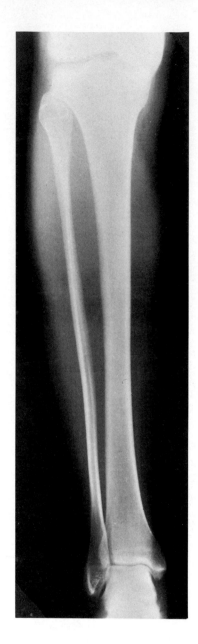

Figure 20

Anteroposterior radiograph of leg
(female aged 32 years).

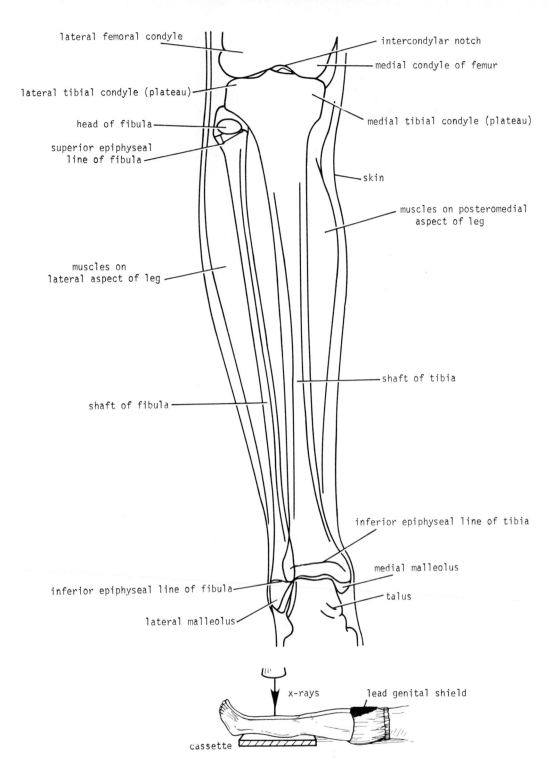

lateral femoral condyle

intercondylar notch

medial condyle of femur

lateral tibial condyle (plateau)

medial tibial condyle (plateau)

head of fibula

superior epiphyseal line of fibula

skin

muscles on posteromedial aspect of leg

muscles on lateral aspect of leg

shaft of tibia

shaft of fibula

inferior epiphyseal line of tibia

medial malleolus

inferior epiphyseal line of fibula

talus

lateral malleolus

x-rays

lead genital shield

cassette

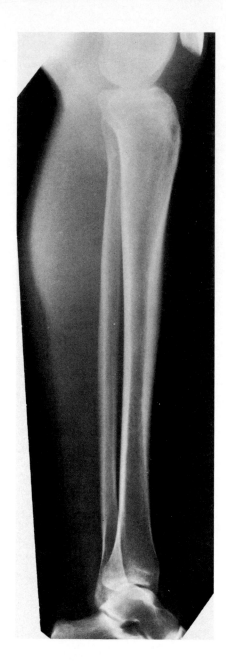

Figure 21

Lateral radiograph of leg
(female aged 32 years).

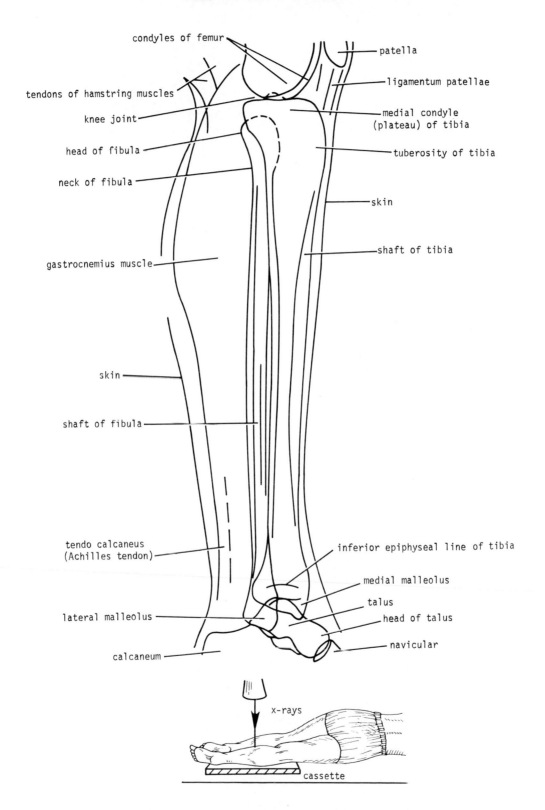

condyles of femur

patella

ligamentum patellae

tendons of hamstring muscles

medial condyle (plateau) of tibia

knee joint

head of fibula

tuberosity of tibia

neck of fibula

skin

shaft of tibia

gastrocnemius muscle

skin

shaft of fibula

tendo calcaneus (Achilles tendon)

inferior epiphyseal line of tibia

medial malleolus

talus

lateral malleolus

head of talus

navicular

calcaneum

x-rays

cassette

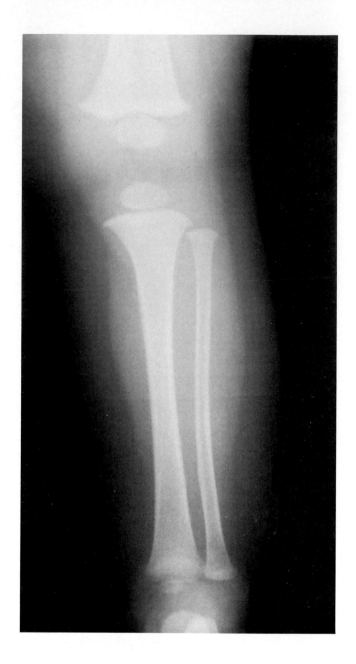

Figure 22

Anteroposterior radiograph of leg
(female aged 7 months).

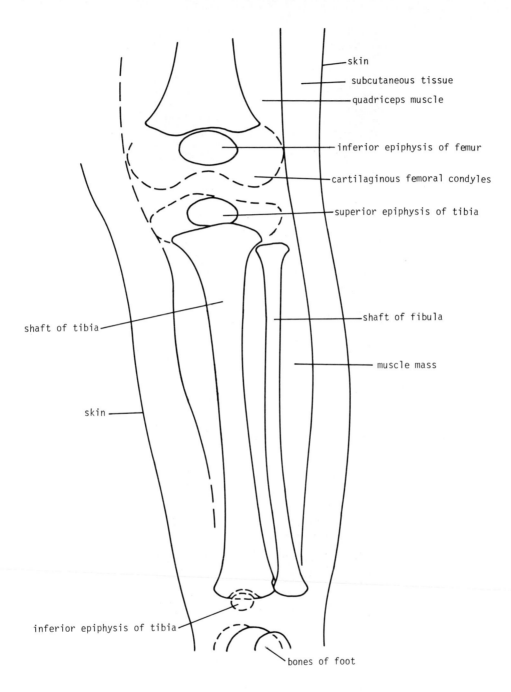

skin

subcutaneous tissue

quadriceps muscle

inferior epiphysis of femur

cartilaginous femoral condyles

superior epiphysis of tibia

shaft of fibula

muscle mass

shaft of tibia

skin

inferior epiphysis of tibia

bones of foot

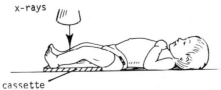

x-rays

cassette

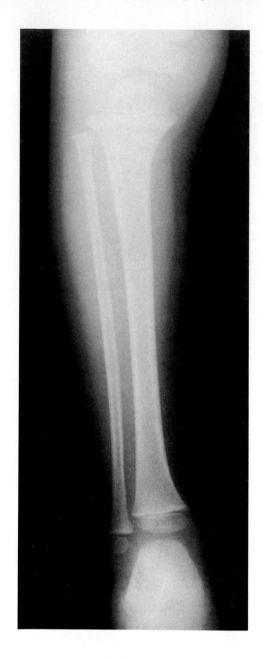

Figure 23

Anteroposterior radiograph of leg
(male aged 2½ years).

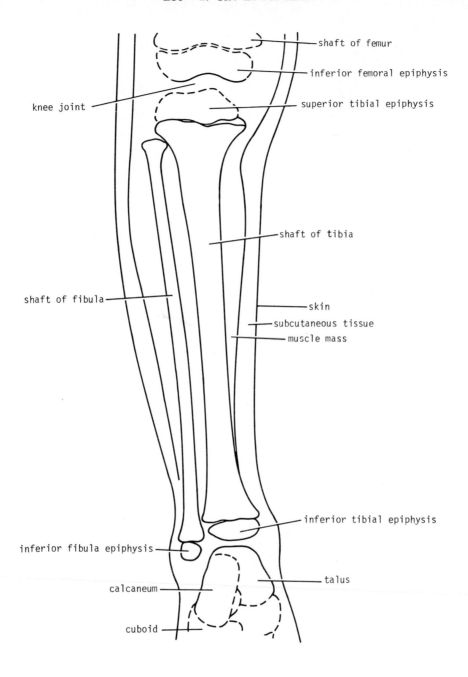

shaft of femur

inferior femoral epiphysis

knee joint

superior tibial epiphysis

shaft of tibia

shaft of fibula

skin

subcutaneous tissue

muscle mass

inferior tibial epiphysis

inferior fibula epiphysis

talus

calcaneum

cuboid

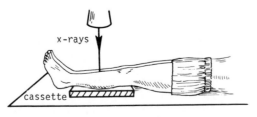

x-rays

cassette

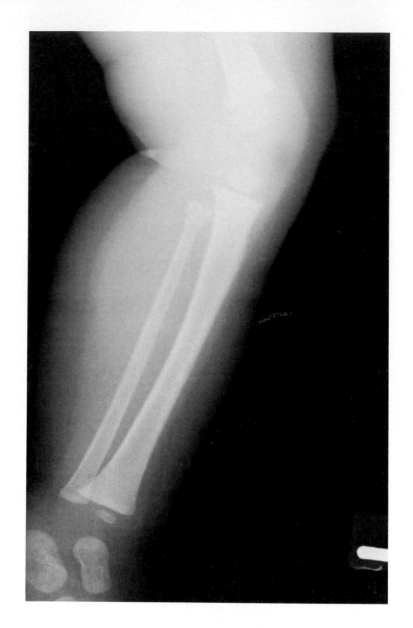

Figure 24

Lateral radiograph of leg
(female aged 7 months).

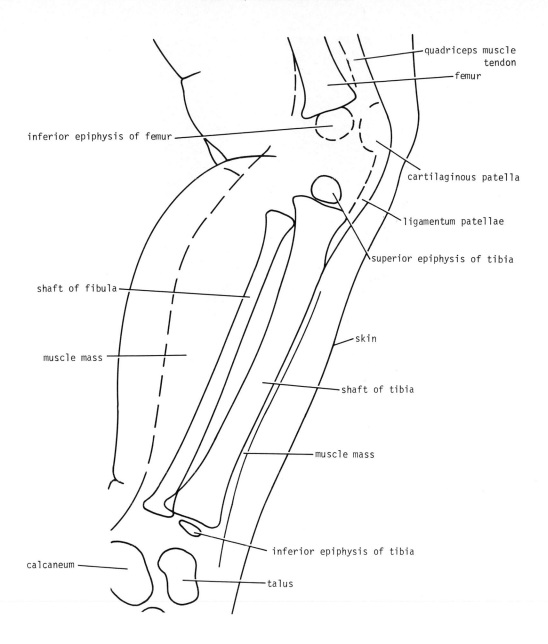

quadriceps muscle tendon

femur

inferior epiphysis of femur

cartilaginous patella

ligamentum patellae

superior epiphysis of tibia

shaft of fibula

skin

shaft of tibia

muscle mass

muscle mass

inferior epiphysis of tibia

calcaneum

talus

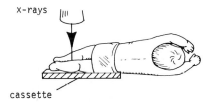

x-rays

cassette

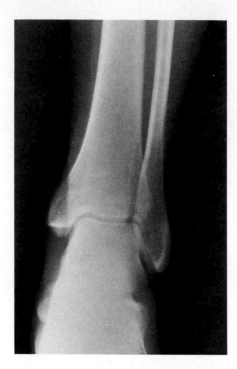

Figure 25

Anteroposterior radiograph of ankle joint
(female aged 32 years).

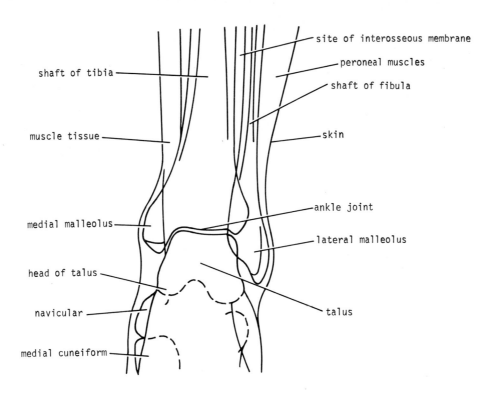

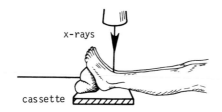

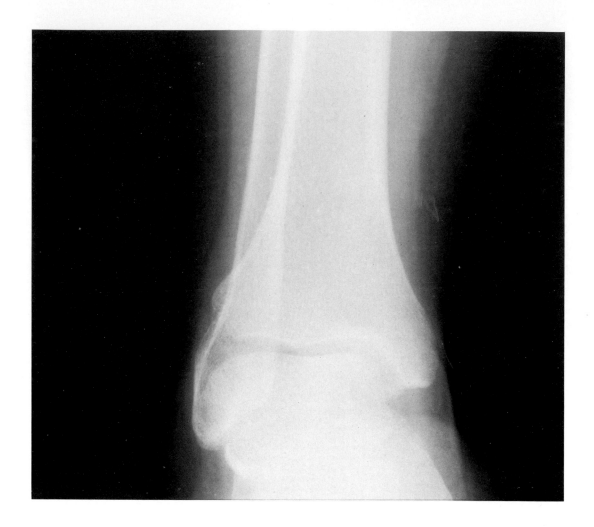

Figure 26

External oblique
radiograph of ankle joint
(female aged 53 years).

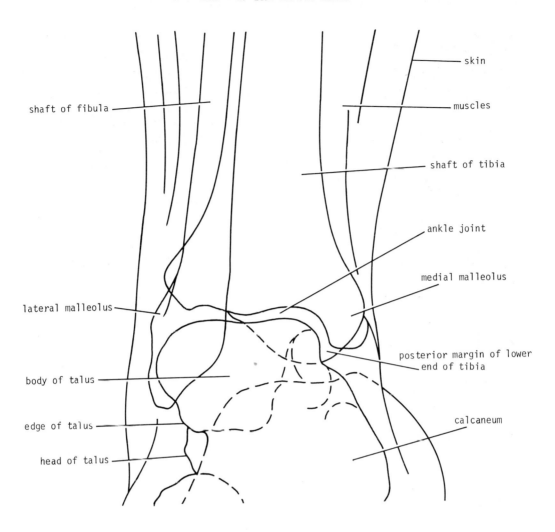

skin

muscles

shaft of fibula

shaft of tibia

ankle joint

medial malleolus

lateral malleolus

posterior margin of lower
end of tibia

body of talus

edge of talus

head of talus

calcaneum

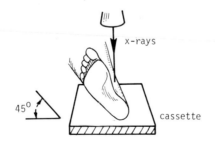

x-rays

45°

cassette

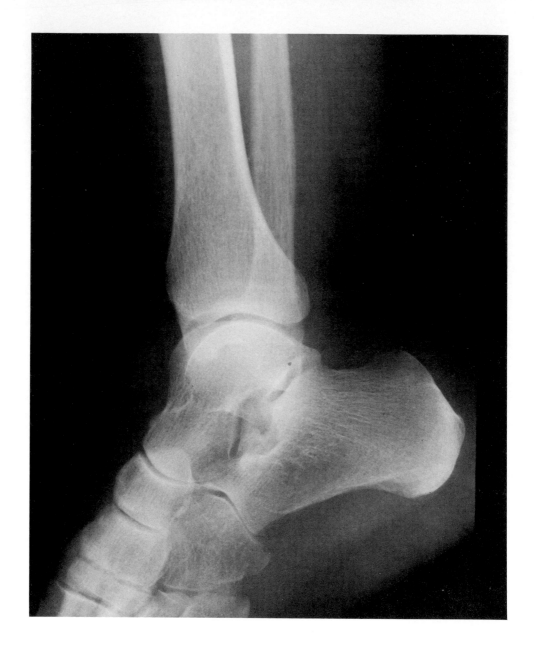

Figure 27

Lateral radiograph of ankle joint
(female aged 53 years).

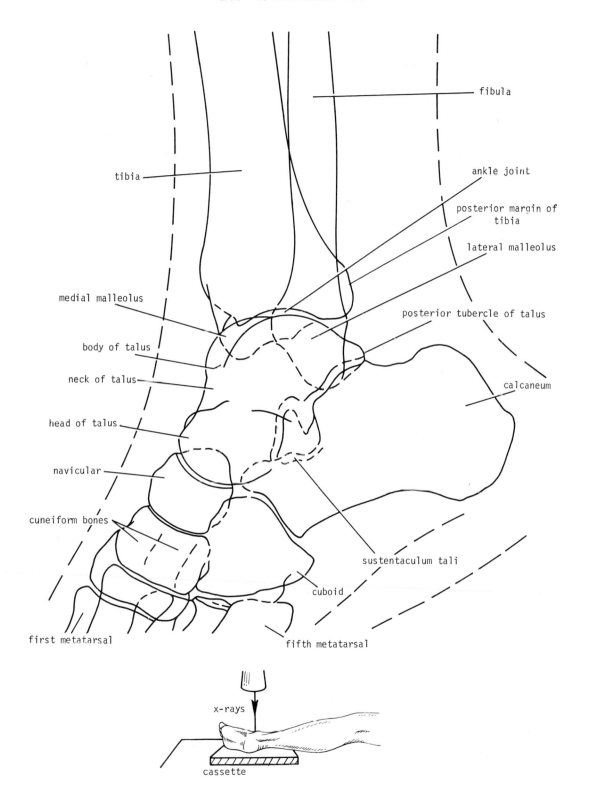

fibula

tibia

ankle joint

posterior margin of
tibia

lateral malleolus

medial malleolus

posterior tubercle of talus

body of talus

neck of talus

calcaneum

head of talus

navicular

cuneiform bones

sustentaculum tali

cuboid

first metatarsal

fifth metatarsal

x-rays

cassette

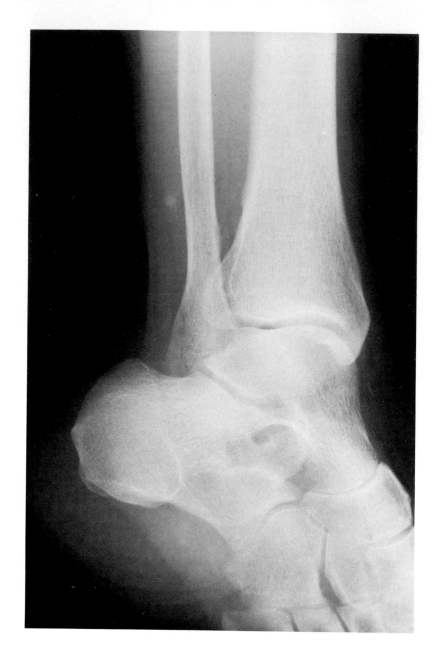

Figure 28

Internal oblique
radiograph of ankle joint
(female aged 53 years).

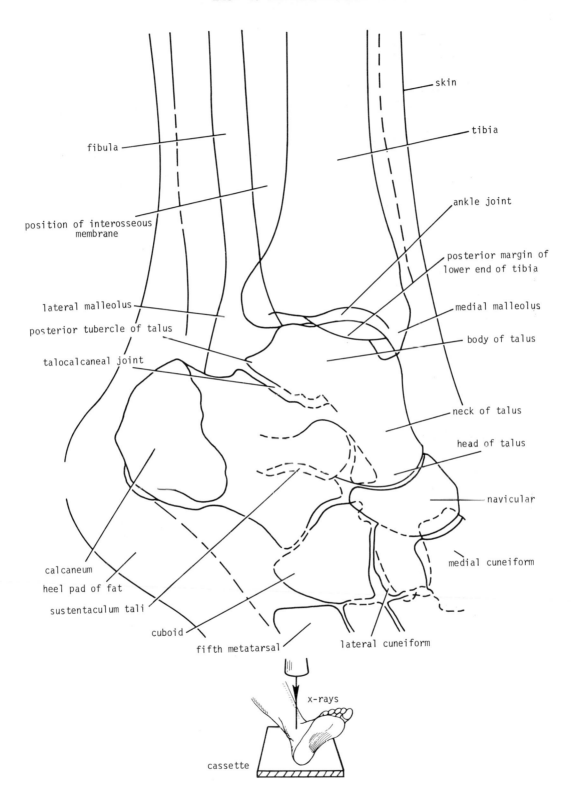

skin

tibia

fibula

ankle joint

position of interosseous
membrane

posterior margin of
lower end of tibia

lateral malleolus

medial malleolus

posterior tubercle of talus

body of talus

talocalcaneal joint

neck of talus

head of talus

navicular

calcaneum

medial cuneiform

heel pad of fat

sustentaculum tali

cuboid

fifth metatarsal

lateral cuneiform

x-rays

cassette

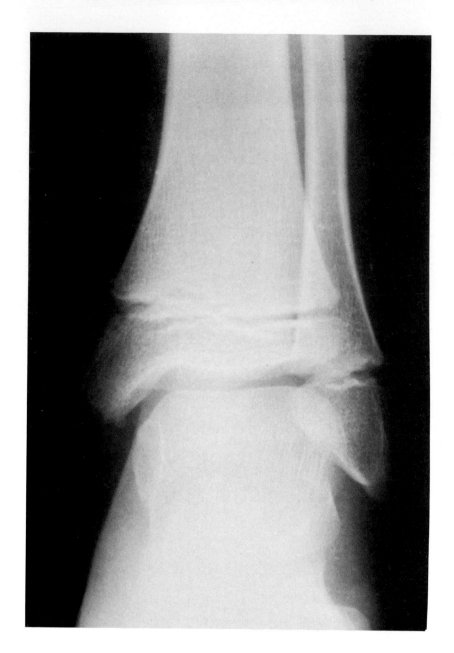

Figure 29

Anteroposterior
radiograph of ankle joint
(male aged 12 years).

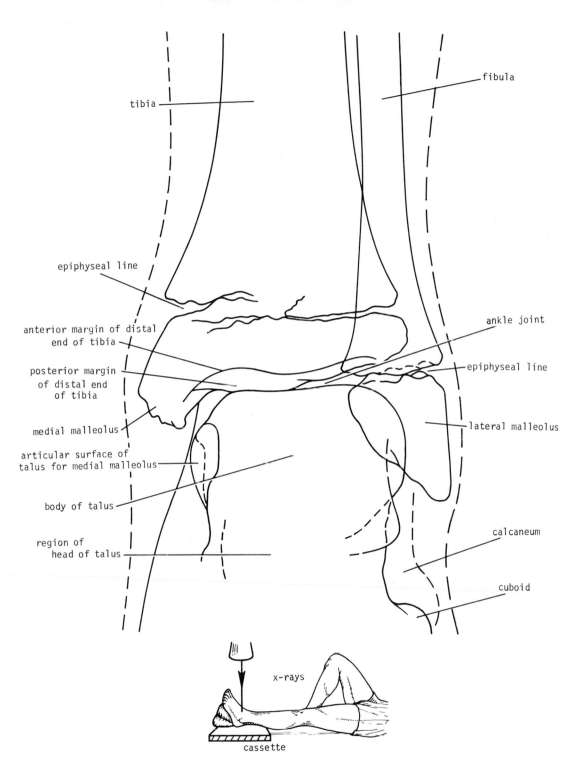

tibia

fibula

epiphyseal line

anterior margin of distal end of tibia

ankle joint

posterior margin of distal end of tibia

epiphyseal line

medial malleolus

articular surface of talus for medial malleolus

lateral malleolus

body of talus

region of head of talus

calcaneum

cuboid

x-rays

cassette

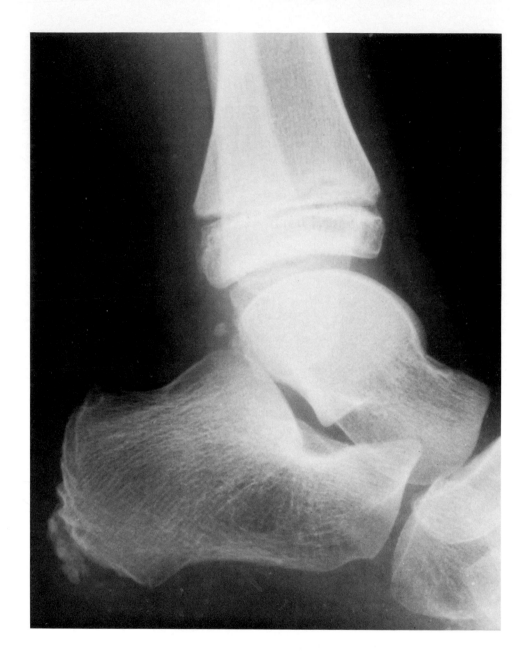

Figure 30

Lateral radiograph of ankle joint
(male aged 12 years).

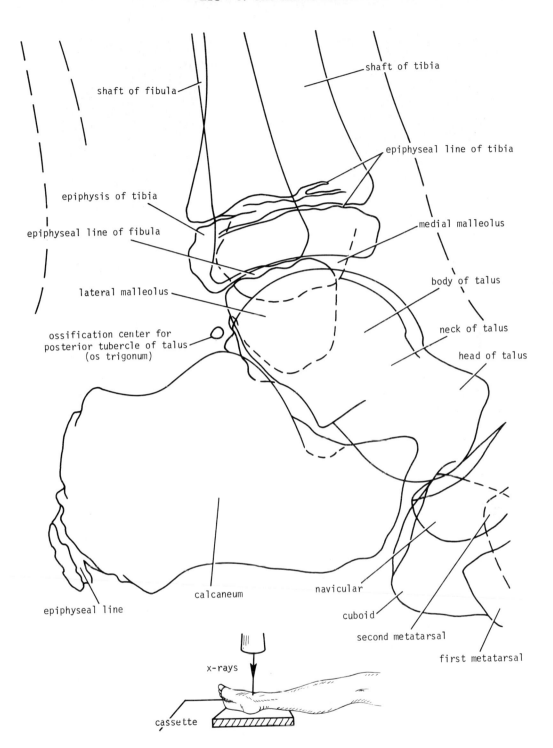

shaft of fibula

shaft of tibia

epiphyseal line of tibia

epiphysis of tibia

medial malleolus

epiphyseal line of fibula

lateral malleolus

body of talus

ossification center for
posterior tubercle of talus
(os trigonum)

neck of talus

head of talus

calcaneum

navicular

epiphyseal line

cuboid

second metatarsal

first metatarsal

x-rays

cassette

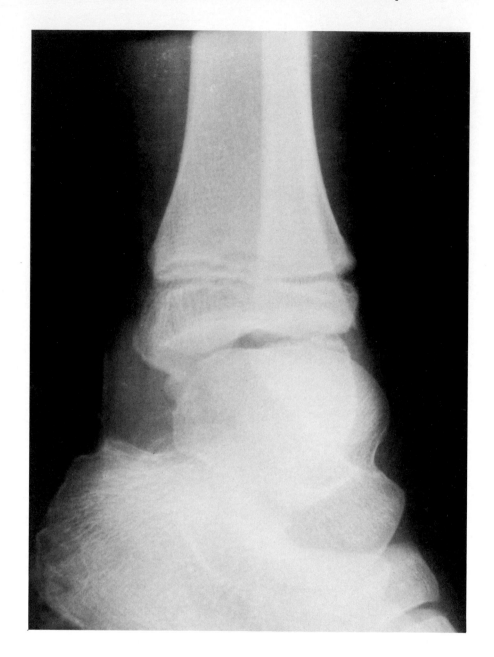

Figure 31

External oblique
radiograph of ankle joint
(male aged 12 years).

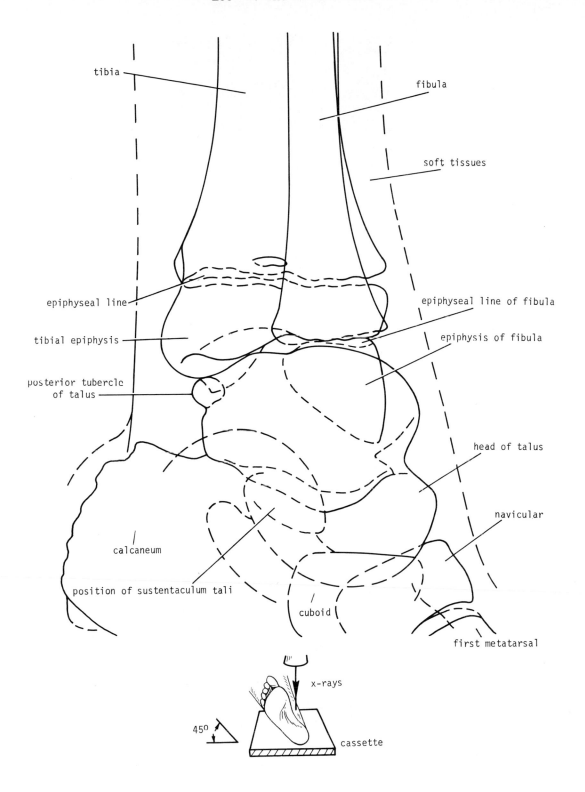

tibia

fibula

soft tissues

epiphyseal line

epiphyseal line of fibula

tibial epiphysis

epiphysis of fibula

posterior tubercle
of talus

head of talus

navicular

calcaneum

position of sustentaculum tali

cuboid

first metatarsal

x-rays

45°

cassette

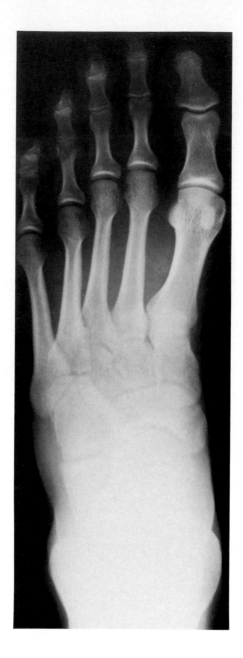

Figure 32

Anteroposterior radiograph of foot
(male aged 17 years).

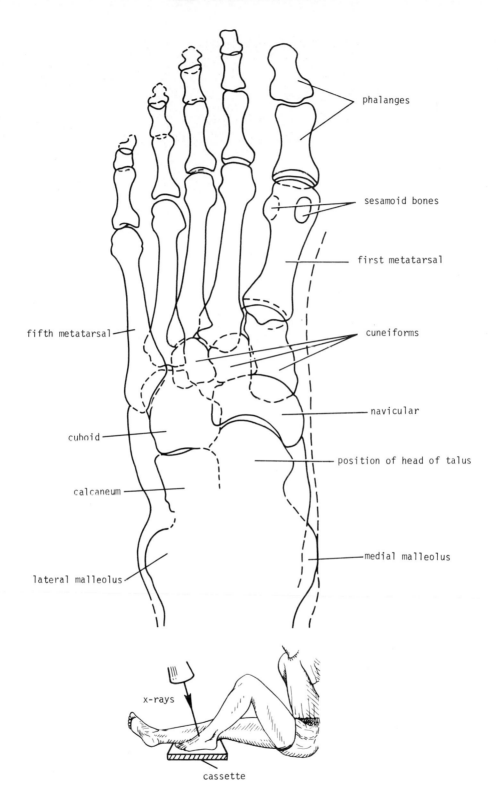

phalanges

sesamoid bones

first metatarsal

fifth metatarsal

cuneiforms

navicular

cuboid

position of head of talus

calcaneum

medial malleolus

lateral malleolus

x-rays

cassette

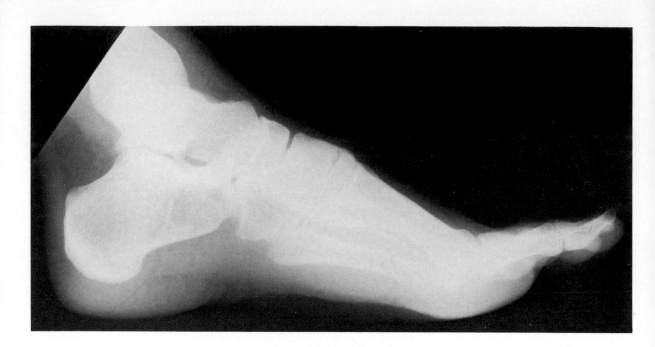

Figure 33

Lateral radiograph of foot
(female aged 15 years).

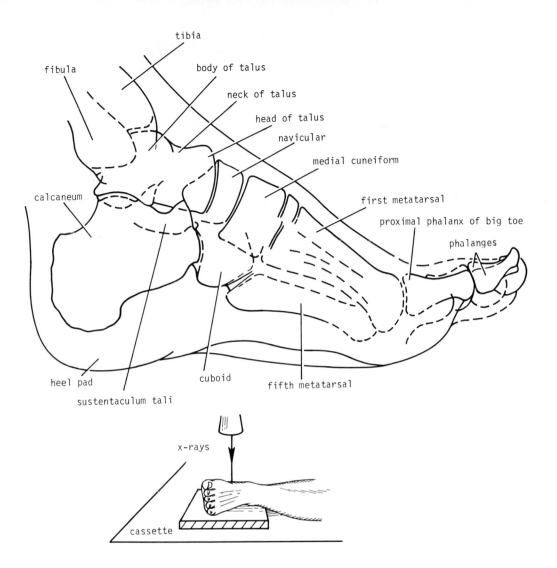

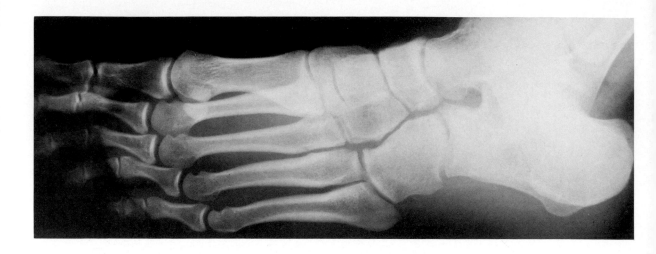

Figure 34

Oblique radiograph of foot
(male aged 17 years).

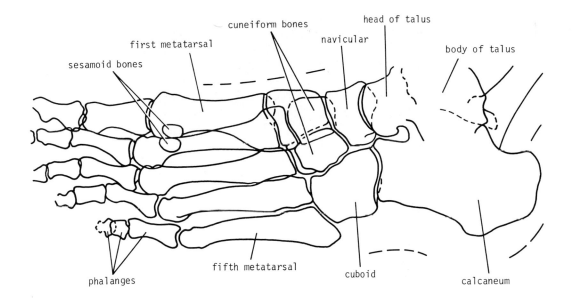

sesamoid bones

first metatarsal

cuneiform bones

navicular

head of talus

body of talus

phalanges

fifth metatarsal

cuboid

calcaneum

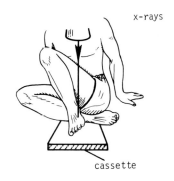

x-rays

cassette

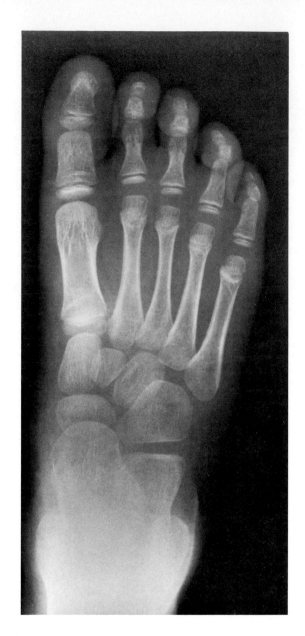

Figure 35

Anteroposterior radiograph of foot
(male aged 10 years).

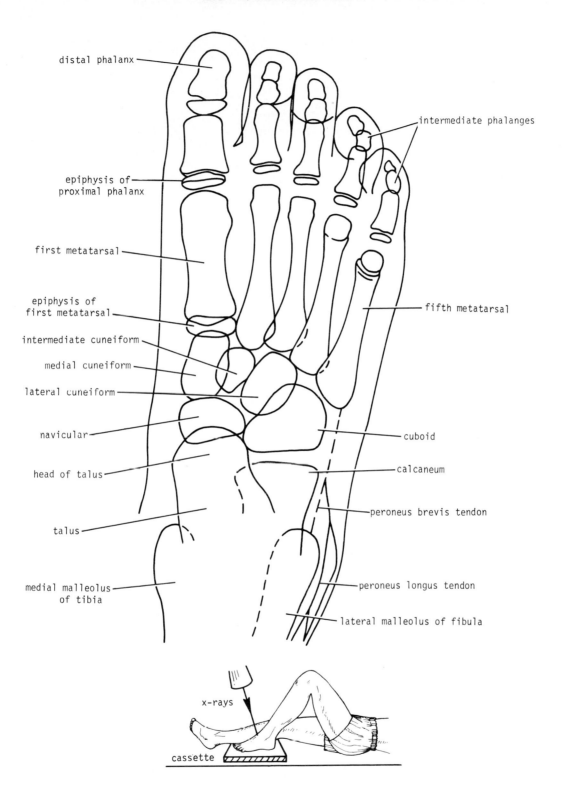

distal phalanx

intermediate phalanges

epiphysis of
proximal phalanx

first metatarsal

epiphysis of
first metatarsal

fifth metatarsal

intermediate cuneiform

medial cuneiform

lateral cuneiform

navicular

cuboid

head of talus

calcaneum

peroneus brevis tendon

talus

medial malleolus
of tibia

peroneus longus tendon

lateral malleolus of fibula

x-rays

cassette

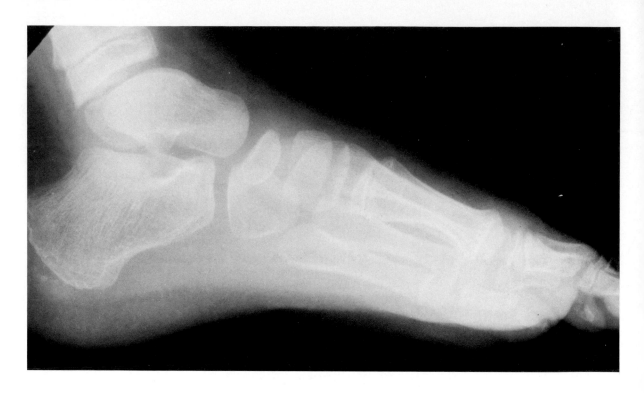

Figure 36

Lateral radiograph of foot
(male aged 10 years).

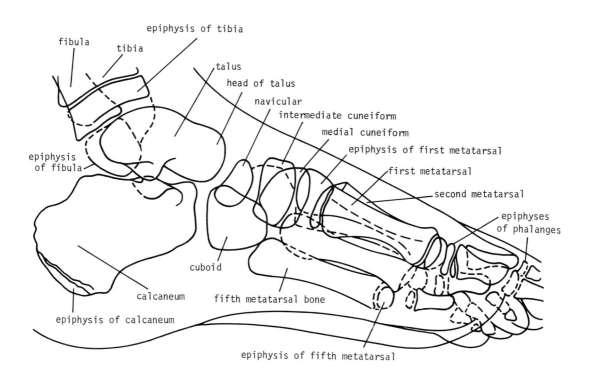

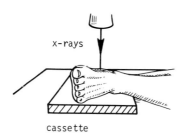

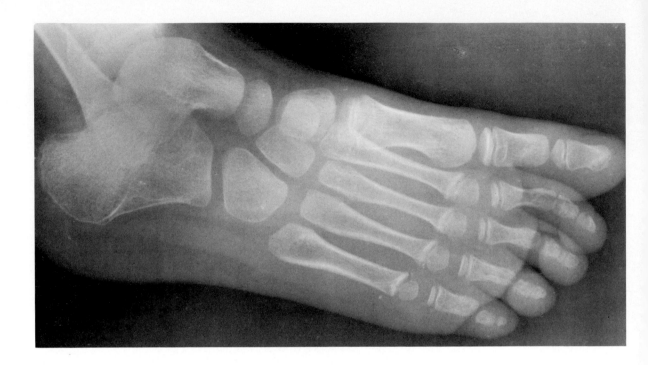

Figure 37

Oblique radiograph of foot
(male aged 10 years).

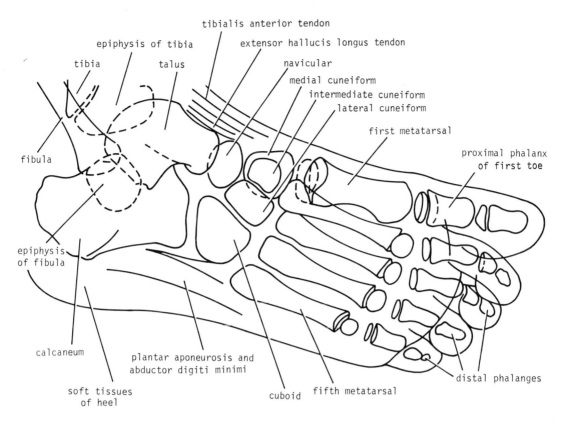

tibialis anterior tendon

epiphysis of tibia

extensor hallucis longus tendon

tibia

talus

navicular

medial cuneiform

intermediate cuneiform

lateral cuneiform

first metatarsal

proximal phalanx
of first toe

fibula

epiphysis
of fibula

calcaneum

plantar aponeurosis and
abductor digiti minimi

distal phalanges

soft tissues
of heel

cuboid

fifth metatarsal

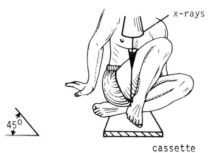

x-rays

45°

cassette

7

THE VERTEBRAL COLUMN

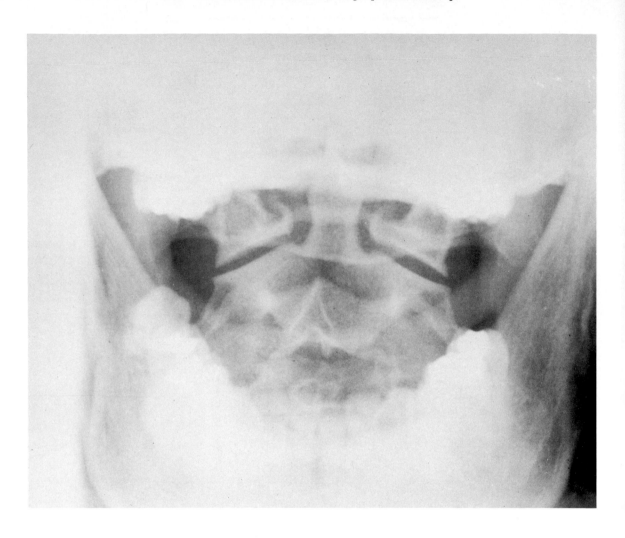

Figure 1

Anteroposterior radiograph of upper
cervical region of vetebral column
with patient's mouth open to
show odontoid process
(male aged 27 years).

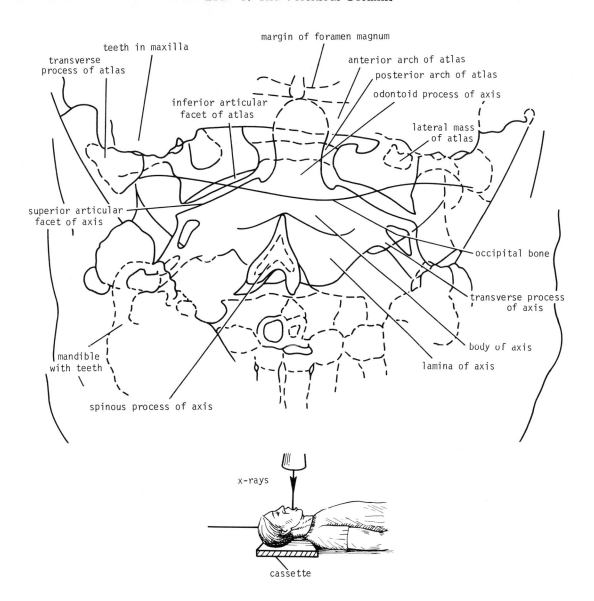

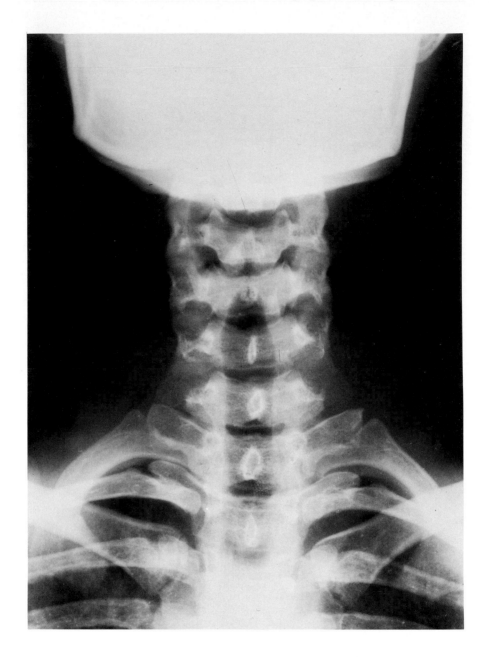

Figure 2

Anteroposterior radiograph of cervical
region of vertebral column
(male aged 21 years).

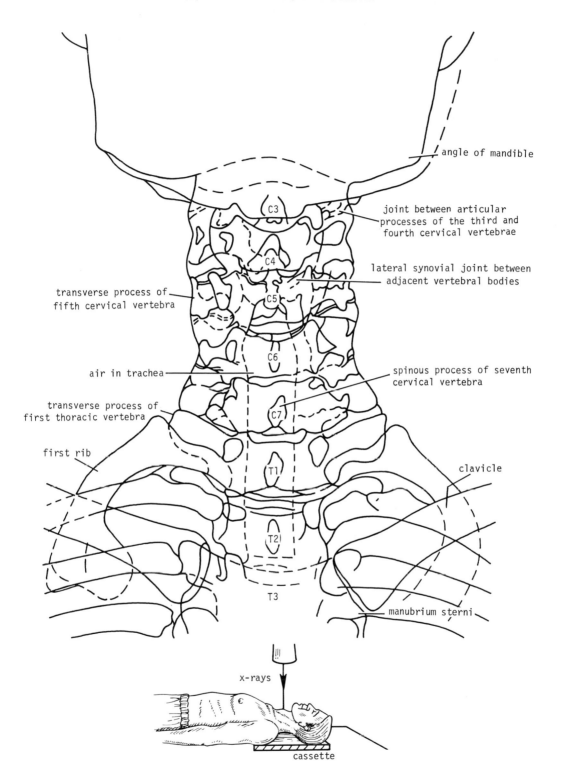

angle of mandible

joint between articular processes of the third and fourth cervical vertebrae

lateral synovial joint between adjacent vertebral bodies

transverse process of fifth cervical vertebra

air in trachea

spinous process of seventh cervical vertebra

transverse process of first thoracic vertebra

first rib

clavicle

manubrium sterni

x-rays

cassette

C3
C4
C5
C6
C7
T1
T2
T3

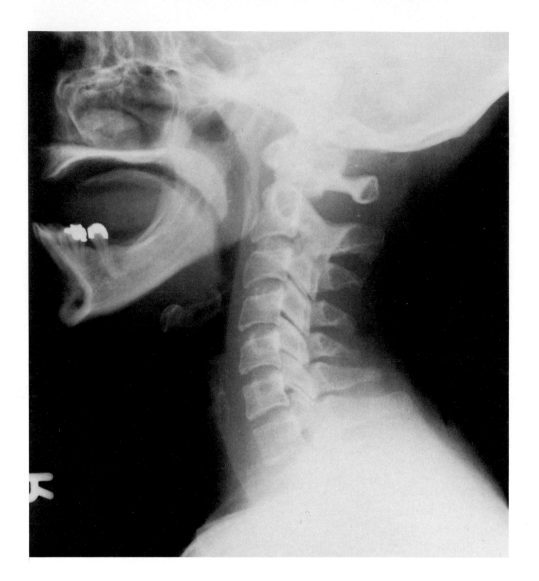

Figure 3

Lateral radiograph of cervical
region of vertebral column
(female aged 42 years).

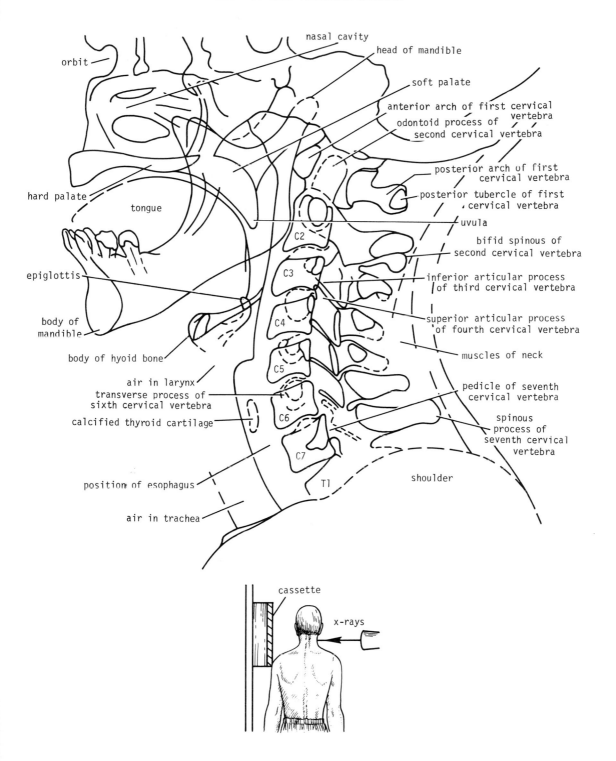

orbit

nasal cavity

head of mandible

soft palate

anterior arch of first cervical vertebra

odontoid process of second cervical vertebra

posterior arch of first cervical vertebra

posterior tubercle of first cervical vertebra

hard palate

tongue

uvula

C2

bifid spinous of second cervical vertebra

inferior articular process of third cervical vertebra

epiglottis

C3

superior articular process of fourth cervical vertebra

body of mandible

C4

muscles of neck

body of hyoid bone

C5

air in larynx

transverse process of sixth cervical vertebra

pedicle of seventh cervical vertebra

calcified thyroid cartilage

C6

spinous process of seventh cervical vertebra

C7

position of esophagus

T1

shoulder

air in trachea

cassette

x-rays

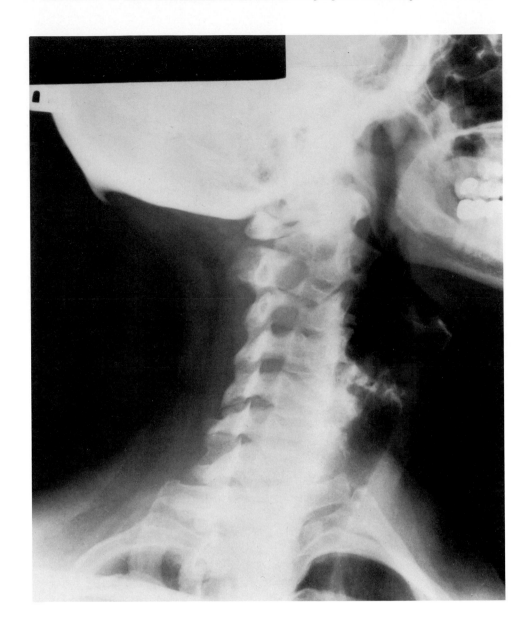

Figure 4

Oblique radiograph of cervical
region of vertebral column
(female aged 45 years).

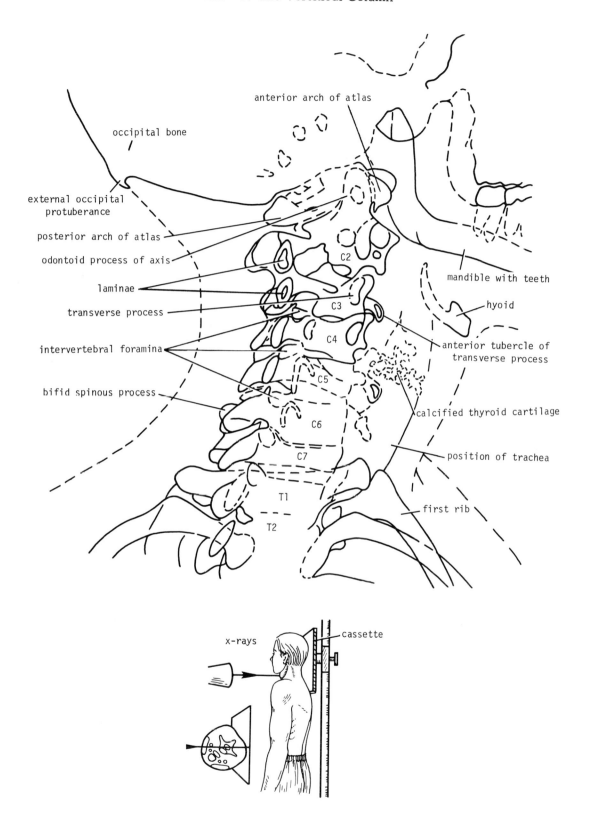

occipital bone

anterior arch of atlas

external occipital protuberance

posterior arch of atlas

odontoid process of axis

laminae

transverse process

intervertebral foramina

bifid spinous process

C2

C3

C4

C5

C6

C7

T1

T2

mandible with teeth

hyoid

anterior tubercle of transverse process

calcified thyroid cartilage

position of trachea

first rib

x-rays

cassette

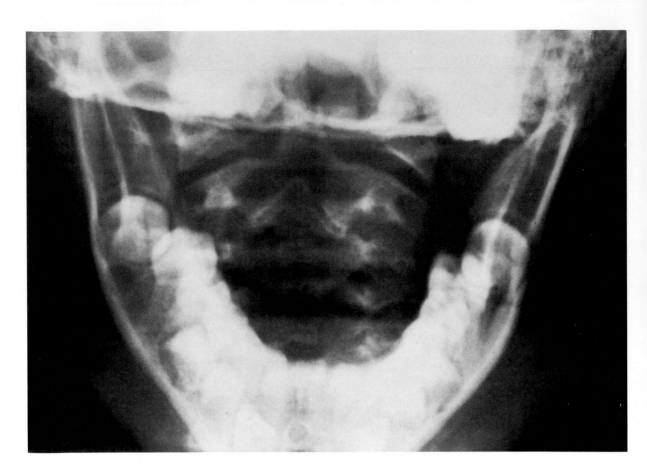

Figure 5

Anteroposterior radiograph of upper
cervical region of vertebral column
with patient's mouth open to
show odontoid process
(male aged 6 years).

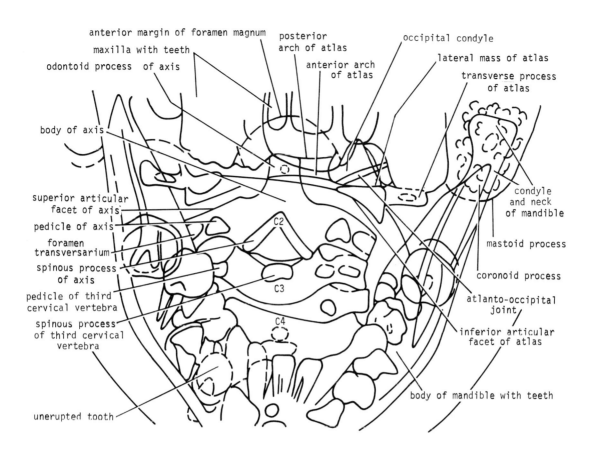

anterior margin of foramen magnum
posterior arch of atlas
occipital condyle
maxilla with teeth
anterior arch of atlas
lateral mass of atlas
odontoid process of axis
transverse process of atlas
body of axis
superior articular facet of axis
pedicle of axis
foramen transversarium
spinous process of axis
pedicle of third cervical vertebra
spinous process of third cervical vertebra
unerupted tooth
condyle and neck of mandible
mastoid process
coronoid process
atlanto-occipital joint
inferior articular facet of atlas
body of mandible with teeth
C2
C3
C4

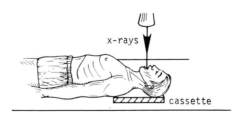

x-rays
cassette

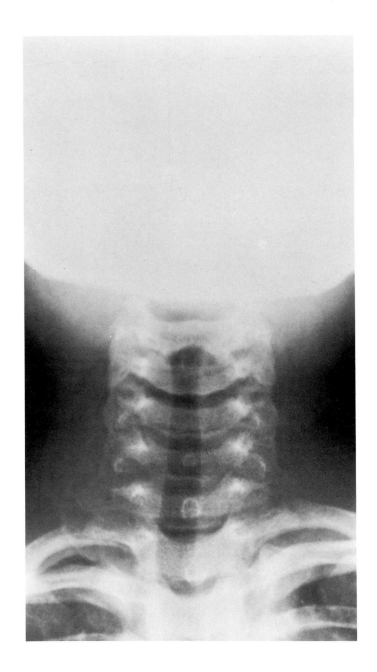

Figure 6

Anteroposterior radiograph of cervical
region of vertebral column
(male aged 6 years).

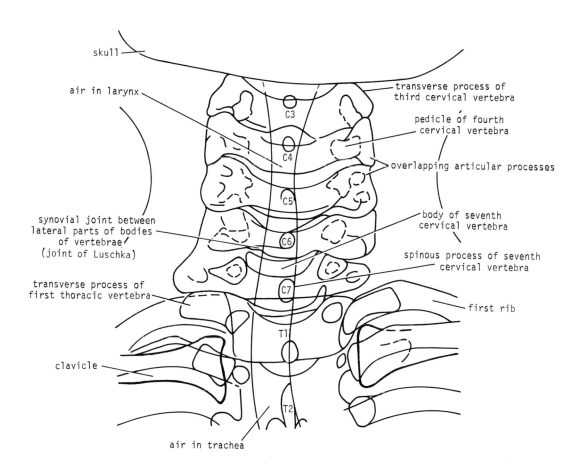

skull

air in larynx

transverse process of
third cervical vertebra

pedicle of fourth
cervical vertebra

overlapping articular processes

C3

C4

C5

C6

C7

body of seventh
cervical vertebra

spinous process of seventh
cervical vertebra

synovial joint between
lateral parts of bodies
of vertebrae
(joint of Luschka)

transverse process of
first thoracic vertebra

first rib

T1

clavicle

T2

air in trachea

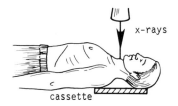

x-rays

cassette

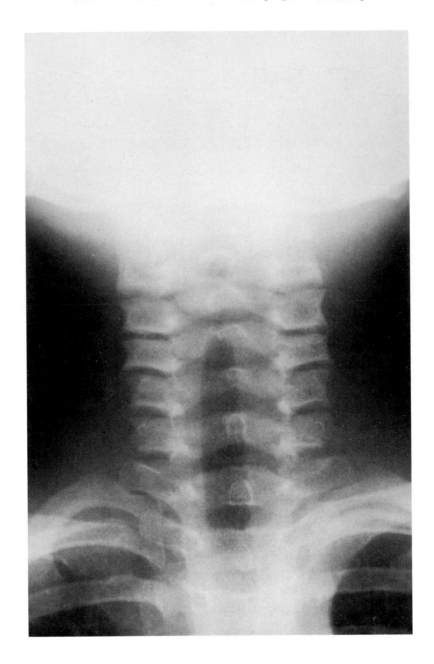

Figure 7

Anteroposterior radiograph of cervical
region of vertebral column
(male aged 7 years).

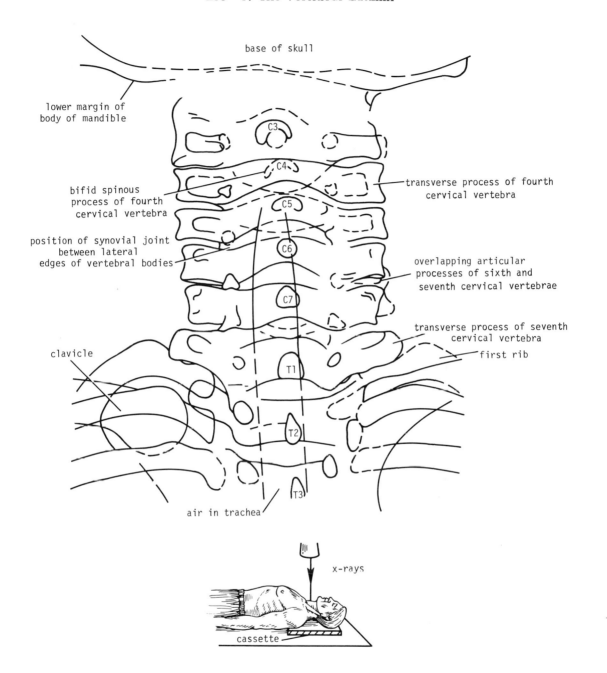

base of skull

lower margin of
body of mandible

bifid spinous
process of fourth
cervical vertebra

transverse process of fourth
cervical vertebra

position of synovial joint
between lateral
edges of vertebral bodies

overlapping articular
processes of sixth and
seventh cervical vertebrae

transverse process of seventh
cervical vertebra

first rib

clavicle

C3

C4

C5

C6

C7

T1

T2

T3

air in trachea

x-rays

cassette

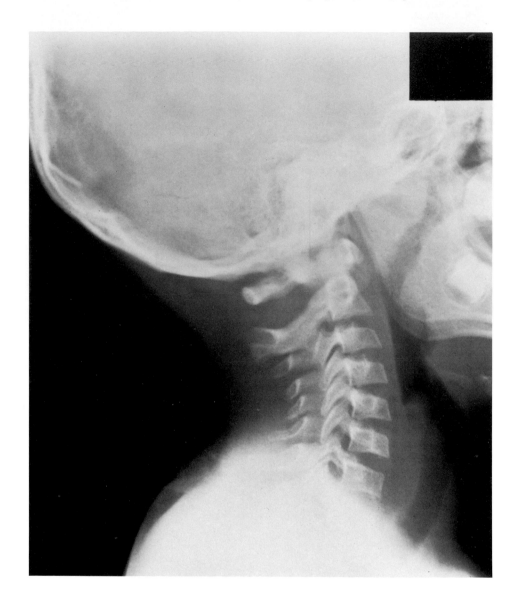

Figure 8

Lateral radiograph of cervical
region of vertebral column
(male aged 6 years).

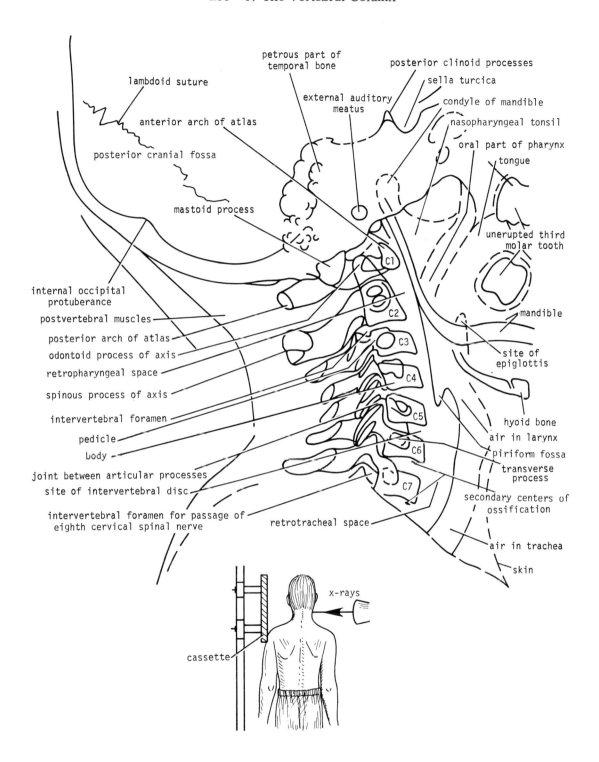

lambdoid suture

anterior arch of atlas

posterior cranial fossa

mastoid process

petrous part of temporal bone

external auditory meatus

posterior clinoid processes

sella turcica

condyle of mandible

nasopharyngeal tonsil

oral part of pharynx

tongue

uneruptedthird molar tooth

internal occipital protuberance

postvertebral muscles

posterior arch of atlas

odontoid process of axis

retropharyngeal space

spinous process of axis

intervertebral foramen

pedicle

body

joint between articular processes

site of intervertebral disc

intervertebral foramen for passage of eighth cervical spinal nerve

mandible

site of epiglottis

hyoid bone

air in larynx

piriform fossa

transverse process

secondary centers of ossification

air in trachea

skin

retrotracheal space

C1
C2
C3
C4
C5
C6
C7

x-rays

cassette

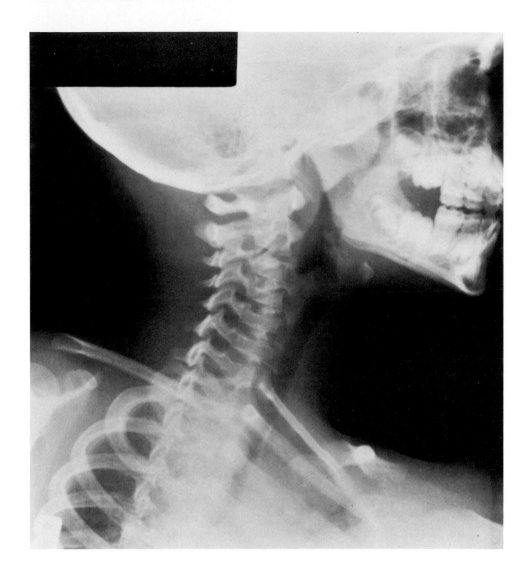

Figure 9

Oblique radiograph of cervical
region of vertebral column
(male aged 5 years).

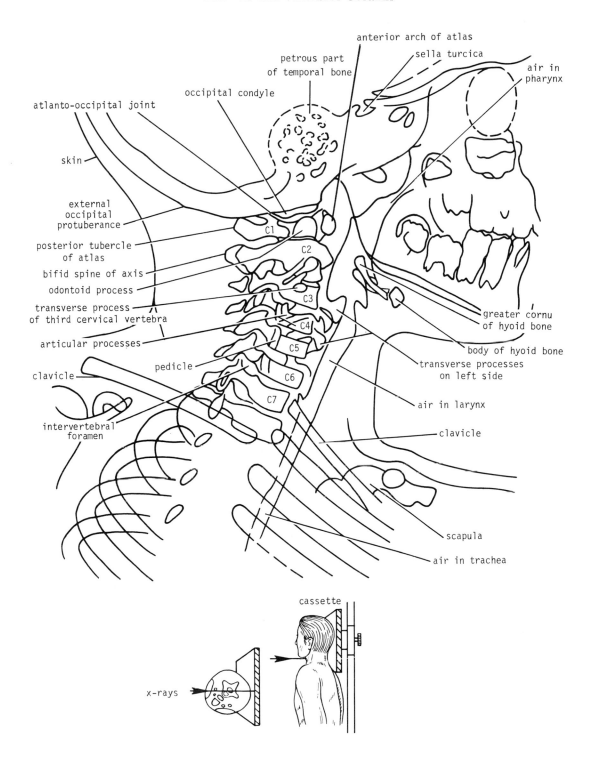

anterior arch of atlas

sella turcica

petrous part
of temporal bone

air in
pharynx

occipital condyle

atlanto-occipital joint

skin

external
occipital
protuberance

posterior tubercle
of atlas

bifid spine of axis

odontoid process

transverse process
of third cervical vertebra

articular processes

clavicle

pedicle

intervertebral
foramen

C1

C2

C3

C4

C5

C6

C7

greater cornu
of hyoid bone

body of hyoid bone

transverse processes
on left side

air in larynx

clavicle

scapula

air in trachea

cassette

x-rays

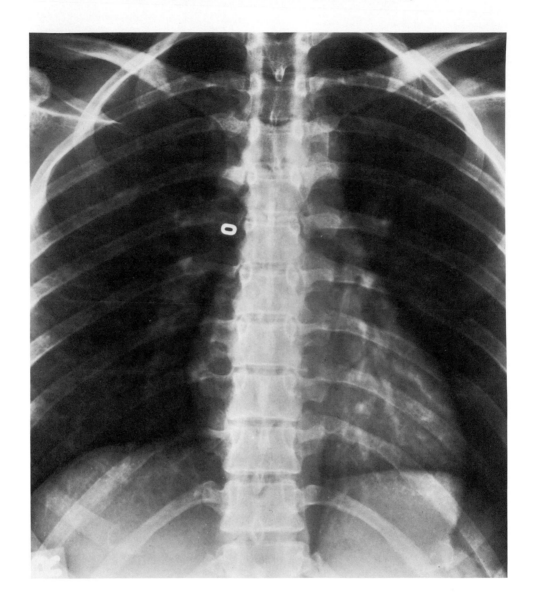

Figure 10

Anteroposterior radiograph of
thoracic region of vertebral column
(female aged 34 years).

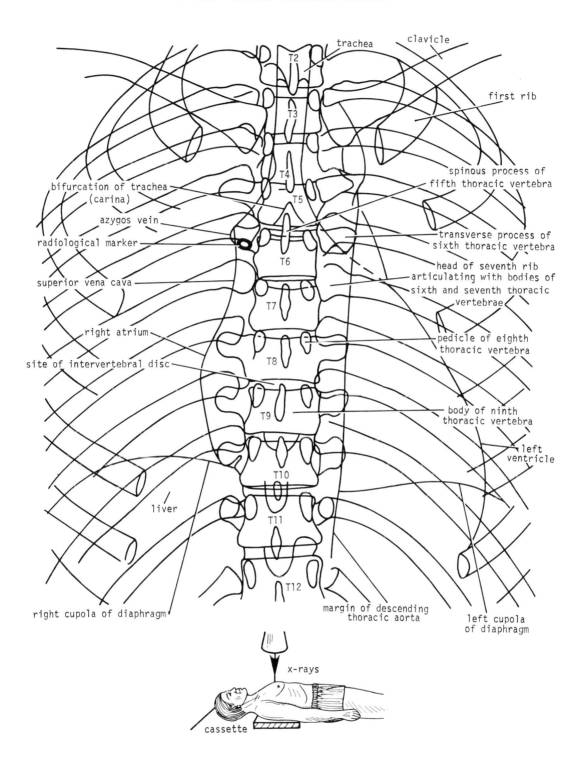

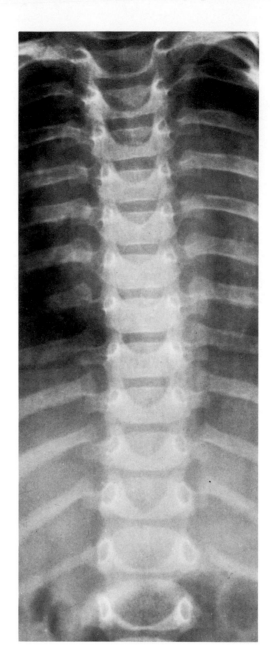

Figure 11

Anteroposterior radiograph of
thoracic region of vertebral column
(male aged 4 years).

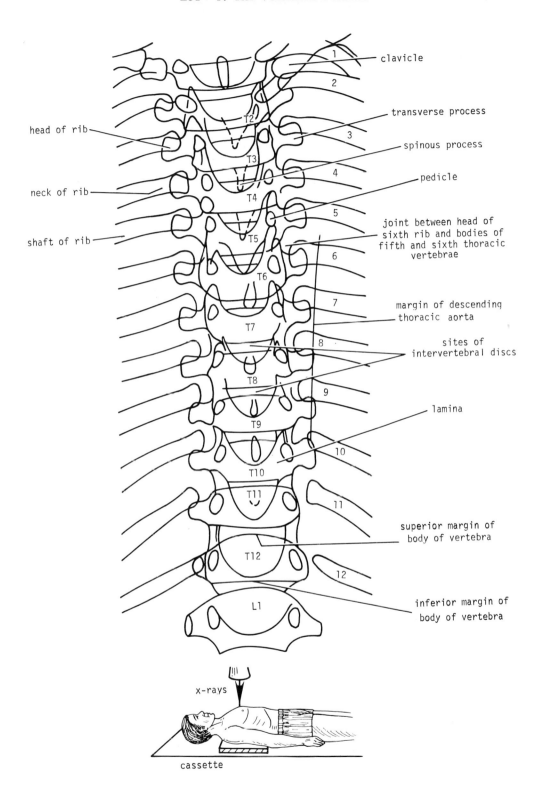

clavicle

transverse process

spinous process

pedicle

joint between head of
sixth rib and bodies of
fifth and sixth thoracic
vertebrae

head of rib

neck of rib

shaft of rib

margin of descending
thoracic aorta

sites of
intervertebral discs

lamina

superior margin of
body of vertebra

inferior margin of
body of vertebra

x-rays

cassette

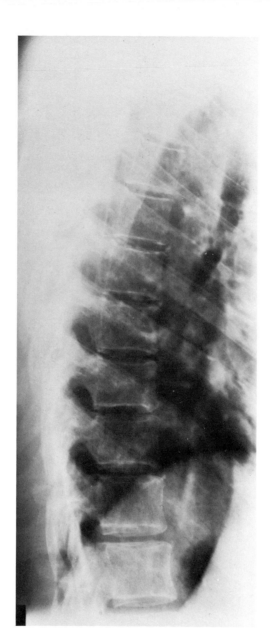

Figure 12

Lateral radiograph of thoracic
region of vertebral column
(male aged 9½ years).

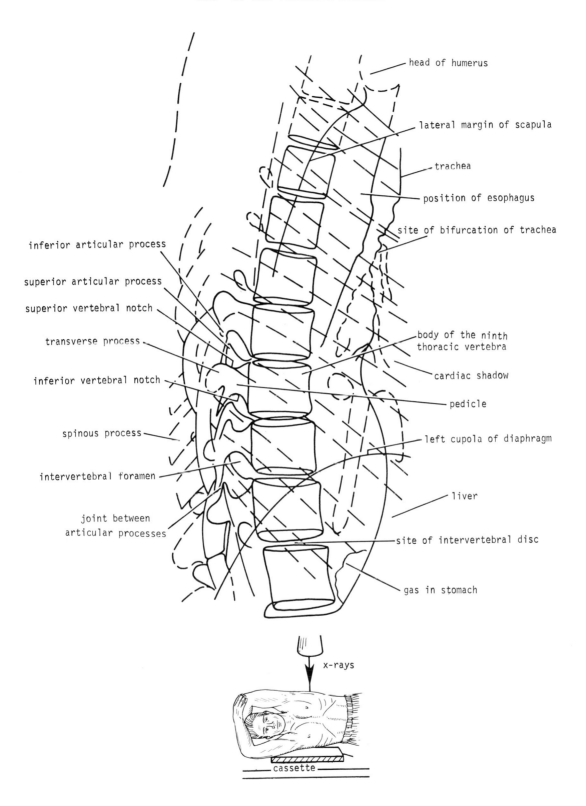

head of humerus

lateral margin of scapula

trachea

position of esophagus

site of bifurcation of trachea

inferior articular process

superior articular process

superior vertebral notch

transverse process

inferior vertebral notch

spinous process

intervertebral foramen

joint between
articular processes

body of the ninth
thoracic vertebra

cardiac shadow

pedicle

left cupola of diaphragm

liver

site of intervertebral disc

gas in stomach

x-rays

cassette

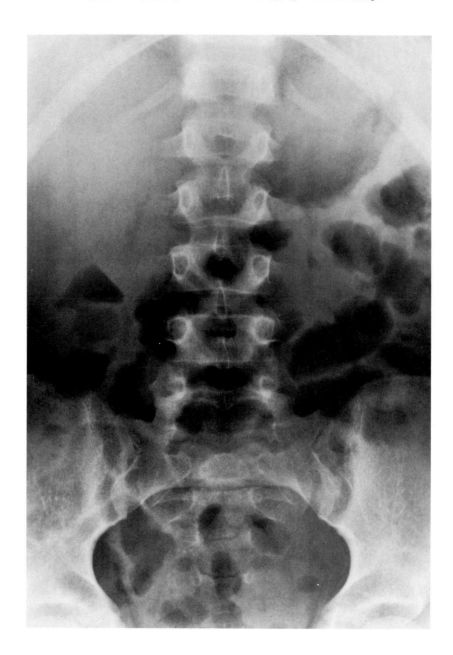

Figure 13

Anteroposterior radiograph of lumbar
region of vertebral column
(male aged 8 years).

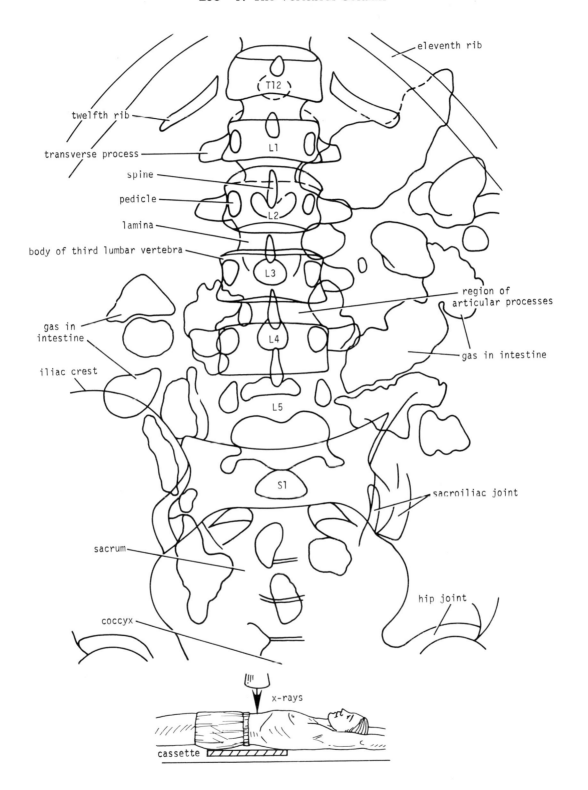

eleventh rib

twelfth rib

transverse process

spine

pedicle

lamina

body of third lumbar vertebra

region of
articular processes

gas in
intestine

gas in intestine

iliac crest

sacroiliac joint

sacrum

hip joint

coccyx

T12

L1

L2

L3

L4

L5

S1

x-rays

cassette

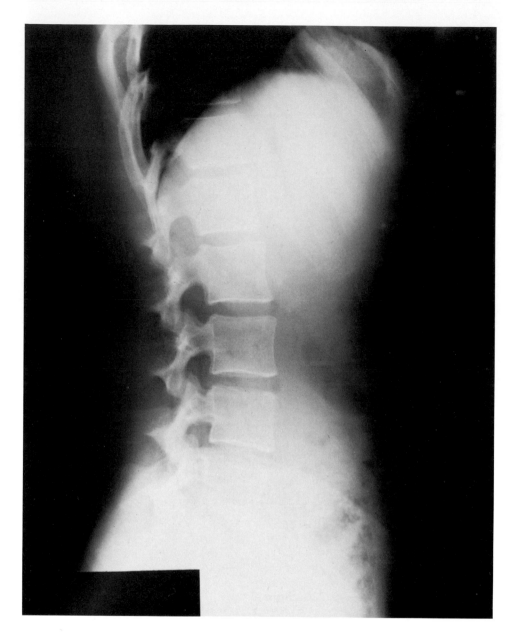

Figure 14

Lateral radiograph of lumbar
region of vertebral column
(female aged 20 years).

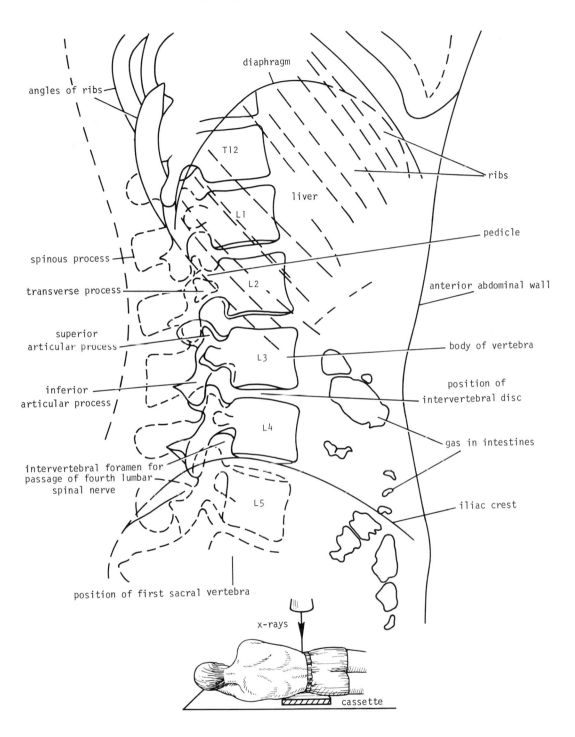

angles of ribs

diaphragm

T12

liver

ribs

L1

pedicle

spinous process

transverse process

L2

anterior abdominal wall

superior
articular process

L3

body of vertebra

position of
intervertebral disc

inferior
articular process

L4

gas in intestines

intervertebral foramen for
passage of fourth lumbar
spinal nerve

L5

iliac crest

position of first sacral vertebra

x-rays

cassette

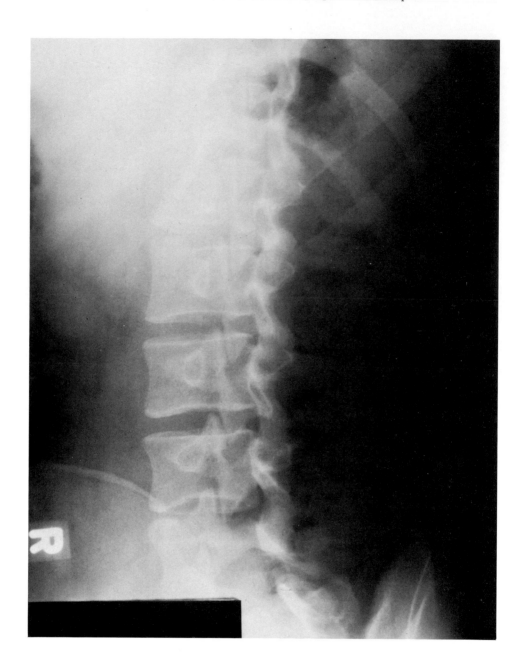

Figure 15

Oblique radiograph of lumbar
region of vertebral column
(female aged 15 years).

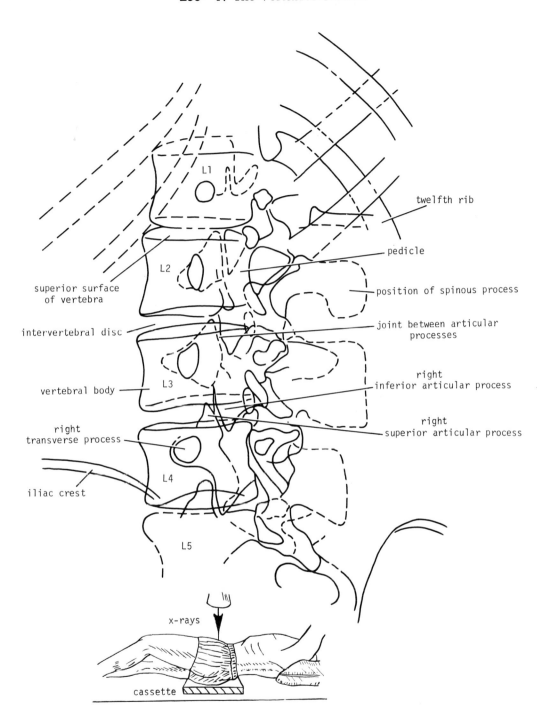

twelfth rib

pedicle

position of spinous process

superior surface of vertebra

intervertebral disc

joint between articular processes

vertebral body

right inferior articular process

right transverse process

right superior articular process

iliac crest

L1

L2

L3

L4

L5

x-rays

cassette

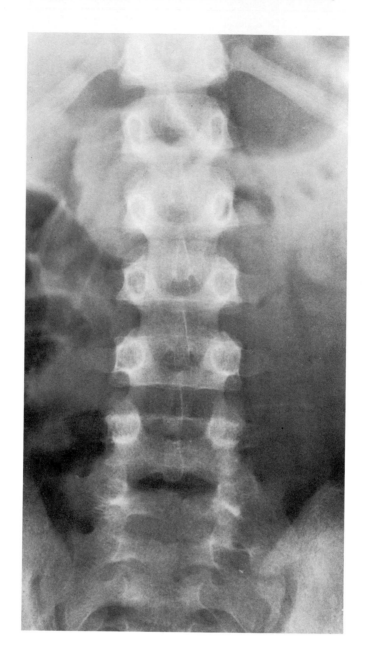

Figure 16

Anteroposterior radiograph of lumbar
region of vertebral column
(male aged 7 years).

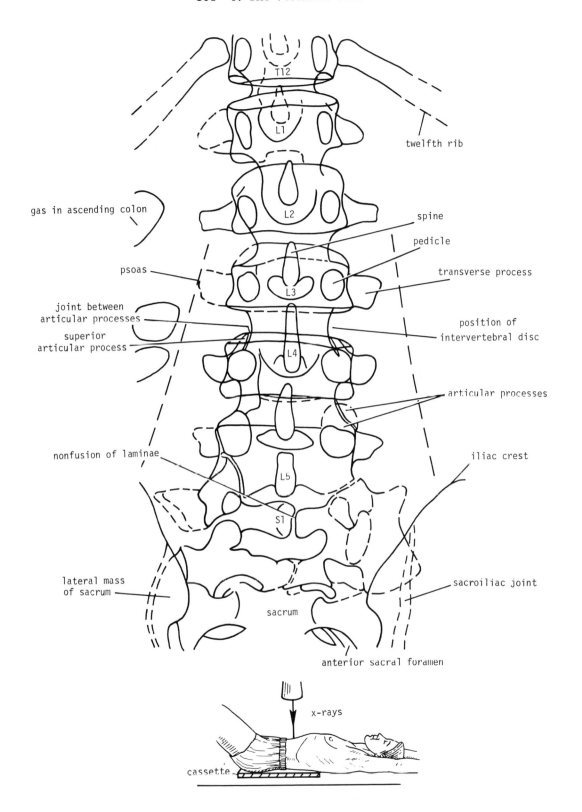

twelfth rib

gas in ascending colon

spine

pedicle

psoas

transverse process

joint between
articular processes

superior
articular process

position of
intervertebral disc

articular processes

nonfusion of laminae

iliac crest

lateral mass
of sacrum

sacroiliac joint

sacrum

anterior sacral foramen

x-rays

cassette

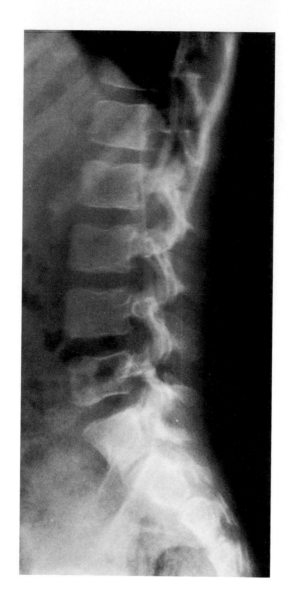

Figure 17

Lateral radiograph of lumbar
region of vertebral column
(male aged 11 years).

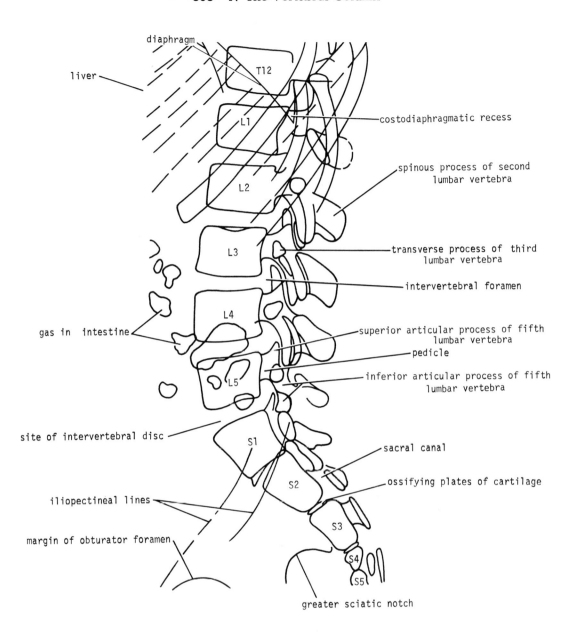

diaphragm

liver

T12

costodiaphragmatic recess

L1

spinous process of second lumbar vertebra

L2

transverse process of third lumbar vertebra

L3

intervertebral foramen

L4

superior articular process of fifth lumbar vertebra

gas in intestine

pedicle

inferior articular process of fifth lumbar vertebra

L5

site of intervertebral disc

S1

sacral canal

S2

ossifying plates of cartilage

iliopectineal lines

S3

margin of obturator foramen

S4

S5

greater sciatic notch

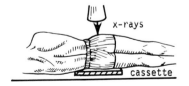

x-rays

cassette

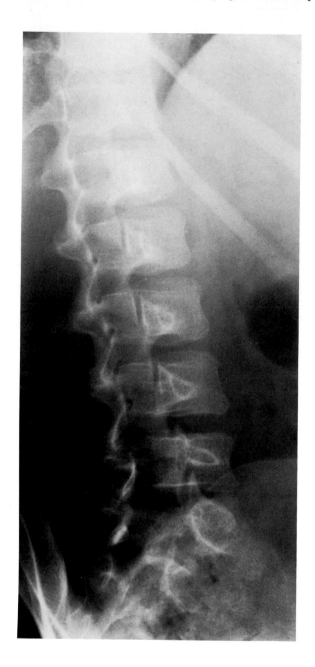

Figure 18

Oblique radiograph of lumbar
region of vertebral column
(male aged 11 years).

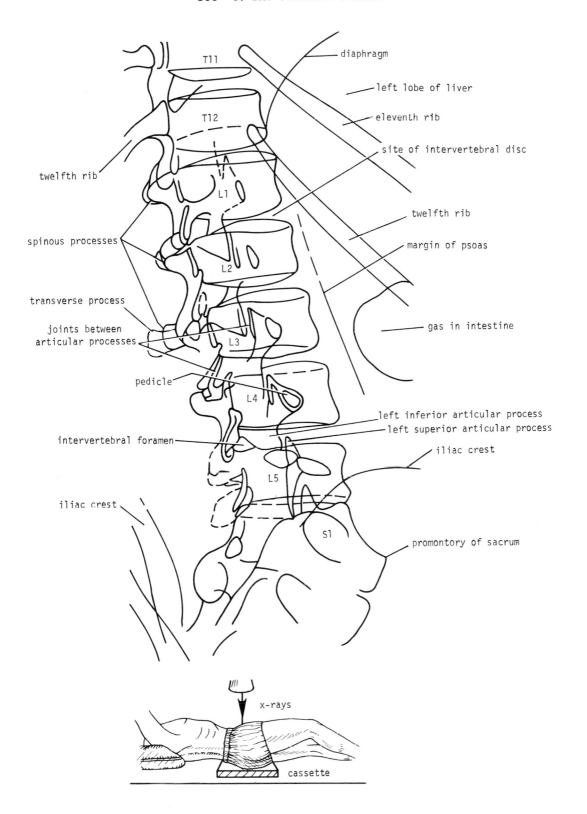

T11

diaphragm

left lobe of liver

T12

eleventh rib

site of intervertebral disc

twelfth rib

L1

twelfth rib

spinous processes

margin of psoas

L2

transverse process

joints between
articular processes

L3

gas in intestine

pedicle

L4

left inferior articular process

left superior articular process

intervertebral foramen

iliac crest

L5

iliac crest

S1

promontory of sacrum

x-rays

cassette

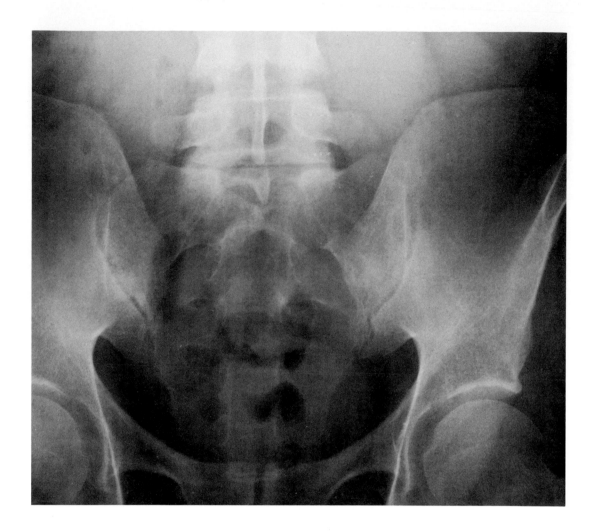

Figure 19

Anteroposterior angled radiograph of
lumbosacral region of vertebral column
(male aged 34 years).

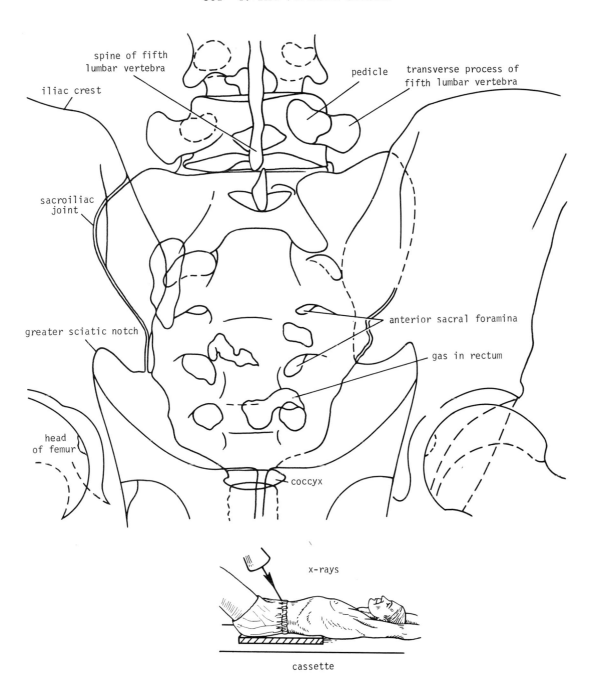

spine of fifth
lumbar vertebra

pedicle

transverse process of
fifth lumbar vertebra

iliac crest

sacroiliac
joint

anterior sacral foramina

gas in rectum

greater sciatic notch

head
of femur

coccyx

x-rays

cassette

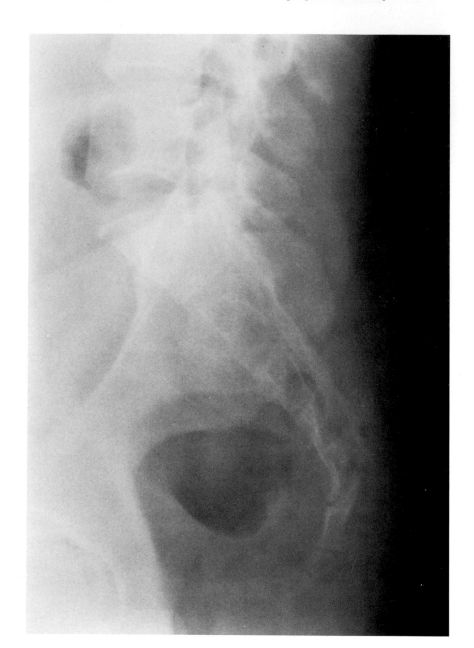

Figure 20

Lateral
radiograph of sacrum and coccyx
(female aged 28 years).

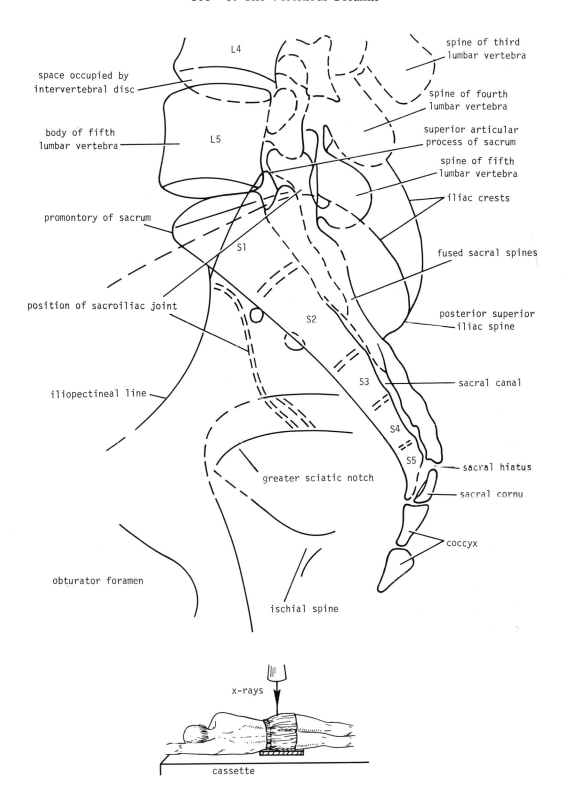

spine of third
lumbar vertebra

space occupied by
intervertebral disc

L4

spine of fourth
lumbar vertebra

superior articular
process of sacrum

body of fifth
lumbar vertebra

L5

spine of fifth
lumbar vertebra

iliac crests

promontory of sacrum

S1

fused sacral spines

position of sacroiliac joint

posterior superior
iliac spine

S2

iliopectineal line

S3

sacral canal

S4

S5

sacral hiatus

sacral cornu

greater sciatic notch

coccyx

obturator foramen

ischial spine

x-rays

cassette

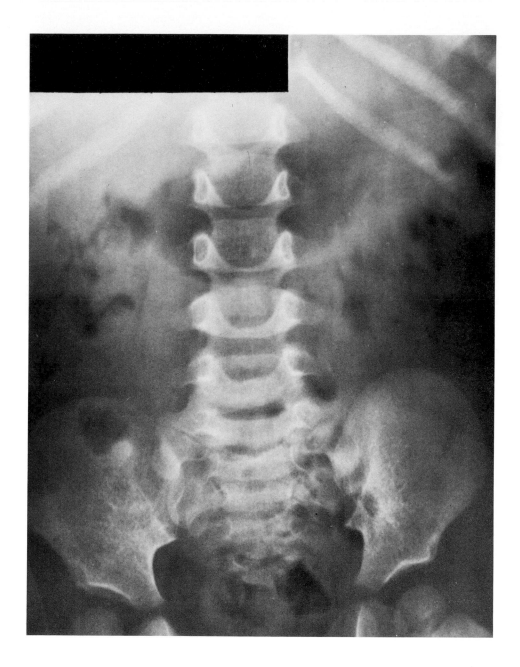

Figure 21

Anteroposterior radiograph of
lumbosacral region of vertebral column
(male aged 2 years).

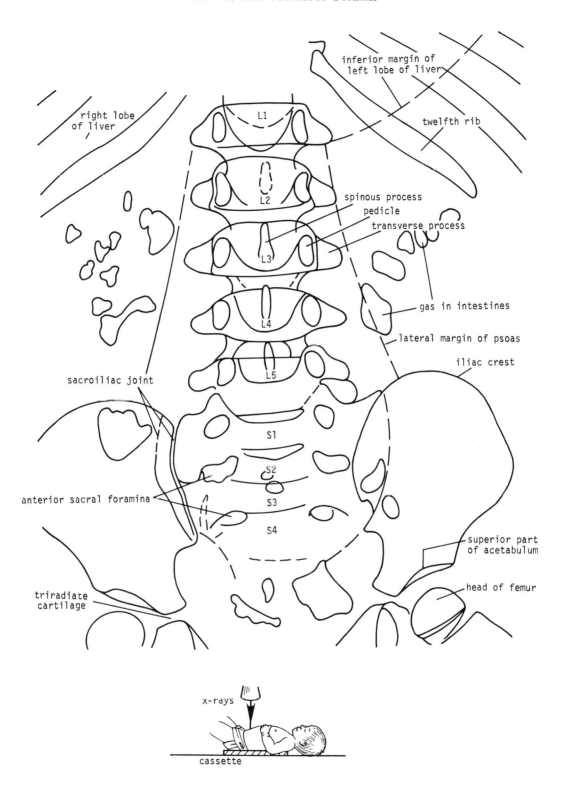

inferior margin of
left lobe of liver

right lobe
of liver

twelfth rib

L1

L2

spinous process

pedicle

transverse process

L3

gas in intestines

L4

lateral margin of psoas

iliac crest

L5

sacroiliac joint

S1

S2

anterior sacral foramina

S3

S4

superior part
of acetabulum

head of femur

triradiate
cartilage

x-rays

cassette

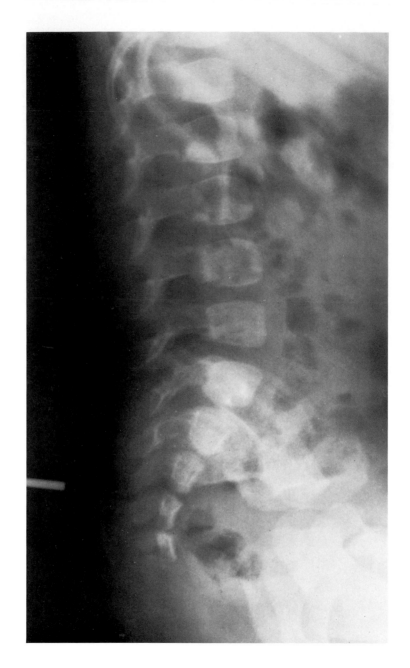

Figure 22

Lateral radiograph
of sacrum and coccyx
(male aged 2 years).

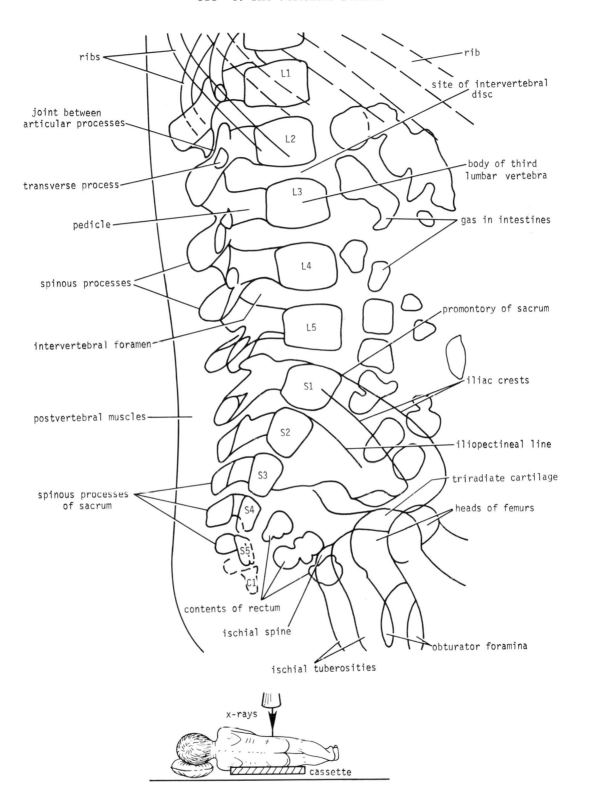

ribs

rib

site of intervertebral
    disc

L1

joint between
articular processes

L2

body of third
lumbar vertebra

transverse process

L3

gas in intestines

pedicle

L4

spinous processes

promontory of sacrum

L5

intervertebral foramen

iliac crests

S1

postvertebral muscles

S2

iliopectineal line

S3

triradiate cartilage

spinous processes
of sacrum

S4

heads of femurs

S5

C1

contents of rectum

ischial spine

obturator foramina

ischial tuberosities

x-rays

cassette

8

PREGNANCY

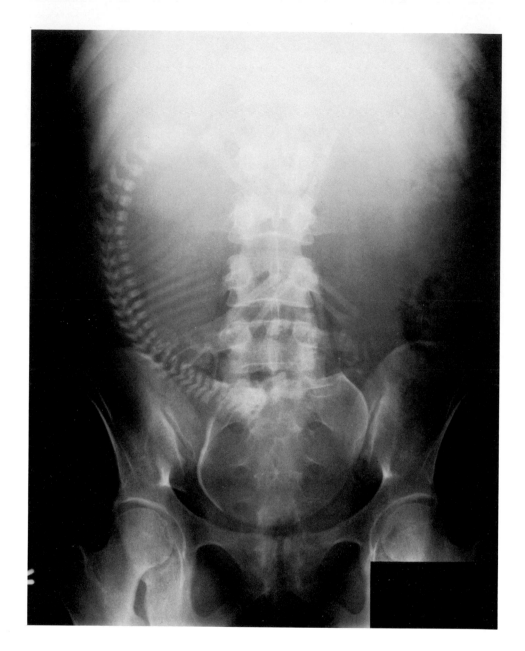

Figure 1

Posteroanterior radiograph of abdomen
and pelvis of pregnant woman aged
27 years. The pregnancy is in
the third trimester.

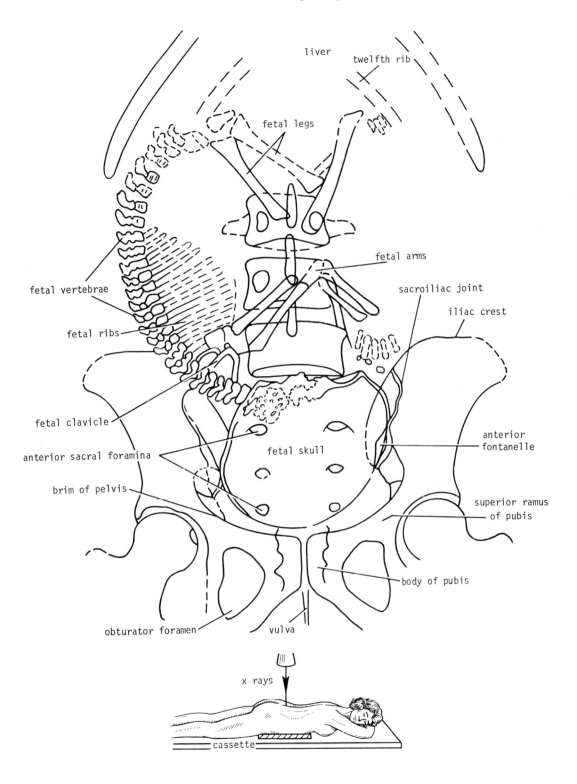

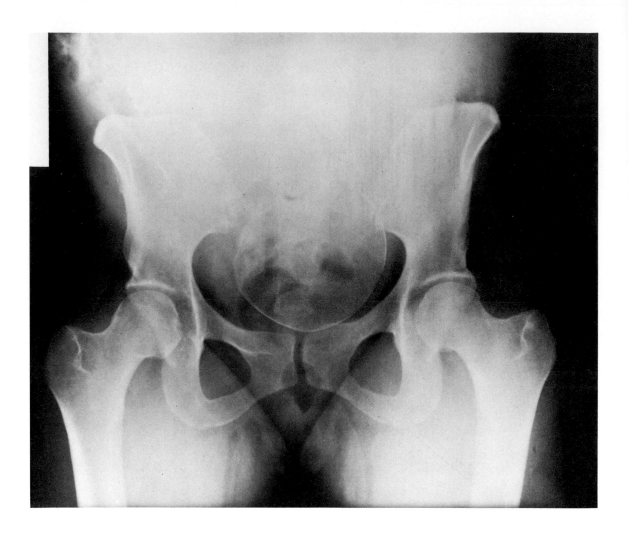

Figure 2

Angled anteroposterior radiograph
of abdomen and pelvis of pregnant
woman aged 27 years. The pregnancy
is in the third trimester.

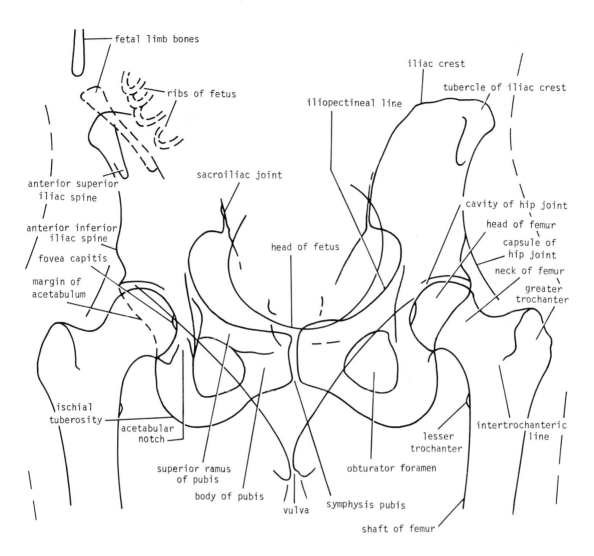

fetal limb bones

ribs of fetus

iliac crest

tubercle of iliac crest

iliopectineal line

sacroiliac joint

anterior superior
iliac spine

anterior inferior
iliac spine

fovea capitis

margin of
acetabulum

head of fetus

cavity of hip joint

head of femur

capsule of
hip joint

neck of femur

greater
trochanter

ischial
tuberosity

acetabular
notch

superior ramus
of pubis

body of pubis

vulva

symphysis pubis

obturator foramen

lesser
trochanter

intertrochanteric
line

shaft of femur

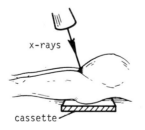

x-rays

cassette

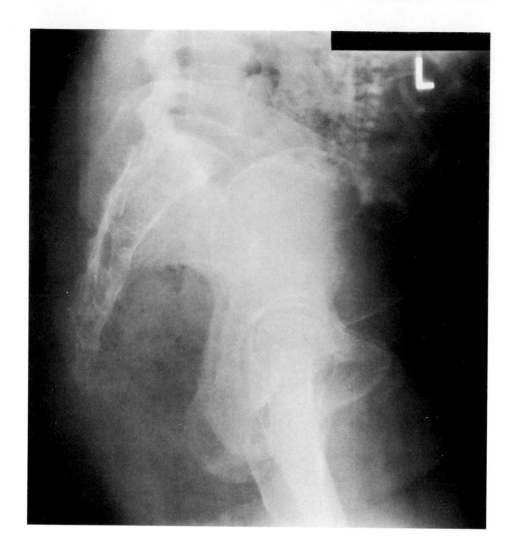

Figure 3

Lateral radiograph of pelvis of pregnant
woman aged 36 years. The pregnancy
is in the third trimester.

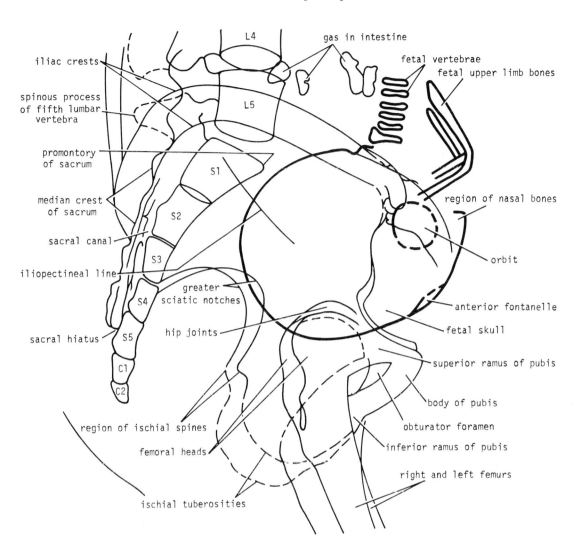

iliac crests

spinous process
of fifth lumbar
vertebra

promontory
of sacrum

median crest
of sacrum

sacral canal

iliopectineal line

sacral hiatus

L4

L5

S1

S2

S3

S4

S5

C1

C2

greater
sciatic notches

region of ischial spines

hip joints

femoral heads

ischial tuberosities

gas in intestine

fetal vertebrae

fetal upper limb bones

region of nasal bones

orbit

anterior fontanelle

fetal skull

superior ramus of pubis

body of pubis

obturator foramen

inferior ramus of pubis

right and left femurs

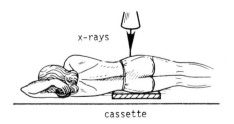

x-rays

cassette

9

ARTERIOGRAPHY
AND VENOGRAPHY

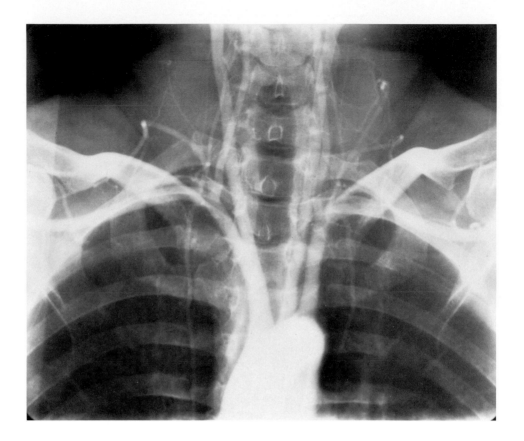

Figure 1

Aortic arch angiogram showing
large arteries at root of neck
(male aged 38 years).

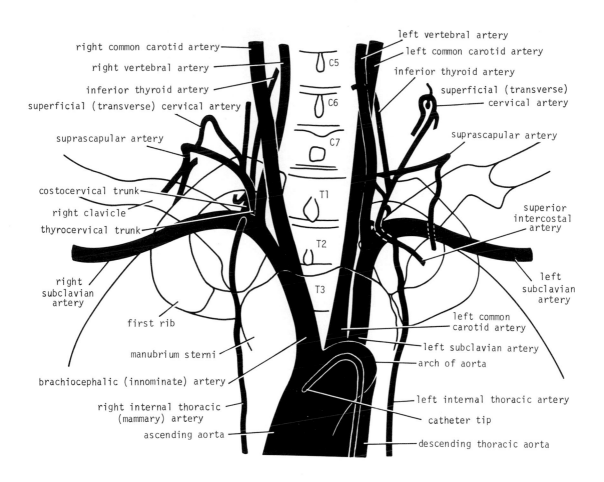

right common carotid artery
right vertebral artery
inferior thyroid artery
superficial (transverse) cervical artery
suprascapular artery
costocervical trunk
right clavicle
thyrocervical trunk
right subclavian artery
first rib
manubrium sterni
brachiocephalic (innominate) artery
right internal thoracic (mammary) artery
ascending aorta

C5
C6
C7
T1
T2
T3

left vertebral artery
left common carotid artery
inferior thyroid artery
superficial (transverse) cervical artery
suprascapular artery
superior intercostal artery
left subclavian artery
left common carotid artery
left subclavian artery
arch of aorta
left internal thoracic artery
catheter tip
descending thoracic aorta

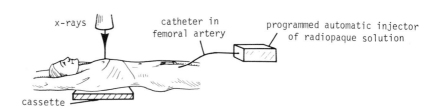

x-rays
catheter in femoral artery
programmed automatic injector of radiopaque solution
cassette

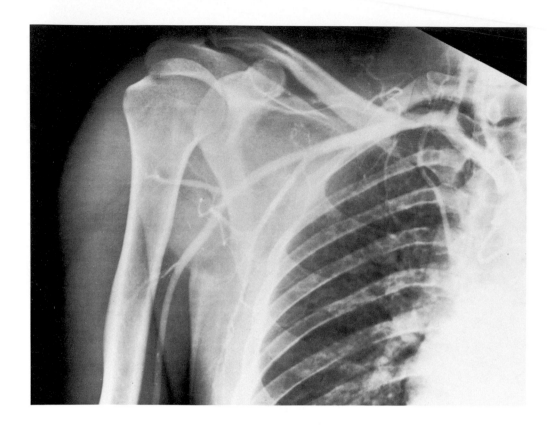

Figure 2

Angiogram of the subclavian,
axillary, and brachial arteries
(male aged 48 years).

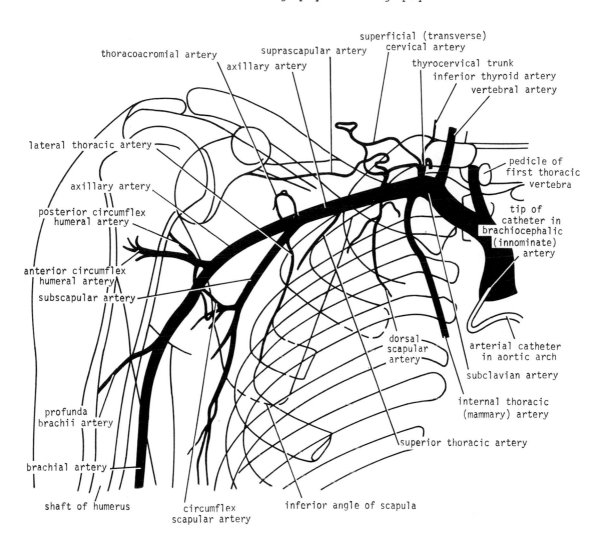

thoracoacromial artery

superficial (transverse) cervical artery

suprascapular artery

axillary artery

thyrocervical trunk

inferior thyroid artery

vertebral artery

lateral thoracic artery

pedicle of first thoracic vertebra

axillary artery

posterior circumflex humeral artery

tip of catheter in brachiocephalic (innominate) artery

anterior circumflex humeral artery

subscapular artery

dorsal scapular artery

arterial catheter in aortic arch

subclavian artery

profunda brachii artery

internal thoracic (mammary) artery

brachial artery

superior thoracic artery

shaft of humerus

circumflex scapular artery

inferior angle of scapula

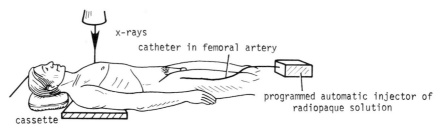

x-rays

catheter in femoral artery

programmed automatic injector of radiopaque solution

cassette

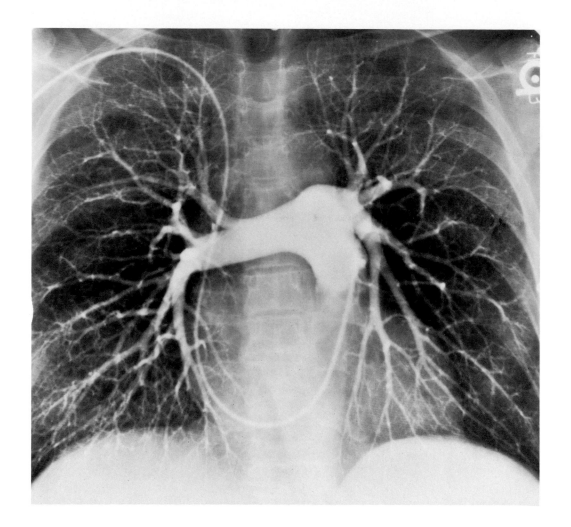

Figure 3

Angiogram of the pulmonary
trunk and pulmonary arteries
(female aged 53 years).

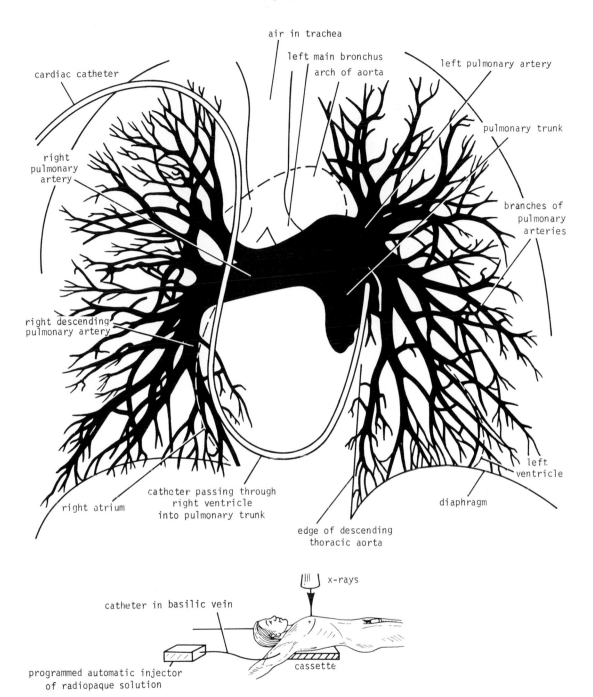

air in trachea

left main bronchus
arch of aorta

left pulmonary artery

cardiac catheter

pulmonary trunk

right pulmonary artery

branches of pulmonary arteries

right descending pulmonary artery

left ventricle

right atrium

catheter passing through right ventricle into pulmonary trunk

diaphragm

edge of descending thoracic aorta

x-rays

catheter in basilic vein

cassette

programmed automatic injector of radiopaque solution

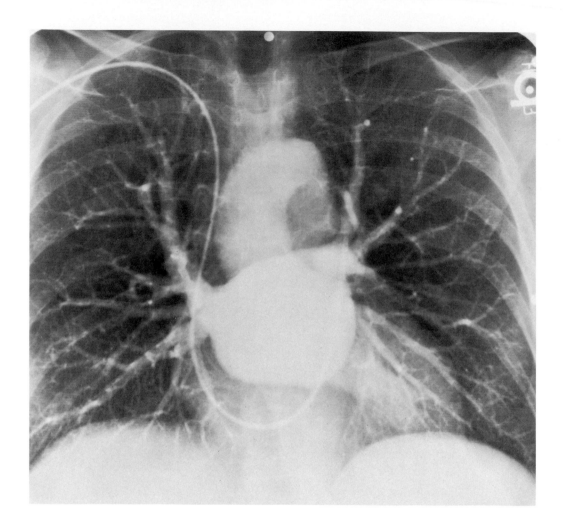

Figure 4

Venogram of the
pulmonary veins and left atrium
(female aged 53 years).

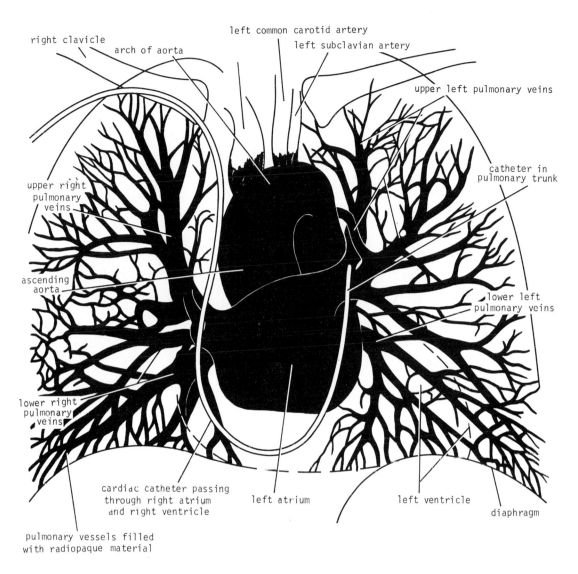

right clavicle

arch of aorta

left common carotid artery

left subclavian artery

upper left pulmonary veins

catheter in pulmonary trunk

upper right pulmonary veins

ascending aorta

lower left pulmonary veins

lower right pulmonary veins

cardiac catheter passing through right atrium and right ventricle

left atrium

left ventricle

diaphragm

pulmonary vessels filled with radiopaque material

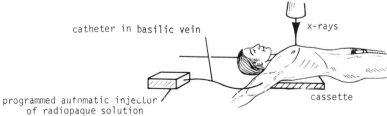

catheter in basilic vein

x-rays

programmed automatic injector of radiopaque solution

cassette

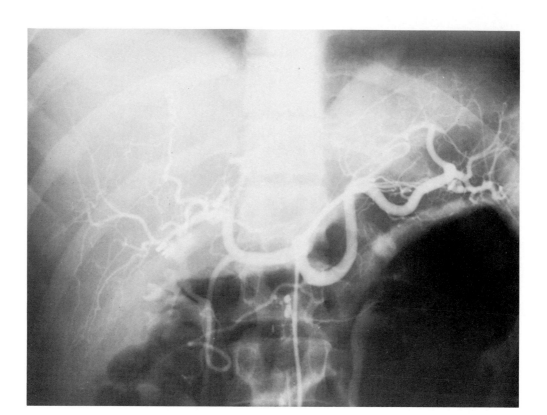

Figure 5

Arteriogram of the celiac
artery and its branches
(male aged 32 years).

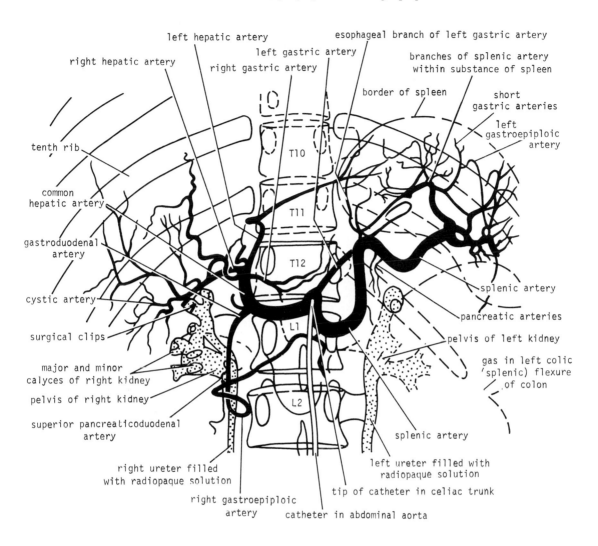

left hepatic artery

esophageal branch of left gastric artery

left gastric artery

right gastric artery

branches of splenic artery
within substance of spleen

right hepatic artery

border of spleen

short
gastric arteries

left
gastroepiploic
artery

tenth rib

T10

common
hepatic artery

T11

gastroduodenal
artery

T12

splenic artery

pancreatic arteries

cystic artery

pelvis of left kidney

L1

surgical clips

gas in left colic
(splenic) flexure
of colon

major and minor
calyces of right kidney

pelvis of right kidney

L2

superior pancreaticoduodenal
artery

splenic artery

right ureter filled
with radiopaque solution

left ureter filled with
radiopaque solution

right gastroepiploic
artery

tip of catheter in celiac trunk

catheter in abdominal aorta

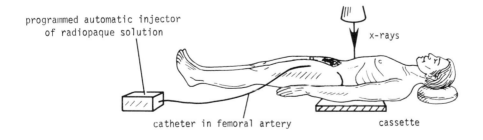

programmed automatic injector
of radiopaque solution

x-rays

catheter in femoral artery

cassette

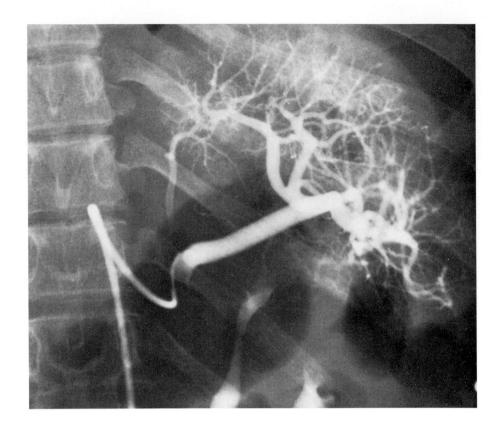

Figure 6

Arteriogram of the splenic
artery and its branches
(female aged 20 years).

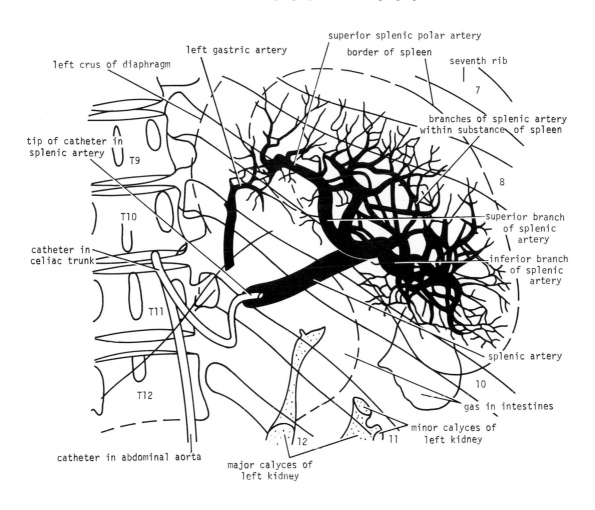

left crus of diaphragm

left gastric artery

superior splenic polar artery

border of spleen

seventh rib

7

branches of splenic artery
within substance of spleen

tip of catheter in
splenic artery

T9

T10

superior branch
of splenic
artery

8

catheter in
celiac trunk

inferior branch
of splenic
artery

T11

splenic artery

10

T12

gas in intestines

minor calyces of
left kidney

11

catheter in abdominal aorta

major calyces of
left kidney

12

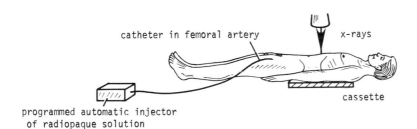

catheter in femoral artery

x-rays

programmed automatic injector
of radiopaque solution

cassette

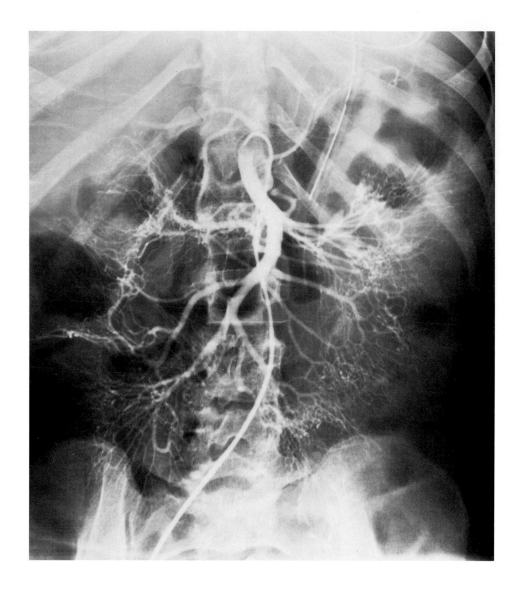

Figure 7

Arteriogram of the superior
mesenteric artery and its branches
(female aged 20 years).

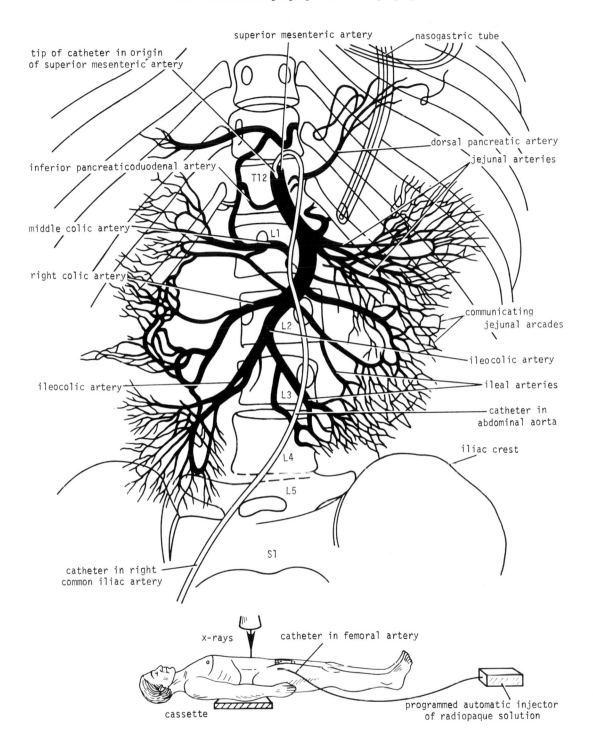

tip of catheter in origin
of superior mesenteric artery

superior mesenteric artery

nasogastric tube

dorsal pancreatic artery

jejunal arteries

inferior pancreaticoduodenal artery

T12

L1

middle colic artery

right colic artery

L2

communicating
jejunal arcades

ileocolic artery

ileal arteries

ileocolic artery

L3

catheter in
abdominal aorta

L4

iliac crest

L5

S1

catheter in right
common iliac artery

x-rays

catheter in femoral artery

cassette

programmed automatic injector
of radiopaque solution

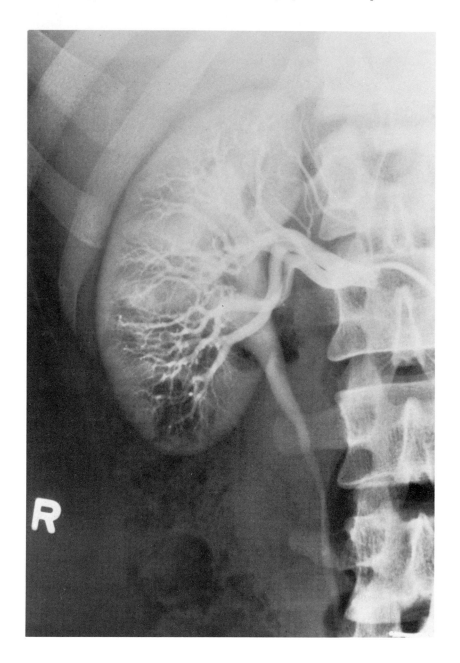

Figure 8

Arteriogram of the right renal artery
(male aged 33 years).

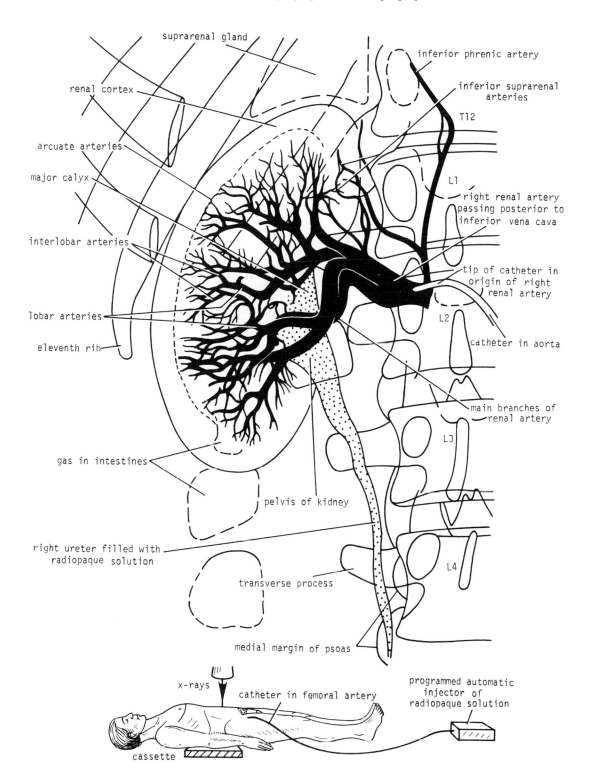

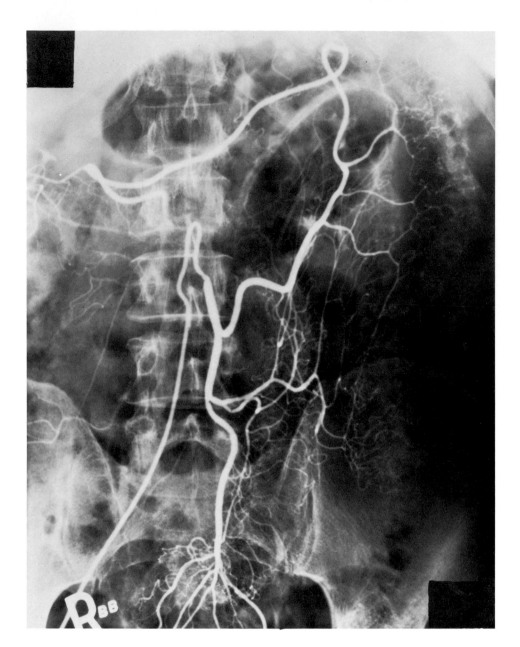

Figure 9

Arteriogram of the inferior
mesenteric artery and its branches
(female aged 63 years).

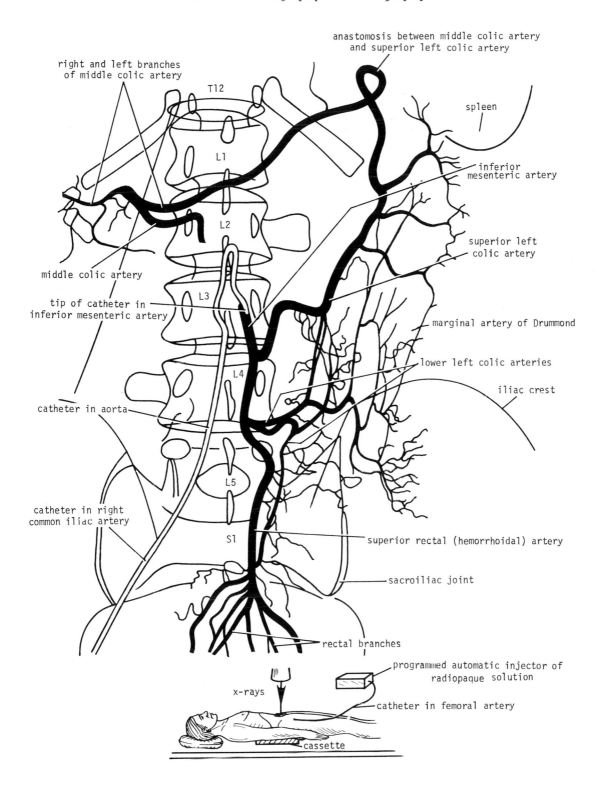

anastomosis between middle colic artery
and superior left colic artery

right and left branches
of middle colic artery

T12

spleen

L1

inferior
mesenteric artery

L2

superior left
colic artery

middle colic artery

L3

tip of catheter in
inferior mesenteric artery

marginal artery of Drummond

lower left colic arteries

L4

iliac crest

catheter in aorta

catheter in right
common iliac artery

L5

S1

superior rectal (hemorrhoidal) artery

sacroiliac joint

rectal branches

programmed automatic injector of
radiopaque solution

x-rays

catheter in femoral artery

cassette

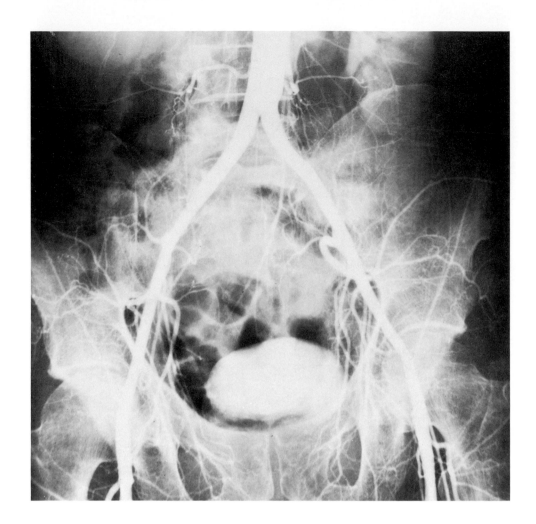

Figure 10

Arteriogram of the lower
part of the abdominal aorta and
iliac and femoral arteries
(male aged 44 years).

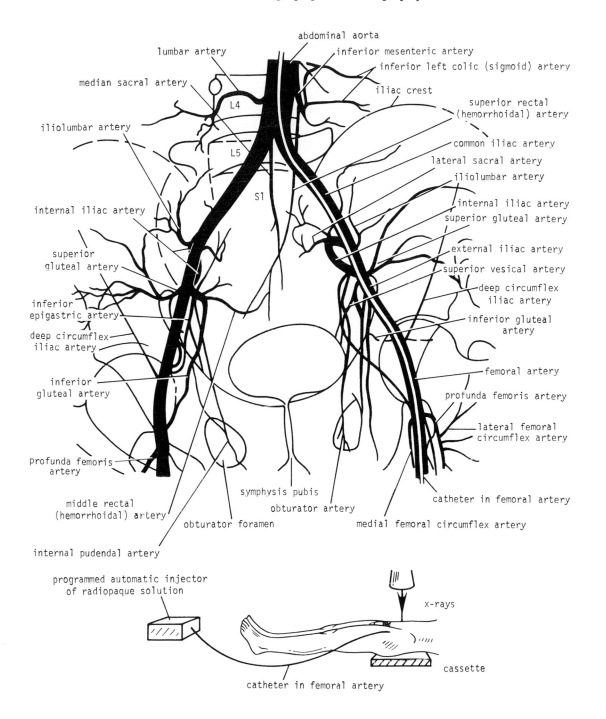

programmed automatic injector
of radiopaque solution

x-rays

cassette

catheter in femoral artery

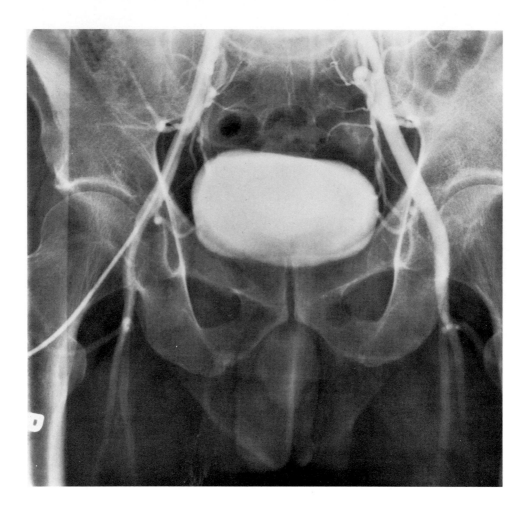

Figure 11

Arteriogram of the
iliac and femoral arteries
(male aged 48 years).

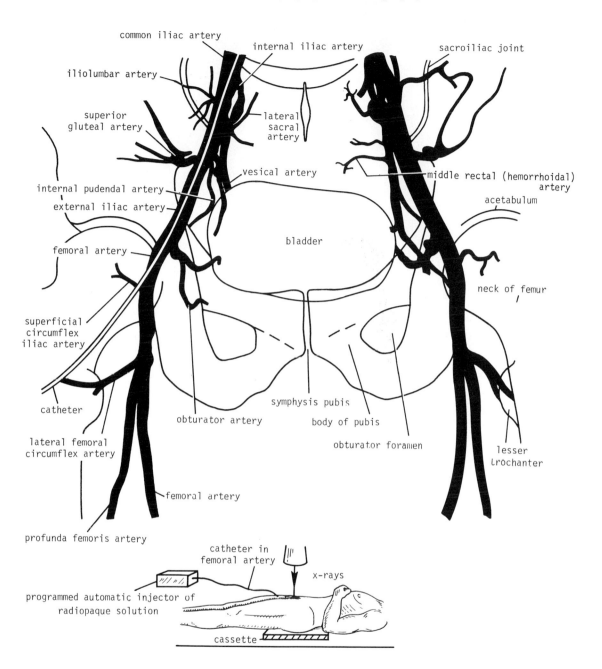

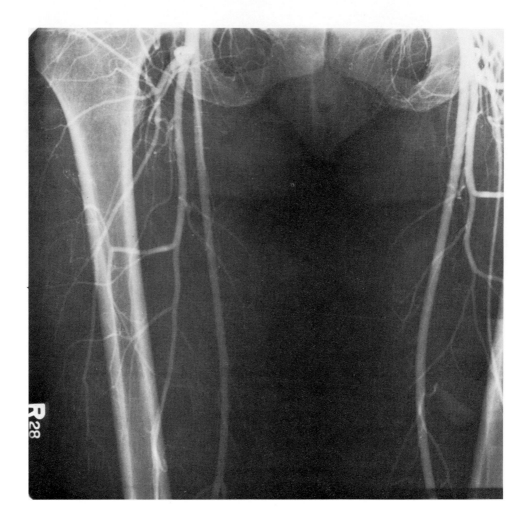

Figure 12

Arteriogram of the
femoral artery and its branches
(female aged 52 years).

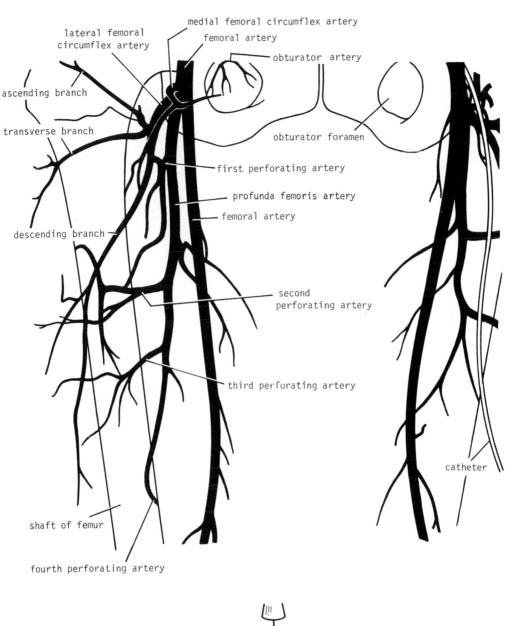

lateral femoral
circumflex artery

medial femoral circumflex artery

femoral artery

obturator artery

ascending branch

transverse branch

obturator foramen

first perforating artery

profunda femoris artery

femoral artery

descending branch

second
perforating artery

third perforating artery

catheter

shaft of femur

fourth perforating artery

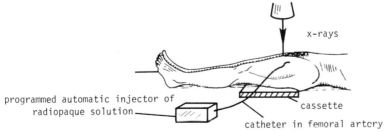

x-rays

programmed automatic injector of
radiopaque solution

cassette

catheter in femoral artery

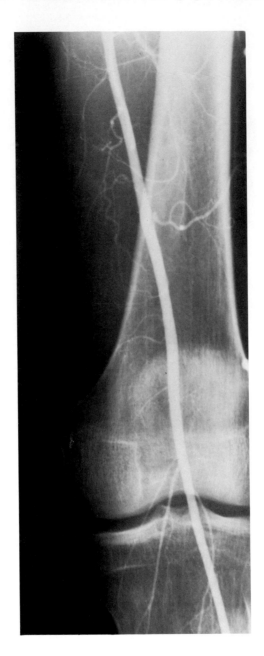

Figure 13

Arteriogram of the femoral and
popliteal arteries and their branches
(male aged 44 years).

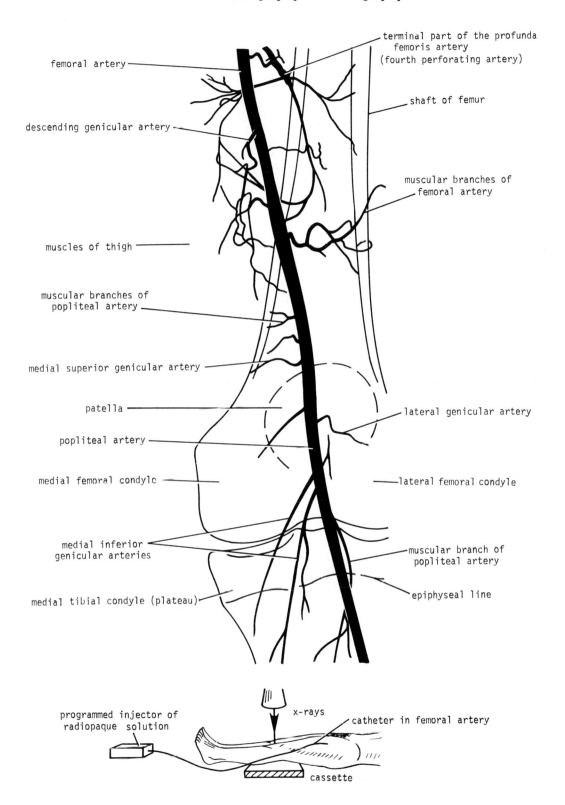

femoral artery

terminal part of the profunda femoris artery (fourth perforating artery)

shaft of femur

descending genicular artery

muscular branches of femoral artery

muscles of thigh

muscular branches of popliteal artery

medial superior genicular artery

patella

lateral genicular artery

popliteal artery

medial femoral condyle

lateral femoral condyle

medial inferior genicular arteries

muscular branch of popliteal artery

medial tibial condyle (plateau)

epiphyseal line

programmed injector of radiopaque solution

x-rays

catheter in femoral artery

cassette

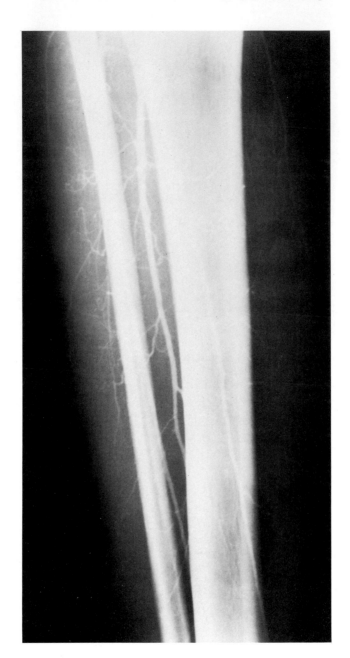

Figure 14

Arteriogram of the
anterior and posterior
tibial arteries and their branches
(male aged 44 years).

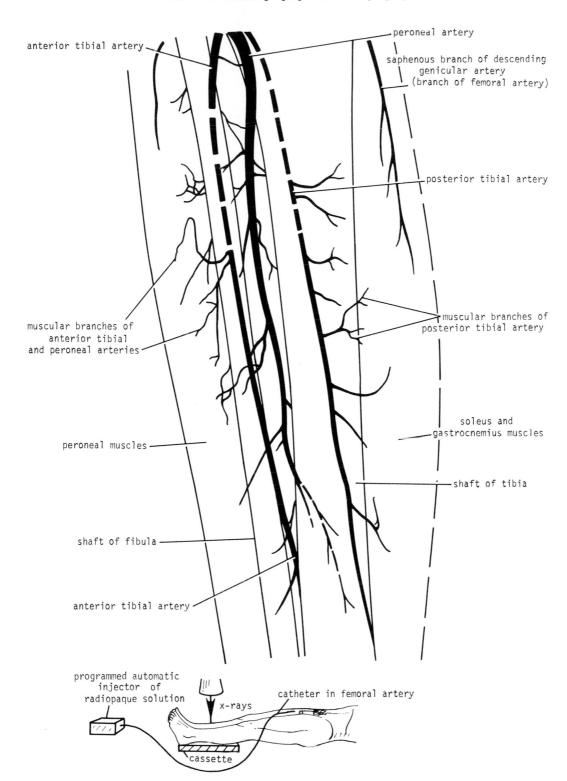

anterior tibial artery

peroneal artery

saphenous branch of descending
genicular artery
(branch of femoral artery)

posterior tibial artery

muscular branches of
posterior tibial artery

muscular branches of
anterior tibial
and peroneal arteries

soleus and
gastrocnemius muscles

peroneal muscles

shaft of tibia

shaft of fibula

anterior tibial artery

programmed automatic
injector of
radiopaque solution

x-rays

catheter in femoral artery

cassette

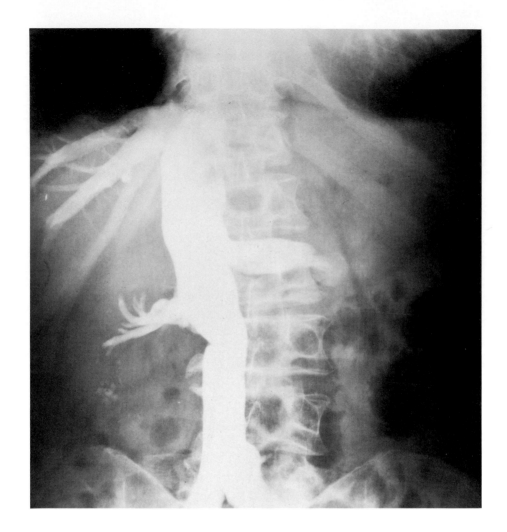

Figure 15

Venogram of the inferior vena cava:
an abnormally high right atrial
pressure has resulted in excessive
filling of the hepatic and renal veins
(male aged 63 years).

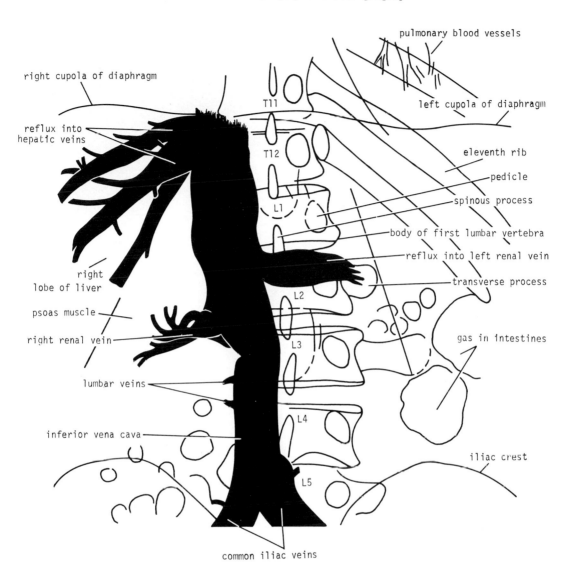

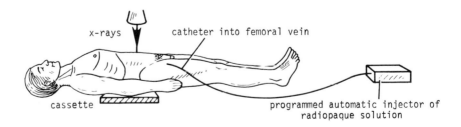

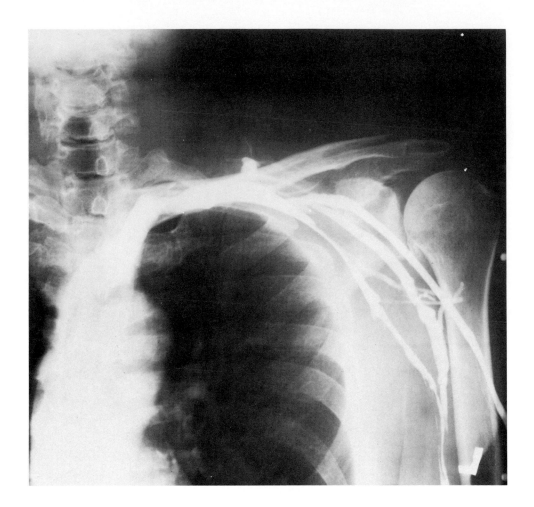

Figure 16

Venogram of the subclavian,
axillary, and brachial veins
(male aged 57 years).

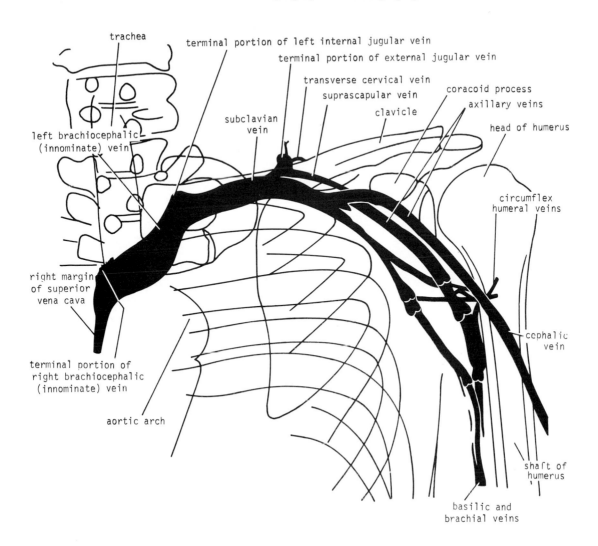

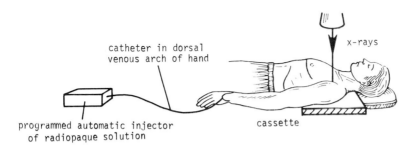

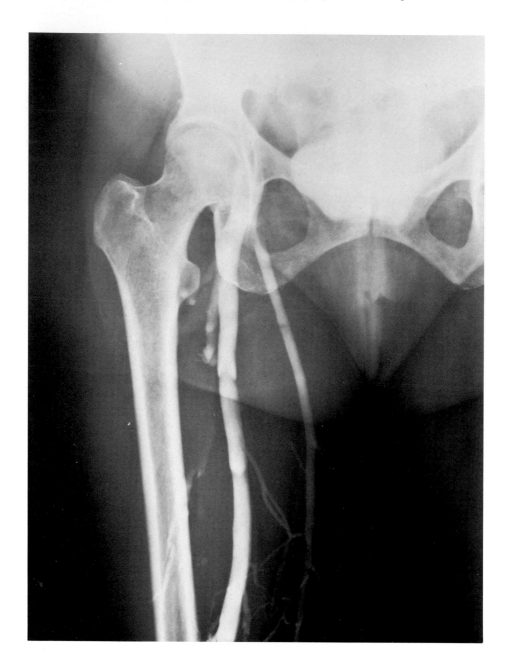

Figure 17

Venogram of the external
iliac vein and the femoral
vein and its major tributaries
(female aged 38 years).

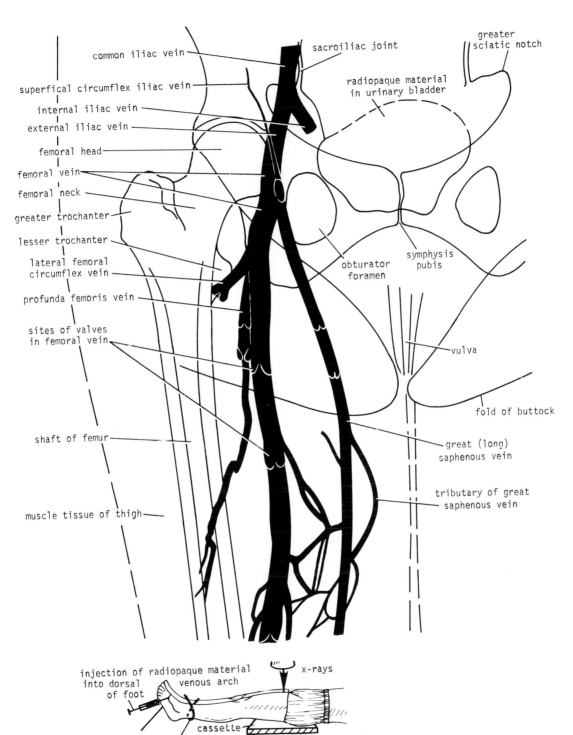

common iliac vein

superfical circumflex iliac vein

internal iliac vein

external iliac vein

femoral head

femoral vein

femoral neck

greater trochanter

lesser trochanter

lateral femoral circumflex vein

profunda femoris vein

sites of valves in femoral vein

shaft of femur

muscle tissue of thigh

sacroiliac joint

greater sciatic notch

radiopaque material in urinary bladder

symphysis pubis

obturator foramen

vulva

fold of buttock

great (long) saphenous vein

tributary of great saphenous vein

injection of radiopaque material into dorsal of foot

venous arch

x-rays

cassette

tourniquet to force radiopaque material into deep veins

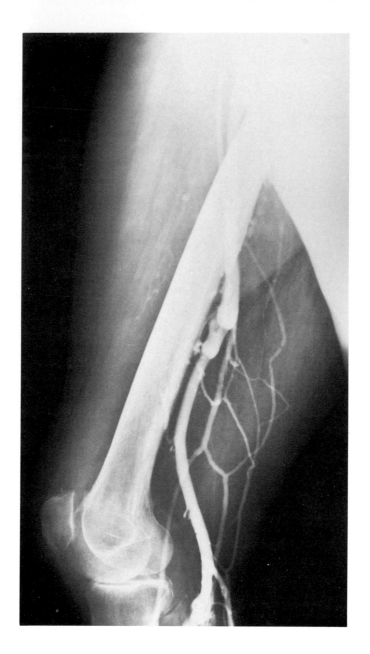

Figure 18

Venogram of the femoral and popliteal
veins and their major tributaries
(male aged 49 years).

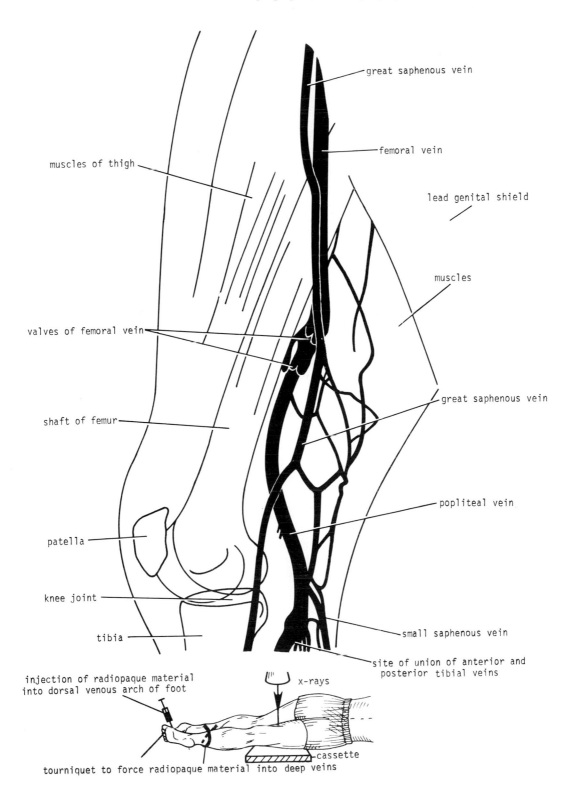

great saphenous vein

femoral vein

muscles of thigh

lead genital shield

muscles

valves of femoral vein

great saphenous vein

shaft of femur

popliteal vein

patella

knee joint

small saphenous vein

tibia

site of union of anterior and posterior tibial veins

injection of radiopaque material into dorsal venous arch of foot

x-rays

cassette

tourniquet to force radiopaque material into deep veins

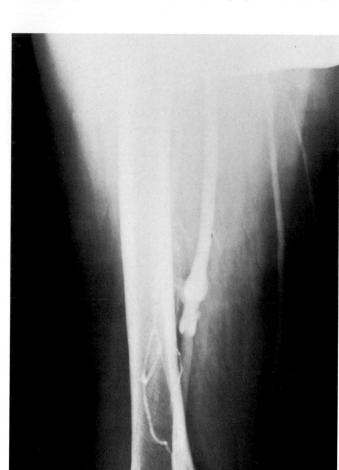

Figure 19

Venogram of the femoral and popliteal
veins and their major tributaries
(male aged 49 years).

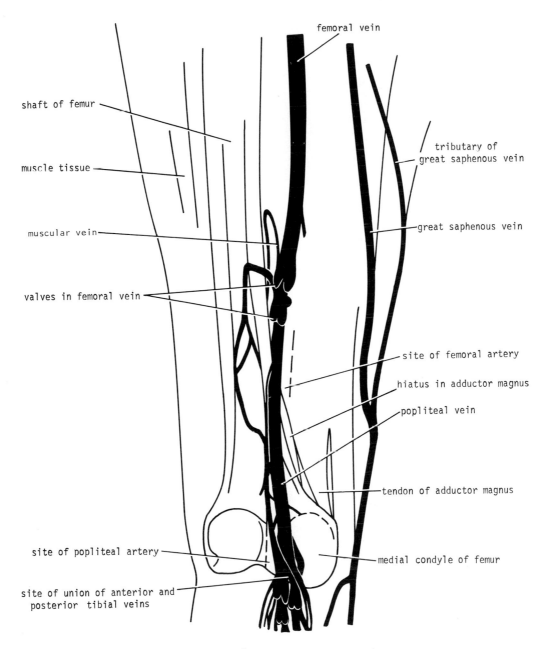

femoral vein

shaft of femur

muscle tissue

muscular vein

valves in femoral vein

tributary of great saphenous vein

great saphenous vein

site of femoral artery

hiatus in adductor magnus

popliteal vein

tendon of adductor magnus

site of popliteal artery

medial condyle of femur

site of union of anterior and posterior tibial veins

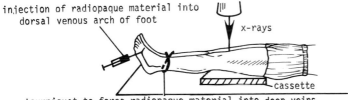

injection of radiopaque material into dorsal venous arch of foot

x-rays

cassette

tourniquet to force radiopaque material into deep veins

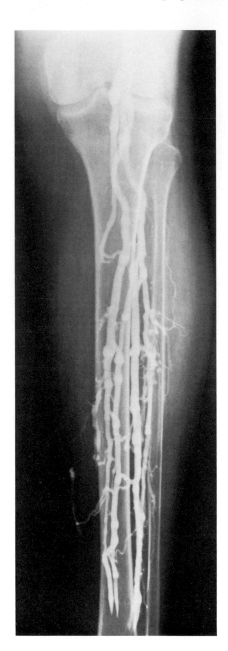

Figure 20

Venogram of the popliteal
and anterior and posterior tibial veins
(male aged 49 years).

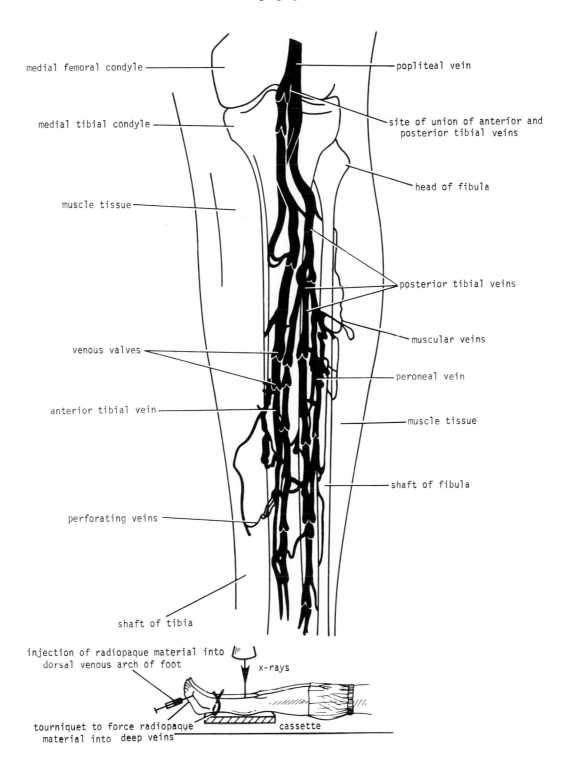

medial femoral condyle

popliteal vein

medial tibial condyle

site of union of anterior and posterior tibial veins

head of fibula

muscle tissue

posterior tibial veins

muscular veins

venous valves

peroneal vein

anterior tibial vein

muscle tissue

shaft of fibula

perforating veins

shaft of tibia

injection of radiopaque material into dorsal venous arch of foot

x-rays

tourniquet to force radiopaque material into deep veins

cassette

LYMPHANGIOGRAPHY

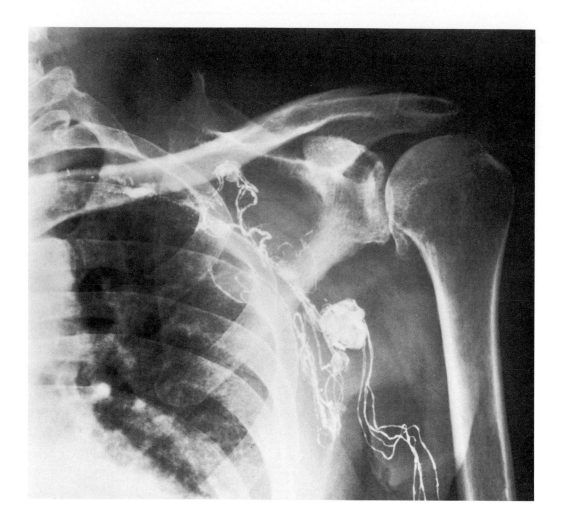

Figure 1

Lymphangiogram of the arm and axilla
(male aged 57 years).

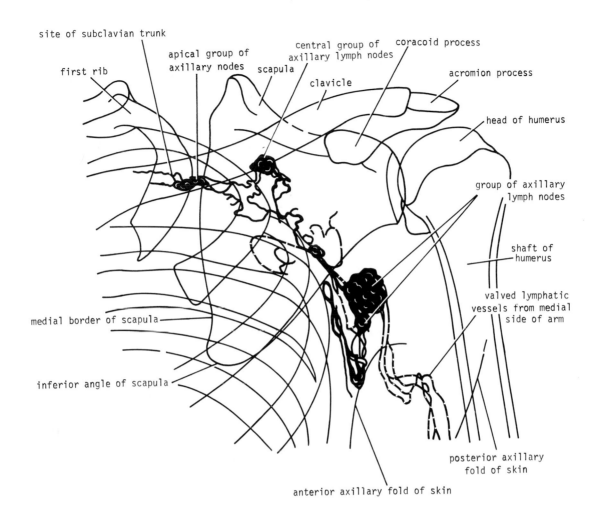

site of subclavian trunk

first rib

apical group of
axillary nodes

scapula

central group of
axillary lymph nodes

coracoid process

clavicle

acromion process

head of humerus

group of axillary
lymph nodes

shaft of
humerus

valved lymphatic
vessels from medial
side of arm

medial border of scapula

inferior angle of scapula

posterior axillary
fold of skin

anterior axillary fold of skin

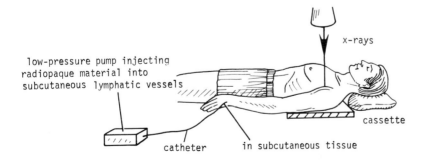

x-rays

low-pressure pump injecting
radiopaque material into
subcutaneous lymphatic vessels

cassette

catheter

in subcutaneous tissue

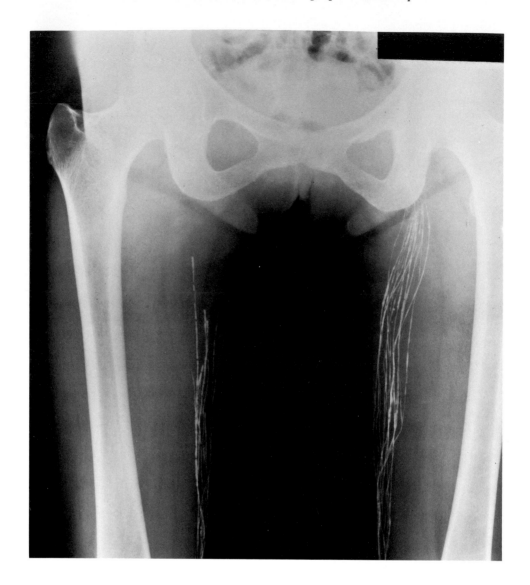

Figure 2

Lymphangiogram of the superficial
lymphatic vessels of the thighs
(female aged 59 years).

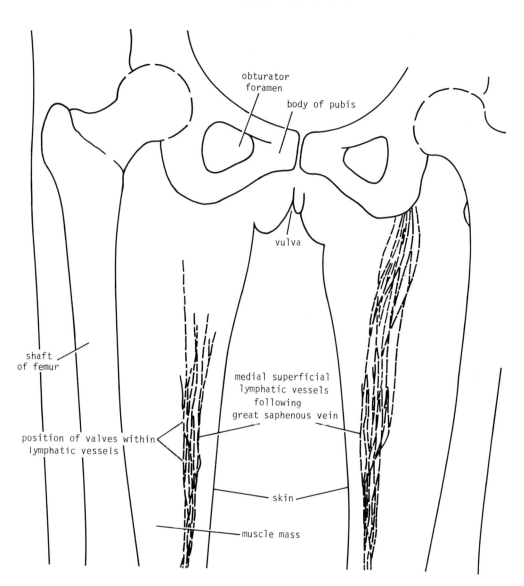

obturator
foramen

body of pubis

vulva

shaft
of femur

medial superficial
lymphatic vessels
following
great saphenous vein

position of valves within
lymphatic vessels

skin

muscle mass

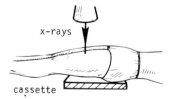

x-rays

cassette

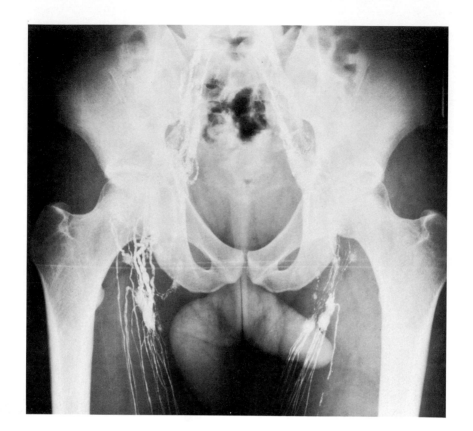

Figure 3

Lymphangiogram
of the thighs and pelvis
(male aged 21 years).

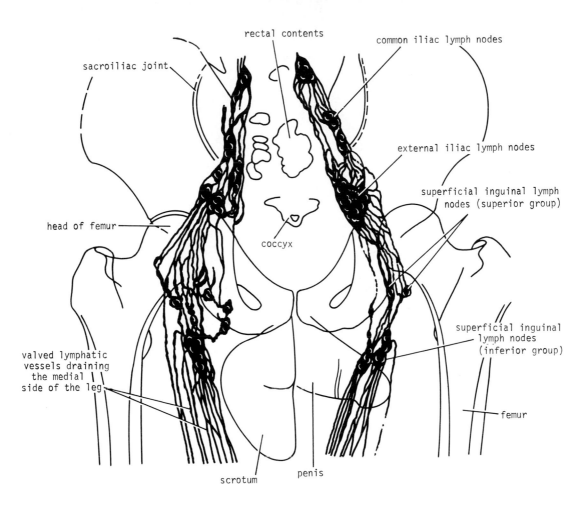

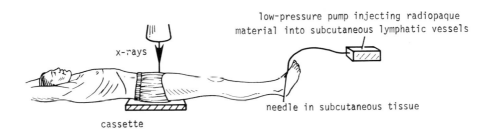

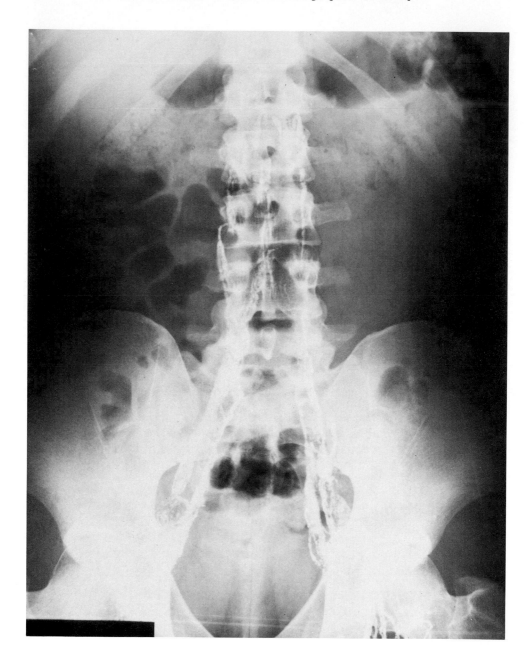

Figure 4

Lymphangiogram
of the pelvis and abdomen
(female aged 21 years).

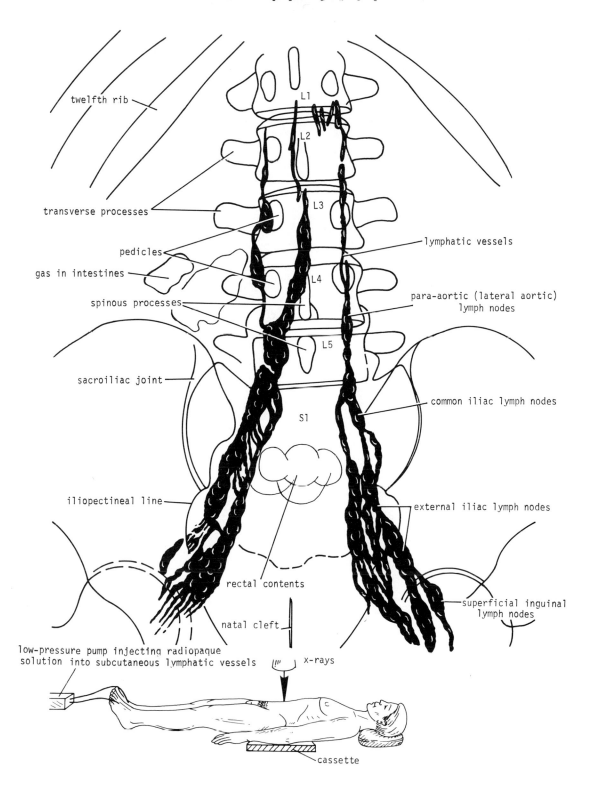

twelfth rib

transverse processes

pedicles

gas in intestines

spinous processes

sacroiliac joint

iliopectineal line

L1

L2

L3

L4

L5

S1

lymphatic vessels

para-aortic (lateral aortic) lymph nodes

common iliac lymph nodes

external iliac lymph nodes

rectal contents

natal cleft

superficial inguinal lymph nodes

low-pressure pump injecting radiopaque solution into subcutaneous lymphatic vessels

x-rays

cassette

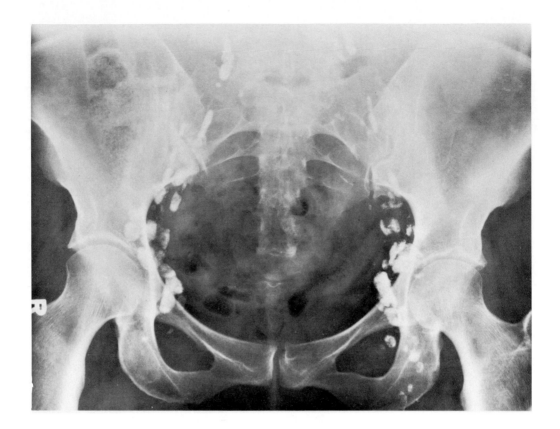

Figure 5

Lymphangiogram showing inguinal and
iliac lymph nodes 24 hours after
injection of radiopaque material
into subcutaneous lymph vessels
on the dorsum of the feet
(female aged 54 years).

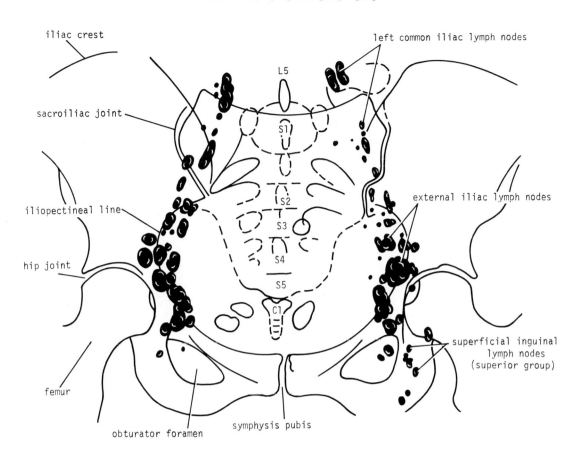

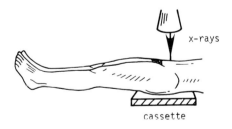

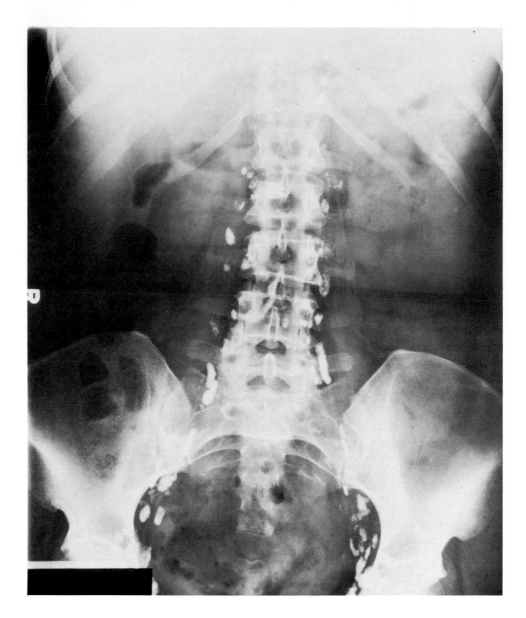

Figure 6

Lymphangiogram showing inguinal,
iliac, and para-aortic lymph nodes
24 hours after injection of radiopaque
material into subcutaneous lymph
vessels on the dorsum of the feet
(female aged 54 years).

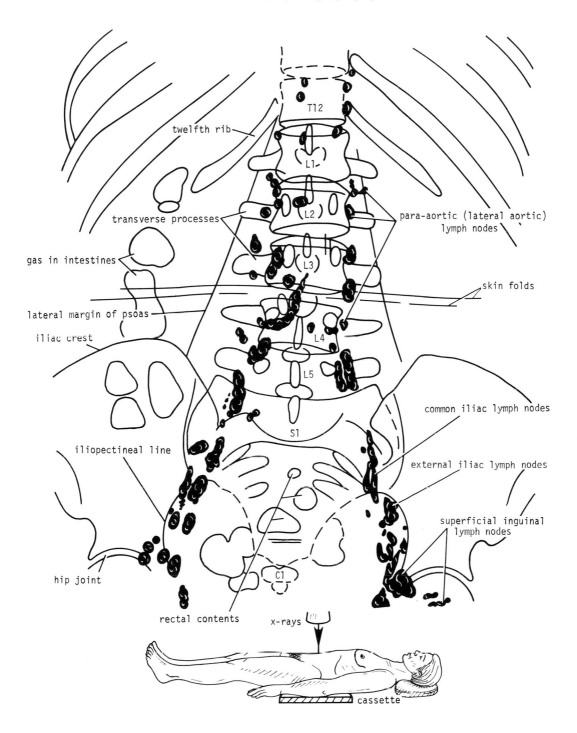

11

THE CENTRAL NERVOUS SYSTEM

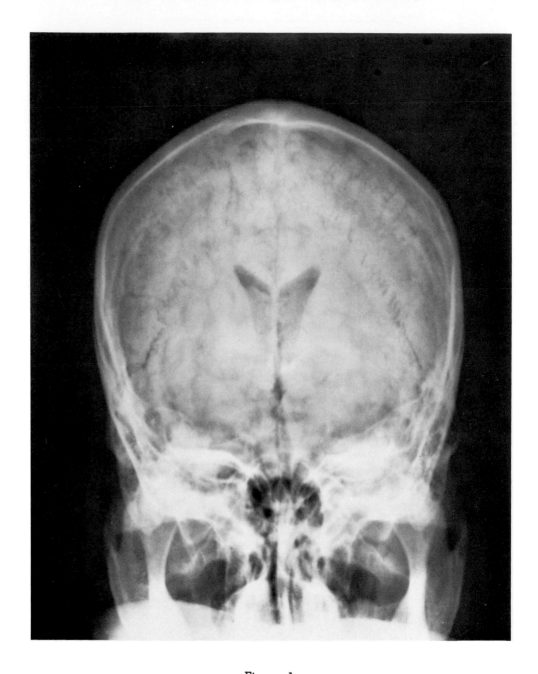

Figure 1

Anteroposterior pneumoencephalogram
(male aged 28 years).

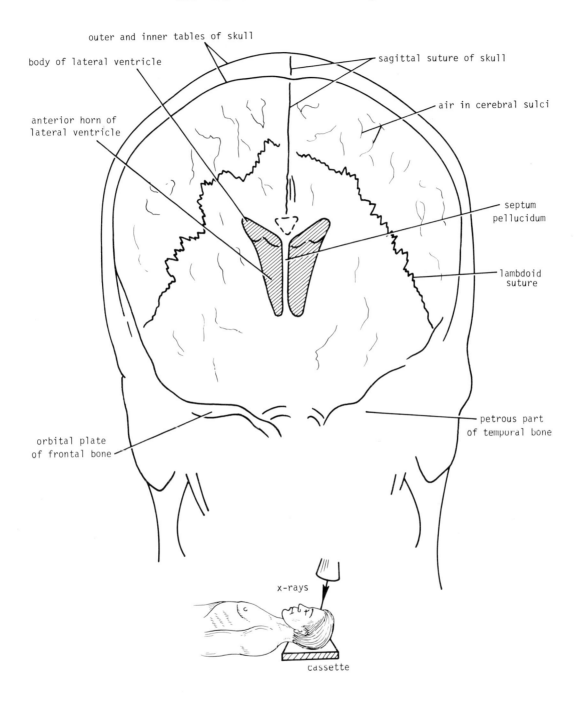

outer and inner tables of skull

body of lateral ventricle

sagittal suture of skull

air in cerebral sulci

anterior horn of
lateral ventricle

septum
pellucidum

lambdoid
suture

petrous part
of temporal bone

orbital plate
of frontal bone

x-rays

cassette

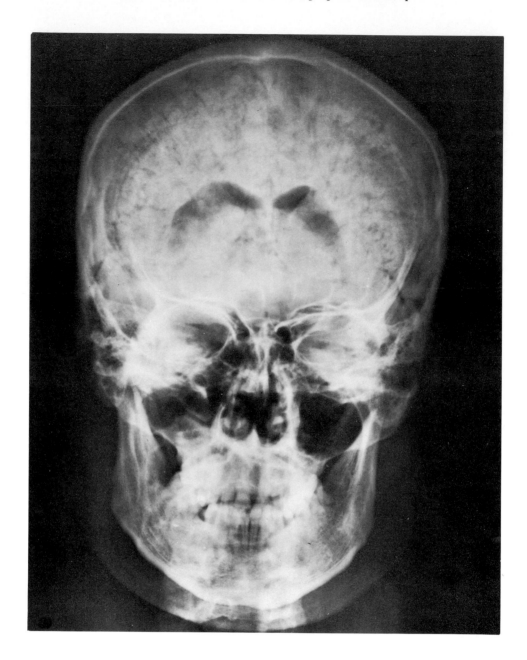

Figure 2

Posteroanterior pneumoencephalogram
(male aged 28 years).

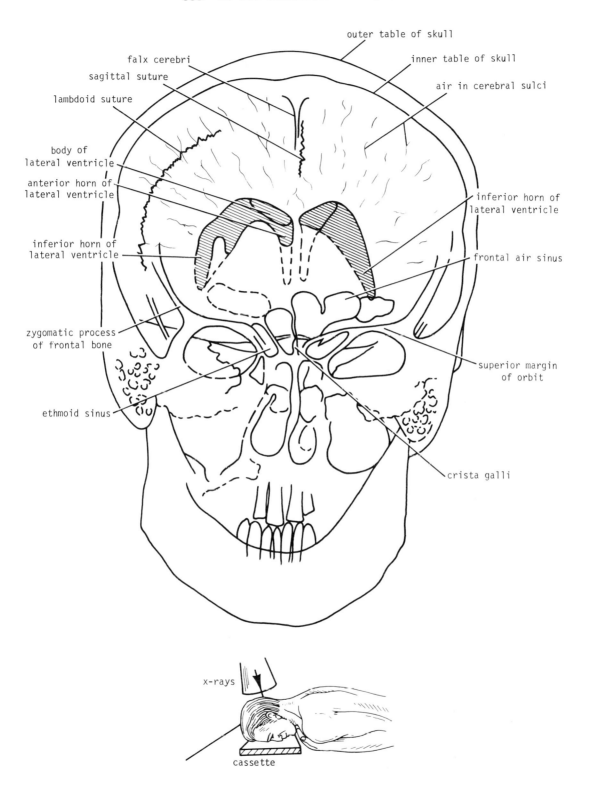

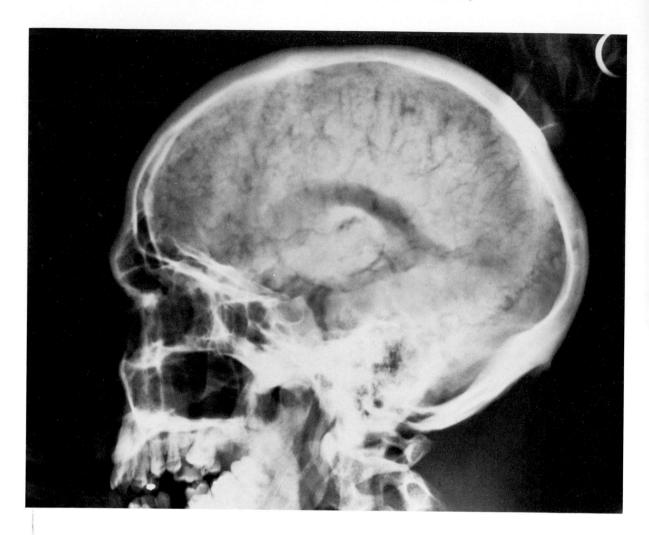

Figure 3

Lateral pneumoencephalogram
(male aged 28 years).

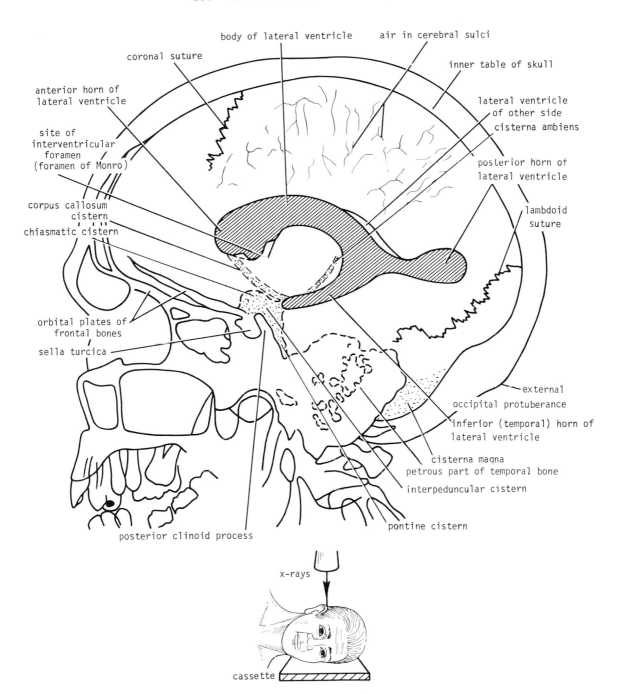

body of lateral ventricle

air in cerebral sulci

coronal suture

inner table of skull

anterior horn of
lateral ventricle

lateral ventricle
of other side
cisterna ambiens

site of
interventricular
foramen
(foramen of Monro)

posterior horn of
lateral ventricle

corpus callosum
cistern

lambdoid
suture

chiasmatic cistern

orbital plates of
frontal bones

external
occipital protuberance

sella turcica

inferior (temporal) horn of
lateral ventricle

cisterna magna
petrous part of temporal bone

interpeduncular cistern

posterior clinoid process

pontine cistern

x-rays

cassette

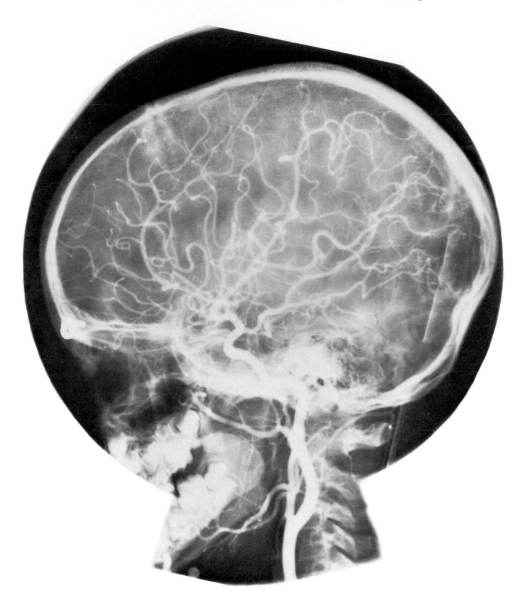

Figure 4

Lateral internal carotid arteriogram
(male aged 20 years).

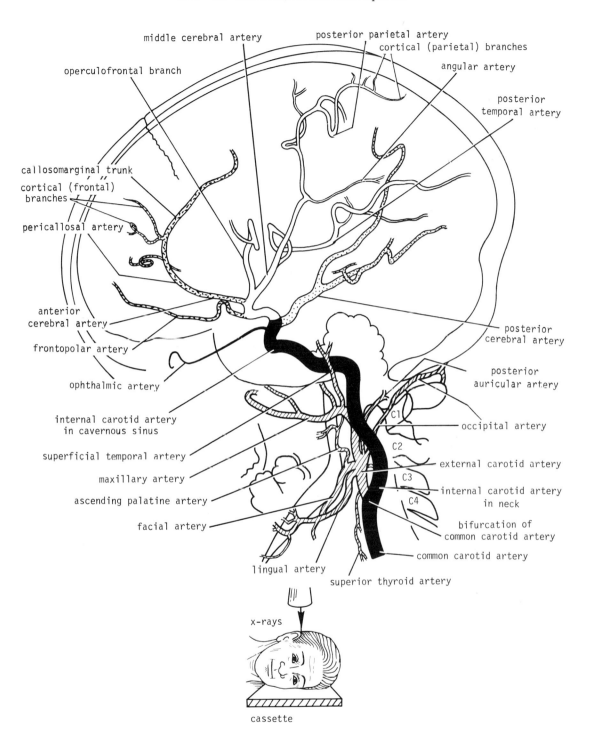

middle cerebral artery

posterior parietal artery

cortical (parietal) branches

operculofrontal branch

angular artery

posterior temporal artery

callosomarginal trunk

cortical (frontal) branches

pericallosal artery

anterior cerebral artery

frontopolar artery

ophthalmic artery

internal carotid artery in cavernous sinus

superficial temporal artery

maxillary artery

ascending palatine artery

facial artery

posterior cerebral artery

posterior auricular artery

occipital artery

external carotid artery

internal carotid artery in neck

bifurcation of common carotid artery

common carotid artery

lingual artery

superior thyroid artery

C1

C2

C3

C4

x-rays

cassette

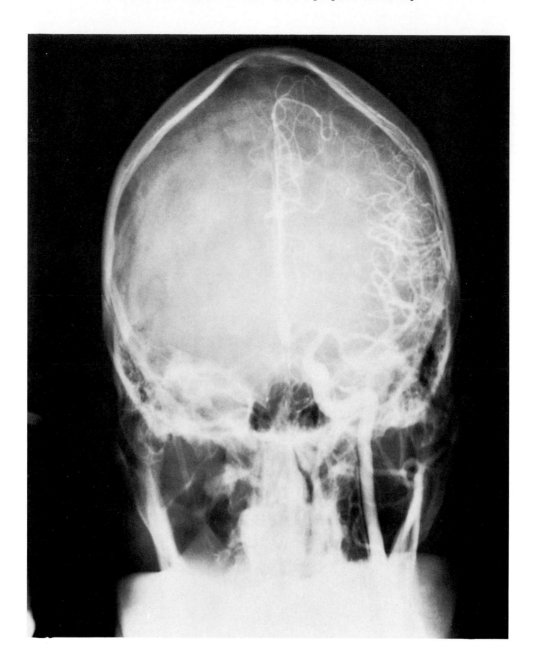

Figure 5

Anteroposterior
internal carotid arteriogram
(male aged 20 years).

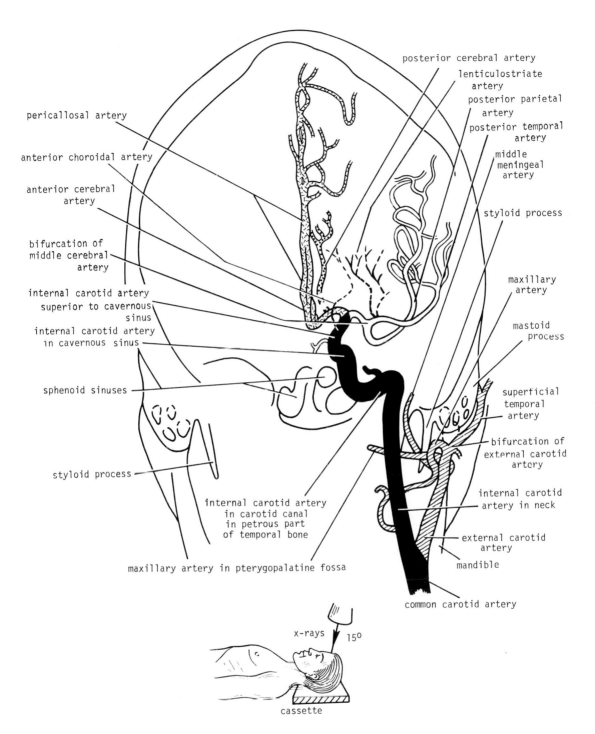

posterior cerebral artery

lenticulostriate artery

posterior parietal artery

posterior temporal artery

middle meningeal artery

styloid process

maxillary artery

mastoid process

superficial temporal artery

bifurcation of external carotid artery

internal carotid artery in neck

external carotid artery

mandible

common carotid artery

pericallosal artery

anterior choroidal artery

anterior cerebral artery

bifurcation of middle cerebral artery

internal carotid artery superior to cavernous sinus

internal carotid artery in cavernous sinus

sphenoid sinuses

styloid process

internal carotid artery in carotid canal in petrous part of temporal bone

maxillary artery in pterygopalatine fossa

x-rays 15°

cassette

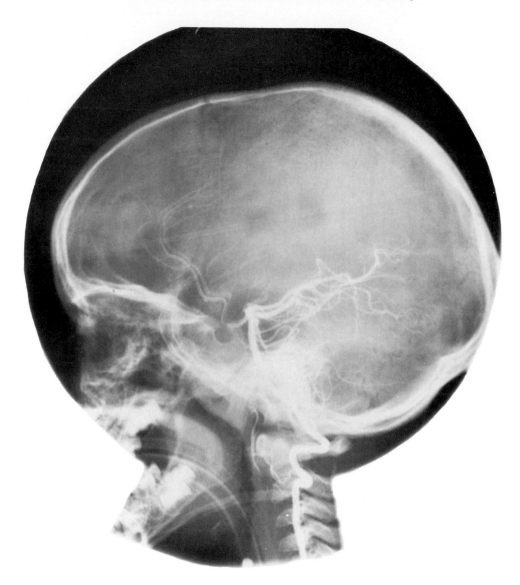

Figure 6

Lateral vertebral arteriogram
(male aged 20 years).

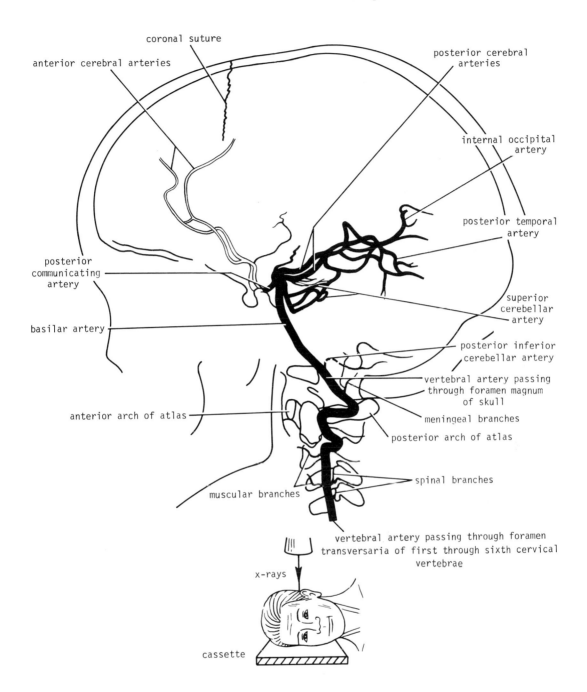

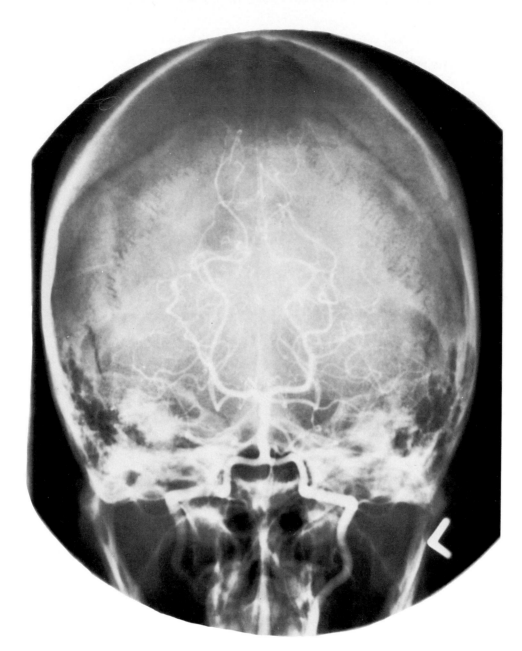

Figure 7

Anteroposterior
(angled) vertebral arteriogram
(female aged 35 years).

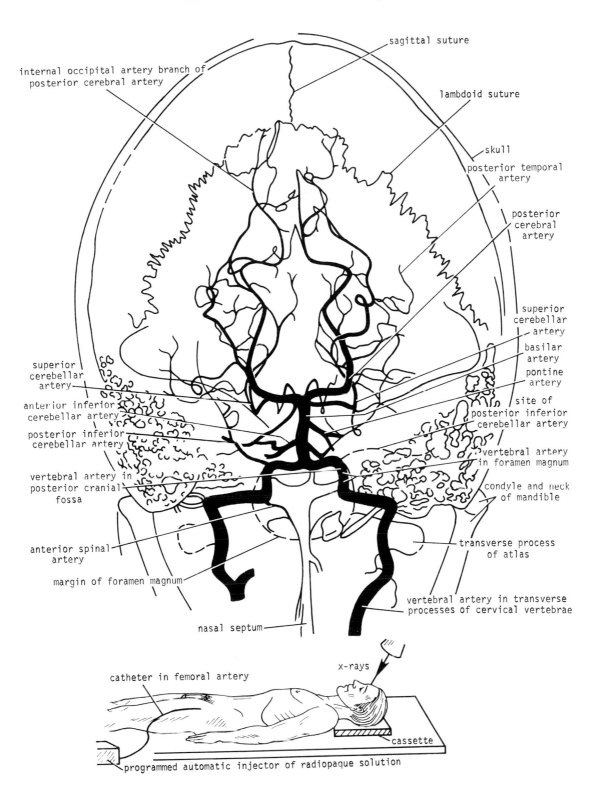

sagittal suture

internal occipital artery branch of posterior cerebral artery

lambdoid suture

skull

posterior temporal artery

posterior cerebral artery

superior cerebellar artery

basilar artery

pontine artery

site of posterior inferior cerebellar artery

vertebral artery in foramen magnum

condyle and neck of mandible

transverse process of atlas

vertebral artery in transverse processes of cervical vertebrae

superior cerebellar artery

anterior inferior cerebellar artery

posterior inferior cerebellar artery

vertebral artery in posterior cranial fossa

anterior spinal artery

margin of foramen magnum

nasal septum

catheter in femoral artery

x-rays

cassette

programmed automatic injector of radiopaque solution

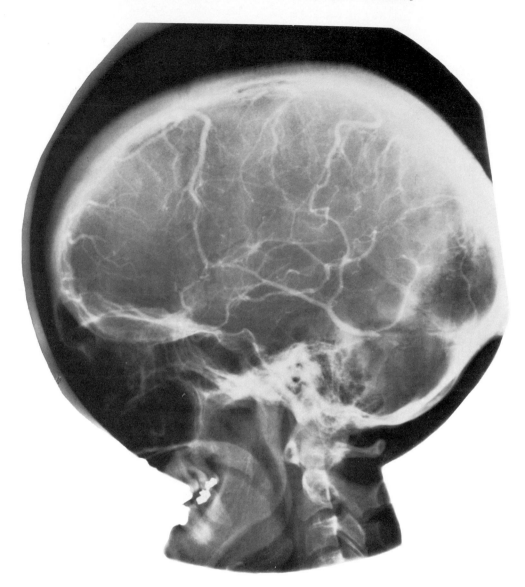

Figure 8

Lateral intracranial venogram
(female aged 32 years).

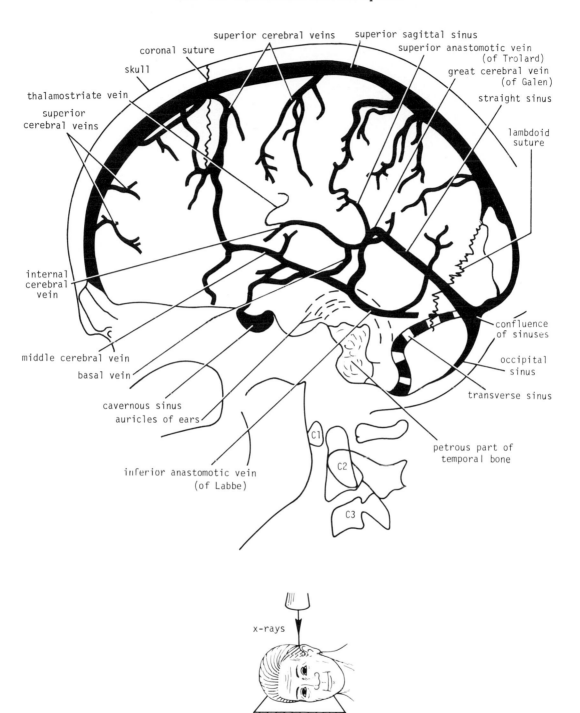

superior cerebral veins   superior sagittal sinus

coronal suture   superior anastomotic vein
(of Trolard)

skull   great cerebral vein
(of Galen)

thalamostriate vein   straight sinus

superior
cerebral veins   lambdoid
suture

internal
cerebral
vein

confluence
of sinuses

middle cerebral vein   occipital
sinus

basal vein

transverse sinus

cavernous sinus
auricles of ears   C1

C2

petrous part of
temporal bone

C3

inferior anastomotic vein
(of Labbe)

x-rays

cassette

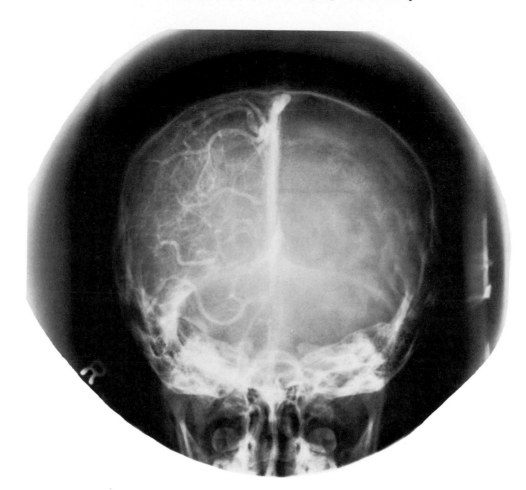

Figure 9

Anteroposterior
intracranial venogram
(male aged 32 years).

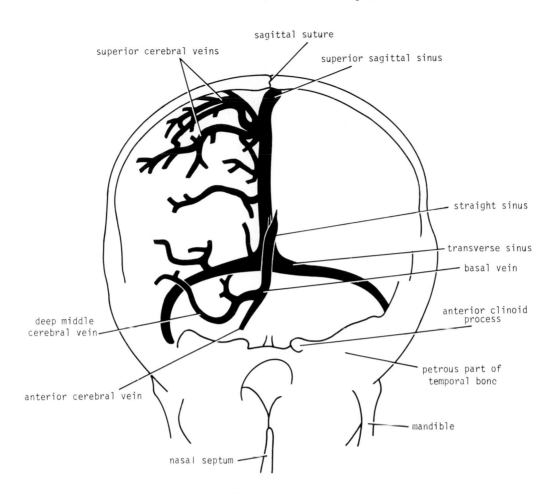

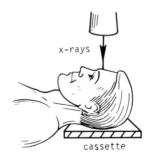

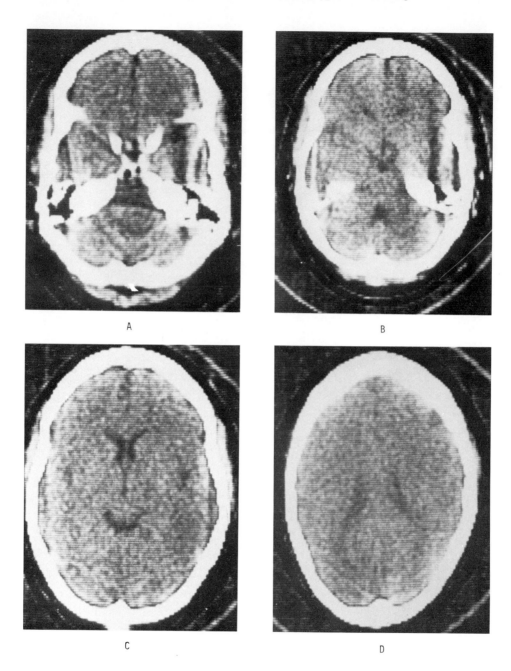

A

B

C

D

Figure 10

Computerized axial tomography of the
brain. A, B, C, and D represent
serial cuts taken progressively
through the skull from the
base toward the vertex
(male aged 52 years).

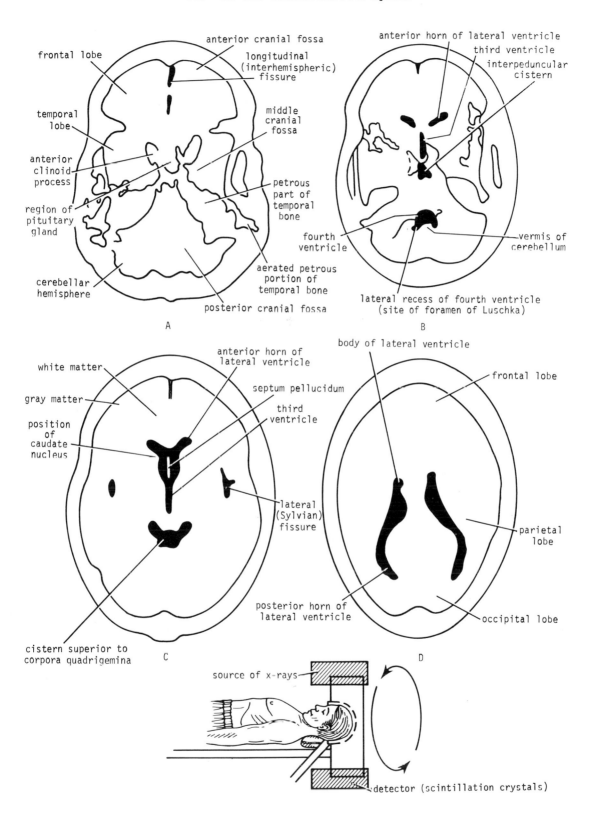

A

frontal lobe

anterior cranial fossa

longitudinal (interhemispheric) fissure

temporal lobe

middle cranial fossa

anterior clinoid process

region of pituitary gland

petrous part of temporal bone

cerebellar hemisphere

aerated petrous portion of temporal bone

posterior cranial fossa

B

anterior horn of lateral ventricle

third ventricle

interpeduncular cistern

fourth ventricle

vermis of cerebellum

lateral recess of fourth ventricle (site of foramen of Luschka)

C

white matter

anterior horn of lateral ventricle

septum pellucidum

gray matter

third ventricle

position of caudate nucleus

lateral (Sylvian) fissure

cistern superior to corpora quadrigemina

D

body of lateral ventricle

frontal lobe

parietal lobe

posterior horn of lateral ventricle

occipital lobe

source of x-rays

detector (scintillation crystals)

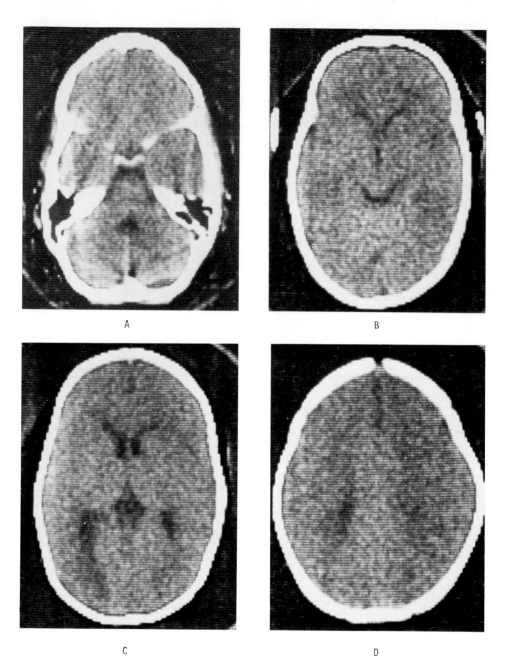

A   B

C   D

Figure 11

Computerized axial tomography of the
brain. A, B, C, and D represent serial
cuts taken progressively through
the skull from the base toward the
vertex (A. male aged 18 years;
B, C, D. male aged 1 year).

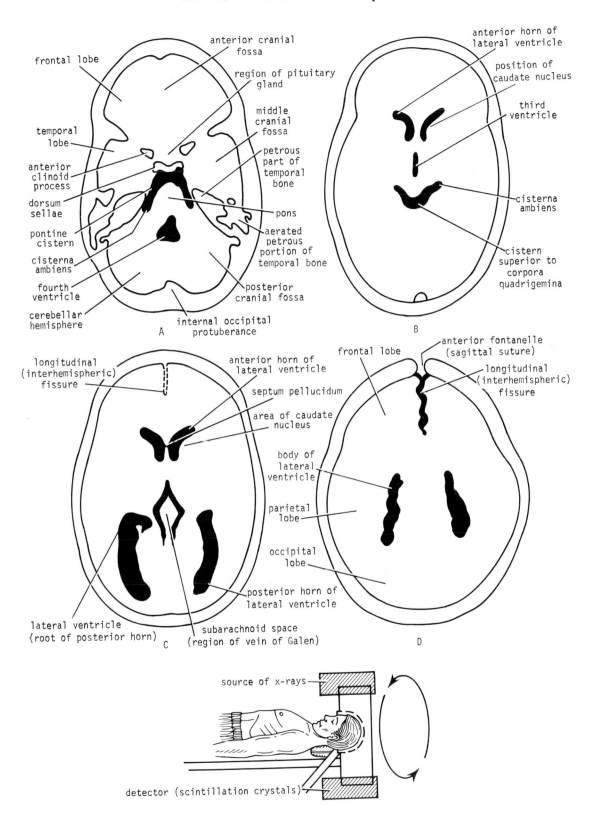

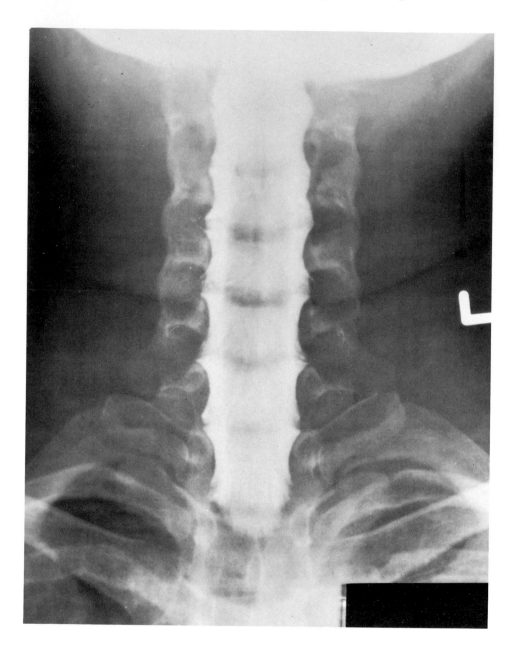

Figure 12

Posteroanterior
myelogram of the cervical region
(female aged 22 years).

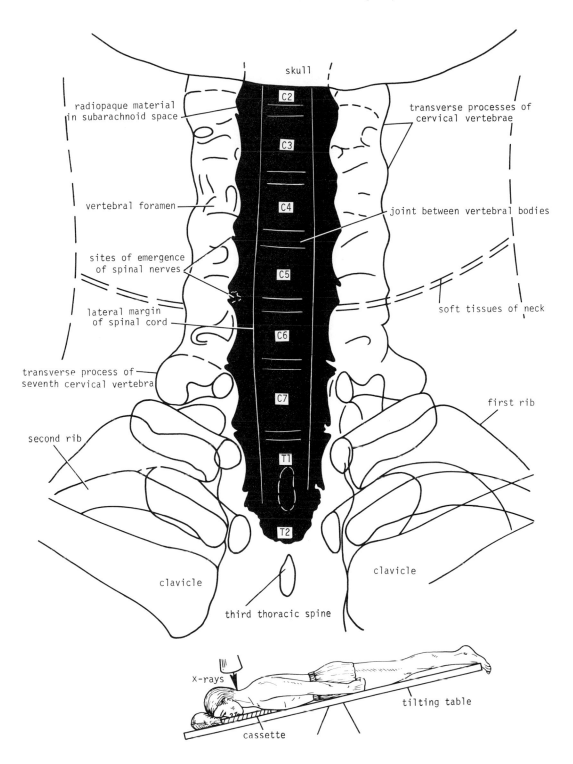

skull

C2

C3

C4

C5

C6

C7

T1

T2

radiopaque material in subarachnoid space

transverse processes of cervical vertebrae

vertebral foramen

joint between vertebral bodies

sites of emergence of spinal nerves

soft tissues of neck

lateral margin of spinal cord

transverse process of seventh cervical vertebra

first rib

second rib

clavicle

clavicle

third thoracic spine

x-rays

tilting table

cassette

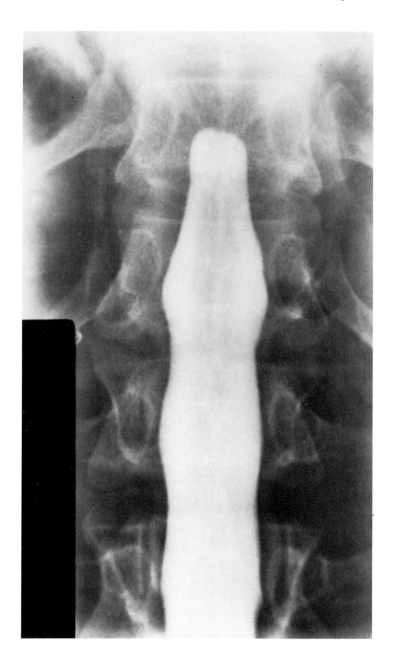

Figure 13

Posteroanterior myelogram
of the lower thoracic and lumbar regions
(male aged 47 years).

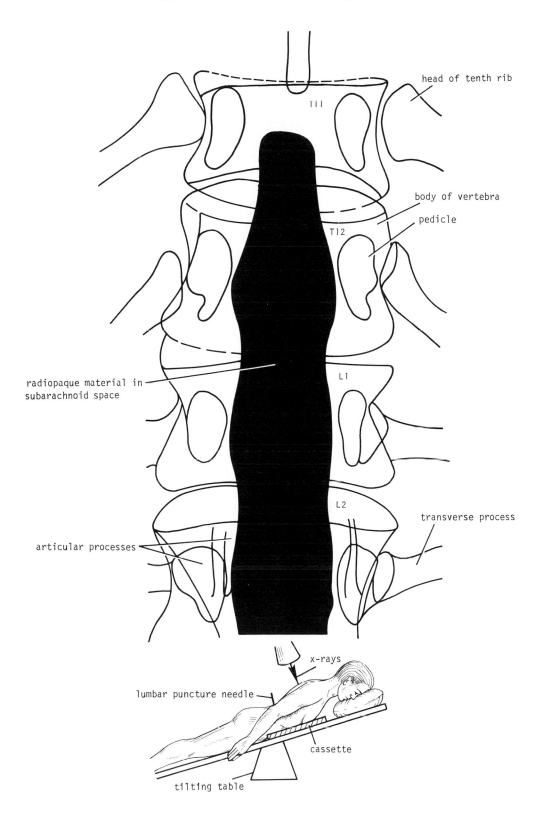

head of tenth rib

body of vertebra

pedicle

TII

TI2

radiopaque material in subarachnoid space

LI

L2

transverse process

articular processes

x-rays

lumbar puncture needle

cassette

tilting table

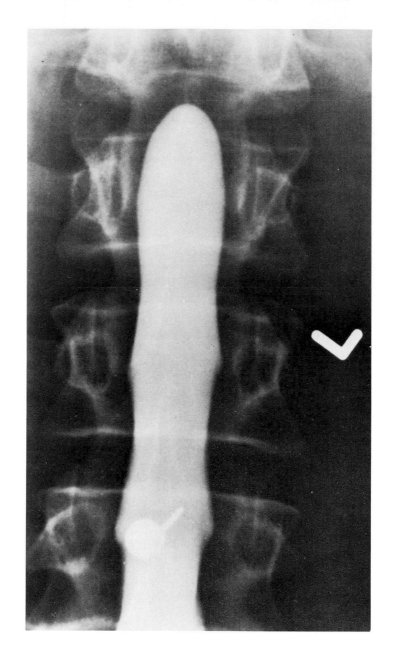

Figure 14

Posteroanterior
myelogram of the lumbar region
(male aged 47 years).

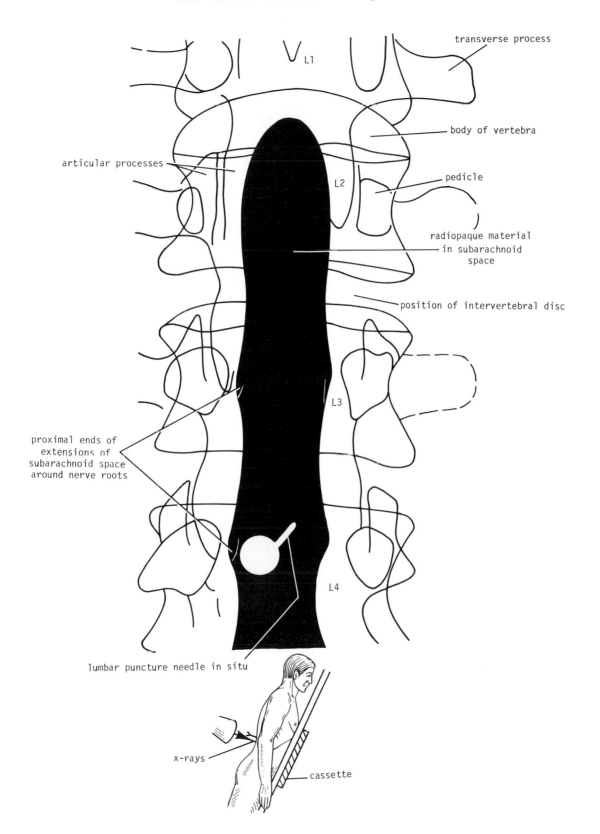

transverse process

body of vertebra

pedicle

radiopaque material
in subarachnoid
space

position of intervertebral disc

articular processes

V_{L1}

L2

L3

L4

proximal ends of
extensions of
subarachnoid space
around nerve roots

lumbar puncture needle in situ

x-rays

cassette

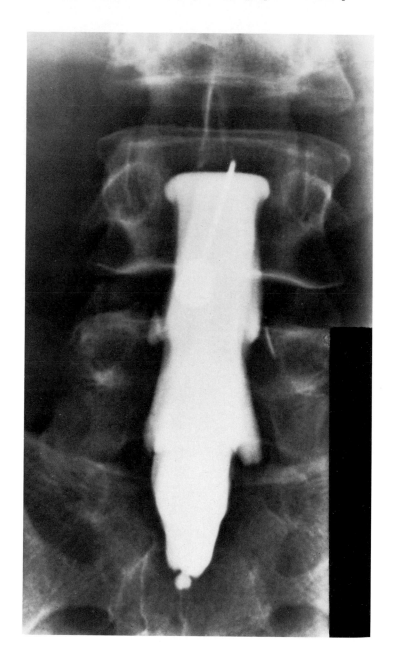

Figure 15

Posteroanterior myelogram
of the lower lumbar and sacral regions
(male aged 47 years).

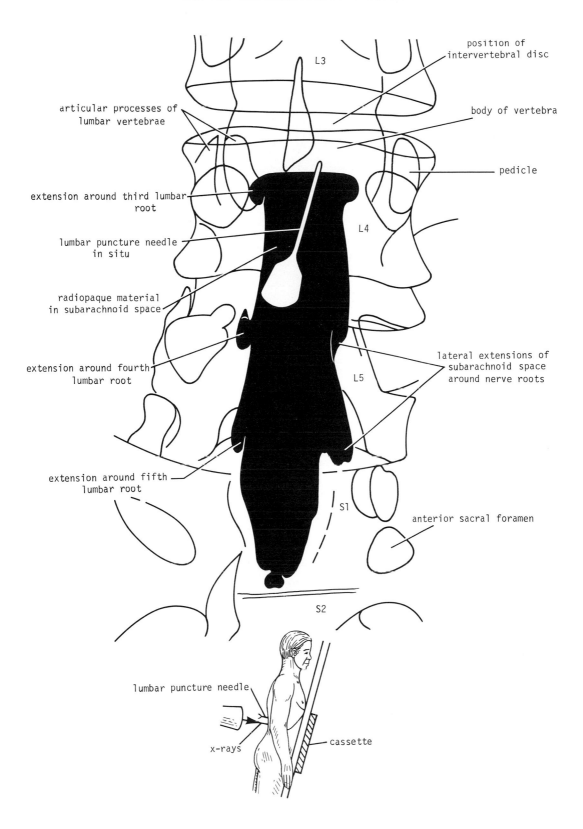

position of
intervertebral disc

body of vertebra

articular processes of
lumbar vertebrae

pedicle

L3

extension around third lumbar
root

L4

lumbar puncture needle
in situ

radiopaque material
in subarachnoid space

lateral extensions of
subarachnoid space
around nerve roots

extension around fourth
lumbar root

L5

extension around fifth
lumbar root

S1

anterior sacral foramen

S2

lumbar puncture needle

x-rays

cassette

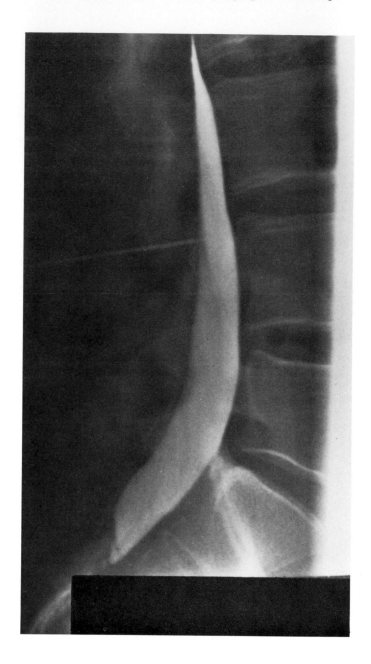

Figure 16

Lateral myelogram of the lower
lumbar and sacral regions
(male aged 47 years).

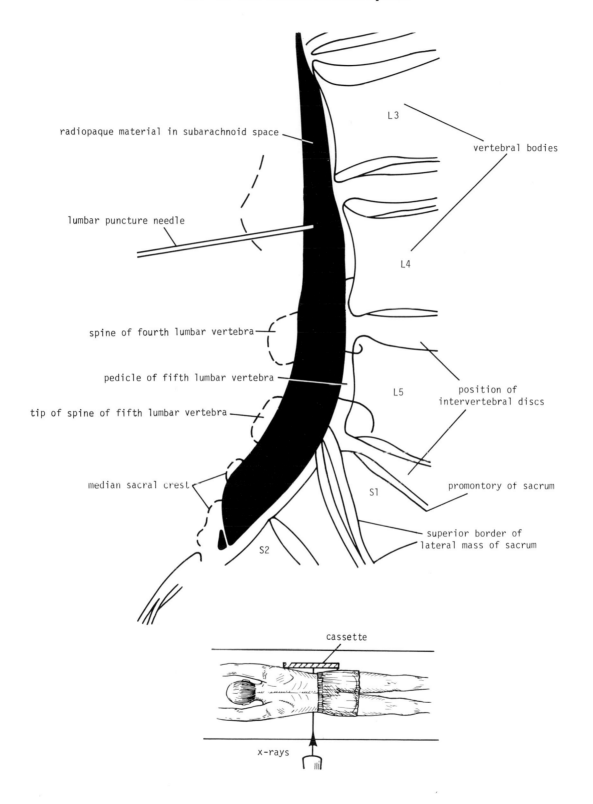

radiopaque material in subarachnoid space

L3

vertebral bodies

lumbar puncture needle

L4

spine of fourth lumbar vertebra

pedicle of fifth lumbar vertebra

position of intervertebral discs

tip of spine of fifth lumbar vertebra

L5

median sacral crest

S1

promontory of sacrum

superior border of lateral mass of sacrum

S2

cassette

x-rays

12

MAMMOGRAPHY

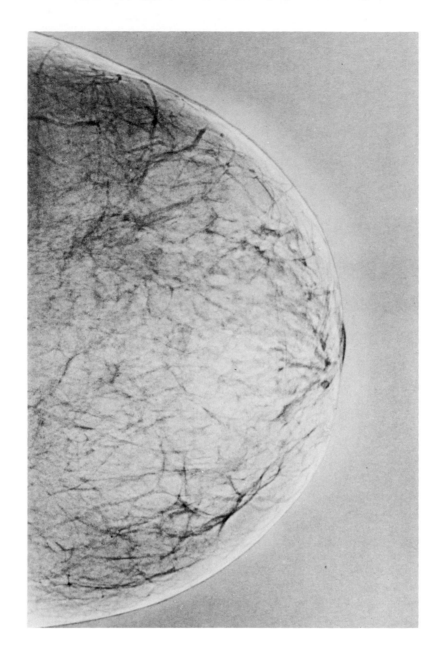

Figure 1

Craniocaudal
xeroradiographic mammogram
(female aged 35 years).

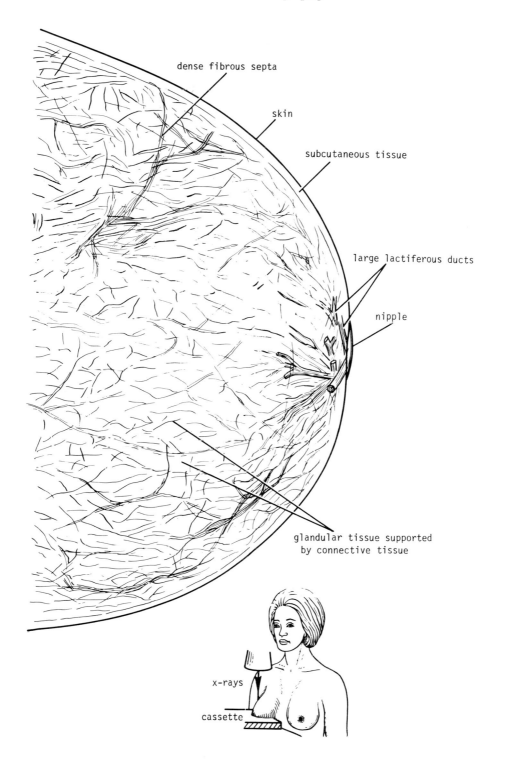

dense fibrous septa

skin

subcutaneous tissue

large lactiferous ducts

nipple

glandular tissue supported
by connective tissue

x-rays

cassette

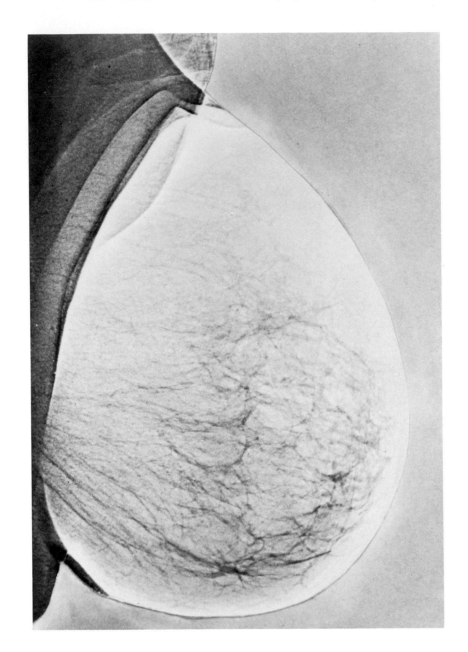

Figure 2

Mediolateral
xeroradiographic mammogram
(female aged 35 years).

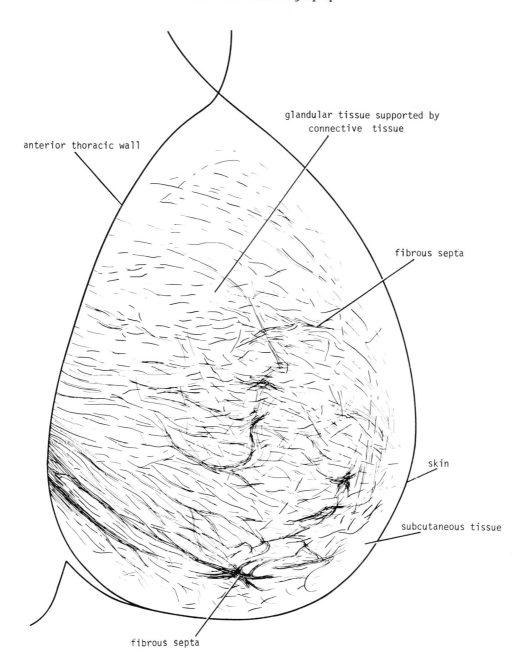

anterior thoracic wall

glandular tissue supported by
connective tissue

fibrous septa

skin

subcutaneous tissue

fibrous septa

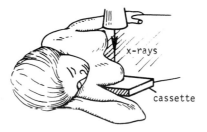

x-rays

cassette

INDEX

INDEX

Abdomen, 122–166. *See also*
    specific structures,
    e.g., Colon
lymphangiogram of, 372
Abdominal cavity. *See also*
    Kidney(s); Liver; Spleen;
    Bladder, urinary
suprarenal glands, 124, 156,
    160, 162
transverse section of, 122
Abdominal wall
anterior, 156, 160, 296
muscles of, 124, 160, 176
Abductor digiti minimi, 266
Acetabulum, 170, 186, 194, 196,
    198, 204, 208, 320, 344
inferior portion, 174, 176,
    200, 206
margins of, 196, 200, 202,
    206, 318
superior portion of, 174, 176,
    200, 206, 310
Ampulla, of vas deferens, 188
Anal canal, 140
Anastomoses, of arteries, middle
    colic and superior
    left, 340
Angle(s)
costophrenic, 88, 100
    posterior, 102
of Louis. *See* sternal *below*
of mandible, 2, 20, 22, 30, 272
of ribs, 102, 296
of scapula, 42, 44, 46, 90,
    96, 326, 366
sternal, 94, 96, 102, 112
Ankle joint, 242, 244, 246, 248,
    250, 252, 254
Antrum, pyloric, of stomach,
    126, 128, 132, 134
Aorta
abdominal, 342
    arteriogram of, 342
    catheter in, 332, 334, 336
arch of, 88, 90, 92, 98, 100,
    116, 126, 330, 354
    angiogram of, 324
    large branches of, 92, 102
ascending, 92, 104, 324, 330
catheter in, 338, 340
descending, 88, 90, 98, 104,
    108, 288, 290, 324, 328
Apex
of left ventricle, 98
of petrous part of temporal
    bone, 26

Appendix
retrocecal, 142
vermiform, 138
Arcades, jejunal, communicating,
    336
Arch
alveolar
    superior, 38
of aorta, 88, 90, 98, 100, 126,
    328, 330, 354
    angiogram of, 324
    branches of, 92, 102, 116
    catheter in, 326
    indentation of, 98
of atlas
    anterior, 4, 8, 12, 26, 38,
        270, 274, 276, 278,
        284, 286, 390
    posterior, 4, 8, 270, 274,
        276, 278, 284, 390
dorsal venous
    of foot, radiopaque material
        in, 356, 360, 362
    of hand, catheter in, 354
zygomatic, 4, 12, 22, 26
Arm(s)
fetal, 316
forearm, 64, 66, 68, 70, 72
medial side of, valved lym-
    phatic vessels from, 366
muscles of. *See under*
    Muscle(s)
upper
    lymphangiogram, 366
    muscles of. *See under*
        Muscle(s)
    skin of, 48, 52, 54, 64, 66, 80
Armpit. *See* Axilla
Arteriography, 324–350, 386–392
Artery(ies). *See also* Trunk,
    arterial
angular, 386
arcuate, 338
auricular, posterior, 386
axillary, 326
    angiogram of, 326
basilar, 390, 392
brachial, 326
    angiogram of, 326
    catheter in, 328, 330
brachiocephalic, 324, 326
of brain, 386, 388, 390, 392
carotid
    common, 386, 388
        bifurcation of, 386
        left, 324, 330
        right, 324
    external, 386, 388
        bifurcation of, 388
    internal
        arteriogram of, 388
        in carotid canal, in petrous
            part of temporal bone,
            388

Artery(ies), carotid, internal
    — *Continued*
    in cavernous sinus, 386
    in neck, 386, 388
    superior to cavernous
        sinus, 388
    lateral internal, arteriogram
        of, 386
celiac, arteriogram of, 332
cerebellar
    anterior, inferior, 392
    posterior, inferior, 390, 392
    superior, 390, 392
cerebral
    anterior, 386, 388, 390
    middle, 386
        bifurcation of, 388
        operculofrontal branch,
            386
        posterior, 386, 388, 390, 392
        internal occipital artery
            branch, 392
cervical, superficial (trans-
    verse), 324, 326
choroidal, anterior, 388
colic
    left
        inferior (lower), 340, 342
        superior, 340
    middle, 336, 340
    right, 336
communicating, posterior, 390
cortical (parietal), branches of,
    386
cystic, 332
epigastric, inferior, 342
facial, 386
femoral, 342, 344, 346,
    348, 360
    arteriograms of, 342, 344,
        346, 348
    branches of, 346
        ascending, 346
        descending, 346
        muscular, 348
        transverse, 346
    catheter in, 324, 326, 332,
        334, 336, 338, 340,
        342, 344, 346, 348,
        350, 392
    lateral circumflex, 342,
        344, 346
    medial circumflex, 342, 346
frontopolar, 386

Artery(ies) — *Continued*
  gastric
    left, 332, 334
      esophageal branch of, 332
    right, 332
    short, 332
  gastroduodenal, 332
  gastroepiploic, 332
  genicular
    descending, 348
      saphenous branch of, 350
    lateral, 348
    medial inferior, 348
    medial superior, 348
  gluteal
    inferior, 342
    superior, 342, 344
  hepatic, 332
  humeral, posterior circumflex, 326
  ileal, 336
  ileocolic, 336
  iliac
    arteriograms of, 342, 344
    common, 342, 344
      right, 336, 340
    deep circumflex, 342
    external, 342, 344
    internal, 342, 344
    superficial circumflex, 344
  iliolumbar, 342, 344
  intercostal, superior, 324
  interlobar, 338
  jejunal, 336
  lenticulostriate, 388
  lingual, 386
  lobar, 338
  lumbar, 342
  marginal, of Drummond, 340
  maxillary, 386, 388
    in pterygopalatine fossa, 388
  meningeal, middle, 388
  mesenteric
    inferior, 340, 342
      catheter in, 340
    superior, catheter in, 336
  of neck, 324, 386
  obturator, 342, 344, 346
  occipital, 386
    internal, 390
  ophthalmic, 386
  palatine, ascending, 386
  pancreatic, 332
    dorsal, 336

Artery(ies) — *Continued*
  pancreaticoduodenal
    inferior, 336
    superior, 332
  parietal, posterior, 386, 388
  perforating
    first, 346
    fourth, 346, 348
    second, 346
    third, 346
  pericallosal, 386, 388
    cortical (frontal) branches, 386
  peroneal, muscular branches of, 350
  phrenic, inferior, 338
  pontine, 392
  popliteal, 348, 360
    arteriogram of, 348
    muscular, branches of, 348
  profunda brachii, 326
  profunda femoris, 342, 344, 346, 348
  pudendal, internal, 342, 344
  pulmonary, 98
    angiogram of, 328
    branches of, 328
    in hilum of lung, 102
    left, 328
    right, 328
      descending, 328
  rectal
    branches of, 340
    middle, 342, 344
    superior, 340, 342
  renal
    main branches of, 338
    right
      arteriogram of, 338
      origin of, 338
      posterior to inferior vena cava, 338
  sacral
    lateral, 342, 344
    median, 342
  scapular
    circumflex, 326
    dorsal, 326
  spinal, anterior, 392
  splenic, 332, 334
    catheter in, 334
    inferior branch of, 334
    superior branch of, 334
  splenic polar, superior, 334
  subclavian, 326
    angiogram of, 326
    left, 104, 324, 330
    right, 324
  subscapular, 326
  suprarenal, inferior, 338
  suprascapular, 324, 326
  temporal
    posterior, 386, 388, 390, 392
    superficial, 386, 388

Artery(ies) — *Continued*
  thoracic
    internal, 326
      left, 324
      right, 324
    lateral, 326
    superior, 326
  thoracoacromial, 326
  thyroid
    inferior, 324, 326
    superior, 386
  tibial, 350
  vertebral, 326
    anteroposterior arteriogram of, 392
    and foramen magnum of skull, 390, 392
    and foramen transversaria of C1–C6, 390
    lateral arteriogram of, 390
    left, 324
    meningeal branches of, 390
    muscular branches of, 390
    in posterior cranial fossa, 392
    right, 324
    spinal branches of, 390
  vesical, 344
    superior, 342
Atlanto-occipital joint, 2, 278, 286
Atlas (first cervical vertebra), 4, 8. *See also* Vertebral column, C1 vertebra
  arch of
    anterior, 4, 8, 12, 26, 38, 270, 274, 276, 278, 284, 286, 390
    posterior, 4, 8, 270, 274, 276, 278, 284, 390
  foramen transversarium(a) of, 28, 390
  inferior articular facet of, 270, 278
  lateral mass of, 10, 14, 270, 278
  transverse process of, 22, 26, 270, 278, 392
Atrium, cardiac
  left, 88, 90, 92, 98, 100, 104, 330
    venogram of, 330
  right, 88, 90, 98, 100, 108, 110, 288, 328, 330
Auricle(s)
  of ears, 4, 8, 394
  left. *See* Atrium, cardiac, left
Auricular appendage. *See* Atrium, cardiac, left

Axilla
  lymph nodes of, 366
  lymphangiogram of, 366
  soft tissues in, 48
Axis (second cervical vertebra).
      See also Vertebral
      column, C2 vertebra
  body of, 270, 278
  lamina of, 270
  odontoid process of, 2, 4, 8,
      14, 22, 26, 28, 270, 274,
      276, 278, 284, 286
  pedicle of, 278
  spines of, 8, 286
  spinous processes of, 270,
      278, 284
  superior articular facet of,
      270, 278
  transverse process of, 270

Barium
  in esophagus, 98, 114, 126
  in stomach, 98, 114, 128, 134
Barium enema
  and colon, 136, 138, 140, 142,
      146, 148
  and rectum, 140
Barium meal
  and duodenum, 128, 130,
      132, 134
  and ileum, 130
  and jejunum, 128, 130, 132,
      134
  and stomach, 128, 130, 132,
      134
Bile duct, common, 152, 154
Bladder, urinary, 122, 124, 158,
      164, 166, 178, 180,
      182, 184, 186, 190
  in female, 158, 164, 178,
      182, 190
  in male, 122, 166, 180, 184,
      186, 194, 344
  neck of, 182
  radiopaque material in, 164,
      166, 178, 180, 182,
      184, 356
  surfaces of, superior, 182
  ureteral catheters in, 166
Blood vessels. See also
      Artery(ies); Vein(s)
  pulmonary, 88, 92, 100, 102,
      108, 156, 330, 352
  cross section of, 100
  thoracic, 88–112

Body(ies)
  of axis, 270, 278
  of cervical vertebrae, 402
  fourth, 284
  seventh, 280
  of hyoid bone, 274, 286
  of lateral ventricle, 398, 400
  of lumbar vertebrae
    fifth, 178, 320
    fourth, 178, 408, 410
    second, 406
    third, 294, 296, 298, 312,
      410
  of mandible, 6, 14, 20, 22, 26,
      28, 30, 34, 36, 38,
      114, 274, 282
    with teeth, 14, 18, 22, 114,
      278
  of penis, 180, 186
  of pubis, 170, 172, 174, 180,
      182, 184, 188, 194,
      196, 198, 200, 208,
      316, 318, 320, 344, 368
  of sphenoid bone, 10
  of sternum, 92, 96, 102
  of stomach, 126, 128, 130,
      132, 134
  of talus, 244, 246, 248, 250,
      252, 258, 260
  of thoracic vertebrae, 290
    T9 vertebra, 288, 292
    T12 vertebra, 404
  of uterus, cavity of, 190
  of ventricle, of brain, 380, 384
Bone(s). See also Joint(s)
  acetabulum. See Acetabulum
  calcaneum. See Calcaneum
  cancellous, trabeculae of, 194
  capitate, 64, 68, 72, 74, 78,
      80, 82, 84
  of carpus, 64, 68, 70, 72, 74,
      76, 78, 80, 82, 84
  clavicles. See Clavicle(s)
  coccyx, 140, 172, 176, 294,
      306, 308, 312, 320,
      370, 374, 376
  compact, 194, 204, 206
  cuboid. See Cuboid bone
  cuneiform. See Cuneiform
      bones
  ethmoid, lateral wall of, 14
  fabella, 214
  femur. See Femur
  fetal limb, 318
  fibula. See Fibula
  of foot, 234, 236, 238, 240,
      242, 244, 246, 248,
      250, 252, 254, 256,
      258, 260, 262, 264,
      266. See also names
      of specific bones, e.g.,
      Metatarsal; Phalanges
  frontal. See Frontal bones

Bone(s) — Continued
  hamate. See Hamate
  of hand, 64, 68, 70, 72, 74, 76,
      78, 80, 82, 84. See also
      names of specific
      bones, e.g., Hamate;
      Metacarpals (metacarpus)
  humerus. See Humerus
  hyoid, 38, 274, 276, 284, 286
  of leg, 232, 234, 236, 238
      240. See also names
      of specific bones, e.g.,
      Femur; Tibia
  lunate, 64, 66, 68, 72, 74, 76,
      78, 80, 82, 84
  malleolus. See Malleolus
  mastoid, 6
  metacarpals. See Metacarpals
      (metacarpus)
  nasal, 16, 18, 22, 28
    of fetus, region of, 172
  navicular. See Navicular
      bone, of foot
  occipital, 6, 10, 12, 26, 270,
      276
    basilar part of, 10, 12
  parietal, 6, 12
  patella, 212, 214, 216, 218,
      224, 226, 228, 230,
      234, 240, 348, 358
  phalanges. See Phalanges
  pisiform, 64, 68, 72, 74,
      78, 80
  pubis. See Pubis
  radius. See Radius
  ribs. See Rib(s)
  sacrum. See Sacrum
  scaphoid. See Navicular
      bone, of hand
  scapula. See Scapula
  sesamoid. See Sesamoid bone(s)
  of skull. See Skull
  sphenoid. See Sphenoid bone
  talus. See Talus
  tarsal, 242, 246, 248, 252,
      254, 256, 258, 260,
      262, 264, 266
  temporal. See Temporal bone(s)
  tibia. See Tibia
  trapezium, 64, 68, 72, 76, 78,
      80, 82, 84
  trapezoid, 64, 68, 72, 74, 76,
      78, 80, 84
  triquetral (triquetrum), 64,
      68, 72, 74, 76, 78, 80,
      82, 84
  ulna. See Ulna

Bone(s) — *Continued*
upper limb(s). *See specific bones, e.g.,* Radius; Ulna
vertebral. *See* Vertebra(e); Vertebral column
zygomatic, 14, 16, 22, 24, 26, 28, 34
Border(s). *See also* Margin(s)
of scapula, 42, 44, 46, 48, 96, 106, 292
of spleen, 332, 334
of thymus
left lobe of, 110
right lobe of, 110
Bowel(s). *See* Intestine(s)
Brain
arteries of, 386, 388, 390, 392
cerebrum, falx cerebri of, 382
parts of, 380, 382, 384, 398, 400
veins of, 394, 396
ventricles of. *See under* Ventricle(s)
Breast(s). *See* Mammary glands
Brim, pelvic, 190, 316
Bronchopulmonary segments, 116, 118
Bronchus
left main, 92, 102, 106, 116, 118, 328
right main, 92, 98, 102, 106, 116, 118
Bursa(e)
popliteus, 220
suprapatellar, 214, 224
Buttocks, 184, 204, 208, 320, 356, 372
skin of, 180, 204

Calcaneum, 234, 238, 240, 244, 246, 248, 250, 252, 254, 256, 258, 260, 262, 264, 266
epiphysis of, 264
Calyces, renal, 158, 160, 162, 164, 166, 332, 334, 338
Calyx. *See* Calyces, renal
Canal(s)
alveolar, inferior, 20, 34, 36, 38
anal, 140
auditory, internal, 12
carotid, 28
site of, 10, 12, 26
cervical, radiopaque material in, 190
condylar, 28

Canal(s) — *Continued*
hypoglossal, 28
inguinal, vas deferens in, 188
mandibular, 2
pyloric, 132
root, of tooth, 36
sacral, 172, 178, 302, 308
semicircular, region of, 12
Canine(s), 20, 34, 36
Capitate, 64, 68, 72, 74, 78, 80, 82, 84
Capitulum (of humerus), 50, 52, 54, 56, 60, 62, 66
Capsule
of hip joint, 318
of knee joint, 220
Cardioesophageal opening, 126
Cardiophrenic recess, 108
Carina. *See* Trachea, bifurcation of
Carotid arteries. *See under* Artery(ies)
Carpus, bones of, 64, 68, 70, 72, 74, 76, 78, 80, 82, 84
Cartilage
articular, 220
arytenoid, region of, 38
costal
calcification of, 136
site of, 112
cricoid, 38
epiphyseal, 48, 174, 176, 182, 184, 200, 202
of femur, inferior, 226, 228, 230
of fibula, superior, 226, 228
of tibia, superior, 226, 228, 230
ossifying plates of, in vertebral column, 302
between pubis and ischial rami, 182
semilunar, 220
thyroid, 38
calcified, 274, 276
triradiate, 174, 176, 184, 200, 202, 310, 312
Catheter(s)
in abdominal aorta, 332, 334, 336
in aorta, 338, 340
arterial, 344, 346
in aortic arch, 326
in brachial artery, 328, 330
in brachiocephalic artery, 326
in celiac trunk, 332, 334
in femoral artery, 324, 326, 332, 334, 336, 338, 340, 342, 346, 348, 350, 392
in inferior mesenteric artery, 340
in pulmonary trunk, 330

Catheter(s), arterial — *Continued*
in right common iliac artery, 340
in right renal artery, 338
in splenic artery, 334
in superior mesenteric artery, 336
cardiac, 328, 330
passing through right atrium and right ventricle, 330
passing through right ventricle, into pulmonary trunk, 328
venous
in dorsal venous arch (of hand), 354
in femoral vein, 352
Caudate nucleus, position of, 398, 400
Cavity(ies)
of elbow joint, 50
glenoid (of scapula), 42, 44, 46, 48
of hip joint, 186, 196, 208, 210, 318
of knee joint, 218, 220
marrow, 204, 206
mouth, 38
nasal, 34, 274
orbital, 8, 18, 20
tympanic, 10
uterine, 190
Cecum, 136, 138, 142, 144, 146, 148
Celiac artery, arteriogram of, 332
Cells, mastoid air, 2, 4, 10, 12, 14, 22, 26, 28, 30
Cerebellum
arteries of, 390, 392
vermis of, 398
Cerebrum
arteries of, 386, 388, 390, 392
veins of, 394, 396, 400
Cervix uteri, canal of, radiopaque material in, 190
Chin, 112
skin fold of, 2, 110
Cholangiogram, 154
Cholecystograms, 150, 152
Cisterna
ambiens, 384, 400
chiasmatic, 384
corpus callosum, 384
interpeduncular, 384, 398
magna, 384
pontine, 384, 400
superior to corpora quadrigemina, 398, 400

Clavicle(s), 42, 44, 46, 48, 112, 114, 116, 118, 126, 286, 288, 290, 354, 366, 402
  fetal, 316
  left, 88, 94, 100, 104, 106, 108, 110, 272, 286, 288
  right, 90, 94, 96, 98, 100, 104, 106, 280, 282, 286, 324, 330
Cleft, natal, 372
Clivus, 4
Coccyx, 140, 172, 176, 294, 306, 308, 312, 320, 370, 374, 376
Cochlea, region of, 12
Colon
  after air double-contrast enema, 144
  ascending, 136, 142, 144, 146, 148
  after barium enema, 136, 138, 140, 142, 146, 148
  descending, 136, 138, 140, 142, 146, 148
  gas in, 128, 134, 152, 158
    ascending colon, 134, 300
    descending colon, 164
    transverse colon, 166
  pelvic (sigmoid), 136, 138, 140, 142, 144, 146, 148
  transverse, 136, 138, 142, 144, 146
Concha(e), 4
  inferior, 2, 6, 14, 20, 24, 38
  middle, 2, 38
  nasal, 16, 22
  superior, 24
Condyle(s)
  of femur. *See under* Femur
  of mandible, 278, 284, 392
  occipital, 2, 26, 28, 278, 286
  of tibia, 212, 214, 216, 218, 220, 226, 228, 230, 232, 234, 348, 362
Contraceptive device, intrauterine (I.U.D.), 182
Cornu, sacral, 308
Cortex
  of femur, 196, 204, 208, 210
  renal, 338
Costophrenic angle, 88, 100
  posterior, 102

Costophrenic recess. *See* Recess, costophrenic
Crest(s)
  frontal, 22, 24
  iliac, 122, 124, 130, 134, 136, 142, 144, 146, 148, 156, 158, 166, 170, 172, 174, 176, 184, 196, 198, 200, 202, 204, 296, 298, 300, 304, 306, 308, 310, 312, 316, 318, 320, 336, 342, 352, 374, 376
    tubercle of, 318
  intertrochanteric, 194, 196, 198, 204, 206, 208
  occipital, 10
    internal, 12, 26
  sacral, median, 172, 410
Crista galli, 4, 14, 24, 382
  position of, 6
Crown, of tooth, 34, 36
Crus, of diaphragm, left, 334
Cuboid bone, 238, 246, 248, 250, 252, 254, 256, 258, 260, 262, 264, 266
Cuneiform bones, 242, 246, 260, 262
  intermediate, 262, 264
  lateral, 248, 262
  medial, 248, 258, 262, 264
Cupola(e), of diaphragm, 88, 90, 92, 102, 106, 108, 110, 126, 154, 288, 292, 352
Cystogram(s), 184
Cystourethrograms, 180, 182, 186

Dental films, 34, 36
Detector in computerized tomography, 398, 400
Diaphragm, 98, 104, 116, 118, 130, 132, 296, 302, 304, 328, 330
  crura of, left, 334
  cupolae of
    left, 92, 102, 106, 108, 110, 126, 288, 292, 352
    right, 88, 90, 92, 102, 106, 108, 126, 154, 288, 352
Disc(s), intervertebral, position of, 174, 178, 284, 288, 290, 292, 296, 298, 300, 302, 304, 308, 312, 406, 408, 410
Dorsum linguae, barium coating on, 38. *See also* Tongue
Dorsum sellae, 4, 12, 38, 400
Duct(s)
  bile, common, 152, 154
    entering duodenum, second part, 154
  cystic, 152
  ejaculatory, 188
  hepatic, 154
  lactiferous, 414

Ductus deferens, 188
Duodenum
  first part of, 126, 128, 130, 132, 134
  second part of, 126, 128, 130, 132, 134
    common bile duct entering, 154
  third part of, 128, 130, 132, 134

Ear(s), 2, 6, 8, 12, 18, 30, 32
  auditory meatus, 6, 8, 10, 18, 30, 32, 38, 284
  auricles of, 4, 8, 394
  mastoid air cells, 2, 4, 10, 12, 14, 22, 26, 28, 30
Elbow joint and region, 50, 52, 54, 56, 58, 60, 62, 64
  cavity of, 50
  and pad of fat, 52, 60
Eminence(s)
  intercondylar, 212, 214, 216, 220, 224, 226, 228
  thenar, 78
    muscle mass of, 80
Enema
  air double-contrast, 144
  barium, 136, 138, 140, 142, 146, 148
Epicondyle(s)
  of femur, 212
  of humerus
    lateral, 50, 54, 56, 58, 62, 64
    medial, 50, 52, 54, 56, 58, 60, 62, 64, 66
  of tibia, 218
Epiglottis, 38, 274, 284
Epiphyseal line(s). *See* Line(s), epiphyseal
Epiphysis(es)
  of calcaneum, 264
  of femur
    head of, 146, 186, 208, 210
    inferior, 222, 224, 226, 230, 236, 238, 240
    superior, 176, 186, 200, 202, 236
  of fibula, 254, 264, 266
    inferior, 238, 240
    superior, 224, 226, 228
  of humerus
    proximal, 108
    superior, 106
  of metacarpal bones, 82, 84
    of fifth metacarpal, 68
    of first metacarpal, 68, 82, 84

Epiphysis(es) — *Continued*
  metatarsal
    of fifth metatarsal, 264
    of first metatarsal, 262, 264
  of phalanges
    of foot, 264
      proximal, 262
    of hand, 68, 82, 84
  of radius, 68
    distal, 82, 84
  of tibia, 252, 254, 264, 266
    inferior, 236, 238, 240
    superior, 222, 224, 226,
      228, 236, 238, 240
  of trochanter, greater, 174,
    184, 200
  of ulna, 68, 70
    distal, 82, 84
Esophagus
  abdominal part of, 134
  barium in, 98, 114, 126
  position of, 102, 104, 106,
    112, 274, 292
Ethmoid bone, lateral wall of, 14

Fabella, 214
Falx cerebri, 382
Fat
  extraperitoneal, 122, 124, 164
  pad of
    associated with elbow joint,
      52, 60
    in heel, 248, 258
    in thoracic wall, 100
Femur, 124, 138, 170, 172, 184,
    196, 202, 204, 206, 208,
    210, 214, 216, 218, 220,
    222, 224, 226, 228, 230,
    232, 234, 236, 238, 240,
    370, 374
  cartilage of, inferior epiphyseal,
    226, 228
    site of former, 230
  condyles of
    cartilaginous, 236
    lateral, 212, 214, 220, 224,
      226, 230, 232, 348
    medial, 214, 216, 220, 224,
      226, 228, 230, 232,
      348, 360, 362
  cortex of, 196, 204, 208, 210
  epicondyle of, 212
  epiphysis of
    inferior, 222, 224, 226,
      230, 236, 238, 240
    superior, 176, 186, 200,
      202, 236

Femur — *Continued*
  fovea capitis, 194, 208, 318
  head of, 122, 124, 144, 146,
    170, 172, 174, 180, 182,
    184, 186, 194, 196, 198,
    204, 206, 208, 210, 306,
    310, 312, 318, 320,
    356, 370
    left, 172, 320
  medial supracondylar ridge,
    216
  medulla of, 196, 208, 210
  metaphysis of
    inferior, 228, 230
  neck of, 170, 176, 184, 186,
    194, 196, 198, 200, 202,
    204, 206, 208, 210, 318,
    320, 344, 356
  popliteal surface of, 216
  right, 172, 320
  shaft of, 140, 176, 186, 194,
    196, 198, 200, 202, 204,
    206, 208, 210, 224, 226,
    228, 230, 238, 318, 320,
    346, 348, 356, 358, 360,
    368
  trochanters of. *See* Trochanters
    of femur
Fetus, in third trimester of preg-
    nancy, 172, 316, 318,
    320
Fibula, 212, 214, 222, 246, 248,
    250, 254, 258, 264, 266
  cartilage of, superior,
    epiphyseal, 226, 228
  epiphyseal line of, 252, 254
    inferior, 232
    superior, 232
  epiphysis of, 254, 264, 266
    inferior, 238, 240
    superior, 224, 226, 228
  head of, 212, 214, 216,
    220, 224, 226, 230,
    232, 234, 362
  lateral malleolus of, 262
  metaphysis of, 228
  neck of, 212, 214, 216,
    230, 234
  shaft of, 216, 224, 226, 228,
    232, 234, 236, 238, 240,
    242, 244, 252, 350, 362
  styloid process of, 214, 216
Filling, dental. *See* Metallic
    objects, on radiogram
Fimbriae, of uterine tube, 190
Fissure(s)
  cerebral
    lateral (Sylvian), 398
    longitudinal (interhemis-
      pheric), 398, 400
  orbital, superior, 6, 14, 24
  pterygomaxillary, 18

Flexure, colic
  gas and fecal material in, 160
  left, 130, 136, 142, 144, 146,
    148, 164
    contents of, 160
    gas in, 332
  right, 136, 142, 144, 146, 148
Fold(s)
  axillary
    anterior, 366
    posterior, 48, 366
  mucosal, of stomach, 132
  of nates, 180, 184, 204, 208,
    320, 356
Fontanelles of skull, anterior, 6,
    172, 316, 400
Foot
  bones of. *See* under Bone(s)
    *and names of specific
    bones, e.g.,* Metatar-
    sal; Phalanges
  dorsal venous arch of, injection
    of radiopaque material,
    356
Foramen (foramina)
  interventricular, 384
  intervertebral, 276, 284, 286,
    292, 296, 302, 304, 312
  jugular, 28
    site of, 10
  lacerum, 28
    site of, 10
  of Luschka, site of, 398
  magnum, 8, 10, 12, 22, 28
    margins of, 270, 392
      anterior, 278
      posterior, 24
    and vertebral artery, 390,
      392
  mandibular, 20
  mental, 2
  of Monro, 384
  obturator, 170, 172, 174, 176,
    180, 182, 184, 186, 194,
    196, 198, 200, 204, 300,
    308, 312, 316, 318, 320,
    342, 344, 346, 356, 368,
    374
  ovale, 26, 28
  rotundum, 6
  sacral, anterior, 122, 170, 174,
    182, 190, 196, 200, 202,
    300, 306, 310, 316, 408
  spinosum, 26, 28

Foramen (foramina) — *Continued*
transversarium(a), 22, 26, 278
of atlas (C1), 28, 390
of C1–C6, and vertebral artery, 390
vertebral, 402
Forearm, 64, 66, 68, 70, 72, 78
Fossa(e)
acetabular, 194, 198, 204
coronoid, of humerus, 54
cranial
anterior, 398, 400
middle, 398, 400
anterior margin of, 4
posterior, 284, 398, 400
vertebral artery in, 392
glenoid, 46, 48, 106
of humerus, olecranon combined with coronoid, 54
intercondylar, 224
intercondyloid, 218
mandibular, 20, 32
of temporal bone, 30, 32, 38
navicularis, 186
olecranon, 50, 54, 56, 58
piriform, 284
barium coating on wall, 38
posterior cranial fossa, vertebral artery in, 392
pterygopalatine, maxillary artery in, 388
radial, position of, 56
Fovea capitis, of femur, 194, 204, 318
Frontal bone(s), 12, 14, 18
nasal process of, 18
orbital plates of, 2, 4, 6, 8, 14, 18, 24, 280, 384
zygomatic processes of, 382
Fundus, of gallbladder, 150

Galen, vein of. *See* Vein(s), cerebral, great (of Galen)
Gallbladder, 150, 152
Gland(s)
mammary, 92, 98, 126, 414–416
pituitary, region of, 398, 400
suprarenal, 338
left, region of, 124, 156, 160, 162
right, region of, 124, 156, 160, 162
thymus, 108, 110, 112
thyroid, cartilage of, 38, 274, 276
Glans penis, 186

Gluteal region
arteries of, 342
muscles of, 124
Gray matter, cerebral, 398
Greater multangular. *See* Trapezium
Groove(s)
bicipital
of humerus, 42, 44
for meningeal vessels, 2
anterior division of middle, 18
middle meningeal, 4
for superior sagittal sinus, 10, 12
for transverse sinus, 2, 12, 28
for transverse venous sinus, 8
vascular, frontal, 8

Hamate, 64, 68, 70, 72, 74, 78, 80, 82
hook of, 64, 72, 78, 84
Hamstrings. *See under* Leg(s), muscles of
Hamulus, pterygoid, 28
Hand, 78, 80, 82, 84
bones of, 64, 68, 70, 72, 74, 76, 78, 80, 82, 84
dorsal venous arch of, catheter in, 354
Head(s), 2–38
of femur, 122, 124, 144, 146, 170, 172, 174, 180, 182, 184, 186, 194, 196, 198, 204, 206, 208, 210, 306, 310, 312, 318, 320, 356, 370
epiphysis of, 146, 186, 208
of fetus, 318, 320
of fibula, 212, 214, 216, 220, 224, 226, 230, 232, 234, 362
of humerus, 46, 48, 126, 292, 354, 366
epiphysis of, 108
of mandible, 2, 6, 8, 10, 12, 18, 20, 22, 28, 30, 32, 38, 274
of radius, 50, 52, 54, 56, 58, 60, 62, 64, 66
of rib, 290
seventh, 288
skin of, 286
skull, 2, 4, 6, 8, 10, 12, 26, 28, 110, 280, 282, 380, 382, 384, 390, 392, 394, 402
of talus, 234, 242, 244, 246, 248, 250, 252, 254, 256, 258, 260, 262, 264
temperomandibular joint, 30, 32
of ulna, 64, 66, 72, 74, 76, 78
Heart
atria of
left, 88, 90, 92, 98, 100, 104, 330

Heart, atria of — *Continued*
right, 88, 90, 98, 100, 108, 110, 288, 328, 330
shadow of (in radiograph of thorax), 114, 292
ventricles of
left, 88, 90, 92, 98, 100, 104, 108, 110, 112, 116, 126, 288, 328, 330
right, 88, 100, 102, 104, 106
Heel
pad of fat on, 248, 258
soft tissues of, 266
Heel bone. *See* Calcaneum
Hemisphere(s), cerebellar, 398, 400
Hemorrhoidal artery, 340, 342, 344
Hepatic ducts, 154
Hepatic flexure, 136, 142, 144, 146, 148
Hiatus
in adductor magnus muscle, 360
sacral, 172, 178, 308
Hilus (hilum)
of kidney, 124, 156, 160
of lung, 98, 102
Hip bones, 174, 176, 178. *See also* Acetabulum
Hip joint, 122, 124, 130, 136, 142, 144, 164, 172, 174, 180, 182, 186, 194, 196, 198, 200, 202, 204, 206, 294, 318, 374, 376
capsule of, 318
cavity of, 186, 196, 208, 210, 318
Horn(s), of lateral ventricle of brain
anterior, 380, 382, 384, 398, 400
inferior (temporal), 380, 382, 384
posterior, 384, 398, 400
Humerus, 42–66, 90, 92, 96, 104, 126, 366
anatomical neck of, 42, 46
bicipital groove of, 42
capitulum of, 50, 52, 54, 56, 60, 62, 66
epicondyles of
lateral, 50, 54, 56, 58, 62, 64
medial, 50, 52, 54, 56, 58, 60, 62, 64, 66
epiphyseal line of, 46, 56, 58, 60

Humerus — *Continued*
  epiphysis of
    proximal, 108
    superior, 106
  head of, 46, 48, 126, 292,
      354, 366
    epiphysis of, 108
  medial rotation of, 44, 48
  medial supracondylar ridge of,
      52, 60, 62
  olecranon fossa of, 50, 56
    combined with coronoid
        fossa, translucency
        produced by, 54
  shaft of, 48, 50, 52, 54, 108,
      110, 326, 354, 366
  surgical neck of, 42, 44, 46, 48
  trochlea of, 50, 52, 54, 56,
      58, 60, 62, 64
  tuberosities of
    greater, 42, 44, 46, 48
    lesser, 42, 44, 48
Hyoid bone, 38, 274, 276, 284,
    286
  body of, 274, 286
  greater cornu of, 286
Hysterosalpingogram, of cervical
    canal, 190

Ileum
  coils of, 130
  gas in, 148
  lymph nodes of, 370, 372,
      374, 376
Ilium, 184, 186, 194, 200, 202,
    208, 210. *See also*
    Crest(s), iliac
  spines of
    anterior inferior, 170, 174,
        180, 194, 196,
        198, 318, 320
    anterior superior, 124, 170,
        184, 194, 196, 318, 320
    posterior superior, 308, 320
Incisors, 20, 34, 36
Inguinal region, lymph nodes,
    superficial, 370, 372,
    374, 376
Innominate artery, 324, 326
Innominate line
  of greater wing of sphenoid
      bone, 22
  of lesser wing of sphenoid
      bone, 24

Intestine(s)
  contents of, 122, 178
  gas in, 96, 100, 102, 112,
      114, 122, 124, 128, 150,
      156, 162, 164, 166, 172,
      178, 180, 182, 184, 186,
      188, 190, 294, 296, 302,
      304, 310, 312, 334, 338,
      352, 372, 376
Ischium, 174, 182
  ramus of, 176, 180, 182, 186,
      194, 198, 200, 202
  spines of, 124, 158, 164, 170,
      172, 178, 194, 196, 198,
      210, 308, 312, 320
  tuberosities of, 140, 170, 172,
      176, 180, 184, 194, 196,
      198, 200, 204, 208, 210,
      312, 318, 320
Isthmus, of uterine tube, 190

Jaw. *See* Mandible; Maxilla
Jejunum, 128
  blood supply of, 336
  coils of, 130, 134
  gas in, 148
  loops of, 132, 134
Joint(s). *See also* Bone(s)
  acromioclavicular, 42, 44
  ankle, 242, 244, 246, 248,
      250, 252, 254
  atlanto-occipital, 2, 278, 286
  between articular processes,
      38, 178, 182, 280, 282,
      292, 298, 300, 402
    C3 and C4 vertebrae, 272
    C4 and C5 vertebrae, 284
    L2 and L3 vertebrae, 312
    L3 and L4 vertebrae, 304
  between atlas and occipital
      condyle (atlanto-occi-
      pital), 2, 278, 286
  capsule of. *See* Capsule
  elbow, 50, 52, 54, 56, 58,
      60, 62, 64
  hip. *See* Hip joint
  knee. *See* Knee joint
  lumbosacral, 178
  of Luschka, 280
  sacroiliac. *See* Sacroiliac joint(s)
  shoulder, 42, 44, 46, 48, 96,
      274
  sternoclavicular, 96
  synovial, 272, 280, 282
  talocalcaneal, 248
  temperomandibular
    with mouth closed, 30
    with mouth open, 32
  of vertebral column, 290, 402
Junction
  cardioesophageal, 134
  cartilaginous, between ischium
      and pubis, 184
  duodenojejunal, 128, 134

Kidney(s), 166
  calyces of
    major, 158, 160, 162, 164,
        166, 332, 334, 338
    minor, 158, 160, 162, 164,
        166, 332, 334
  fetal lobulation of, 160
  hilum of, 124, 156, 160
  left, 122, 124, 160, 162
    opacified, 156
    pelvis of, 332
  margins of, lateral, 158, 164
  parenchyma of, 156, 160
  pelvis of, 158, 160, 162, 164,
      166, 332, 338
  poles of, 158
  right, 122, 124, 160, 162
    opacified, 156
    pelvis of, 332
Knee joint, 212, 214, 216, 222,
    224, 226, 228, 230,
    234, 238, 358
  capsule of, 220
  cavity of, 218, 220
  soft tissues around, 218

Labia majora, 182
Lamina(e), vertebral, 162, 276,
    290, 294
  of axis, 270
  nonfusion of, 300
Lamina papyracea, 14
Larynx, 26, 88, 100
  air in, 274, 280, 284, 286
Leg(s)
  bones of, 232, 234, 236,
      238, 240
  fetal, 316
  medial side of, valved lympha-
      tic vessels draining, 370
  muscles of, 236, 238, 240, 244
    gastrocnemius, 230, 234,
        350
    hamstring, 234
    lateral aspect of, 232
    peroneal, 242
    posterior, 216, 228
    on posteromedial aspect, 232
    quadriceps femoris, 224,
        230, 236, 240
    tissue of, 242, 362
  skin of, 232, 234, 236, 238,
      240, 242, 244, 248
Lesser multangular, 64, 68, 72,
    74, 76, 78, 80, 84

Ligament(um)
of knee joint, medial, 220
patellae, 230, 234, 240
sacrococcygeal, posterior, 178
of Treitz, position of, 128
Limb(s)
fetal, 316, 318
lower, 194–266. *See also specific structures, e.g.*, Femur; Knee joint
upper, 42–84. *See also specific structures, e.g.*, Elbow joint and region; Hand
Line(s)
epiphyseal, 46, 56, 58, 60, 62, 70, 104, 210, 254
of femur, 208, 210, 224
of fibula, 232, 252, 254
of radius, 70
of tibia, 220, 224, 232, 234, 250, 252, 348
of ulna, 66, 70
iliopectineal, 172, 182, 186, 188, 194, 198, 302, 308, 312, 318, 320, 372, 374, 376
intertrochanteric, 194, 204, 206, 318
Lingulae, of bronchopulmonary segments, 116
Liver, 88, 92, 96, 98, 100, 102, 104, 108, 112, 114, 124, 160, 162, 288, 292, 296, 302, 316
lobes of
caudate, 154
left, 110, 154, 304, 310
quadrate, 154
right, 110, 154, 156, 162, 310, 352
tributaries of left hepatic duct from, 154
shadow of (in pyelogram), 158
Lobe(s)
frontal, 398, 400
of liver, 110, 154, 156, 162, 304, 310, 352
of lungs, 116, 118
occipital, 398, 400
parietal, 398, 400
temporal, 398, 400
of thymus, 110

Lower limb(s), 194–266. *See also* Foot; Hip joint; Leg(s); Thigh(s)
Lumen
duodenal, radiopaque solution in, 154
of vas deferens, 188
Lunate, 64, 66, 68, 72, 74, 76, 78, 80, 82, 84
Lung(s)
bronchopulmonary segments of, 116, 118
hilum of, 98, 102
pulmonary arteries in, 102
left, 98
roots of, 92, 106, 108
Luschka
foramen of, 398
joint of, 280
Lymphangiography, 366–376
Lymphatic system
of axilla, 366
iliac nodes, 370, 372, 374, 376
inguinal region, 370, 372, 374, 376
para-aortic (lateral aortic), lymph nodes, 372, 376
of thigh
lymph nodes, superficial inguinal (superior and inferior groups), 370, 372, 374, 376
lymphangiograms of, 368, 370
of upper limbs, 366, 368
Lymphatic vessels
abdomen and pelvis, 372
from medial side of arm, valved, 366
of thigh
medial superficial, 368
position of valves in, 368, 370
subcutaneous, radiopaque material in, 372, 376

Malleolus
lateral, 232, 234, 242, 244, 246, 248, 250, 252, 256, 262
medial, 232, 234, 242, 244, 246, 248, 250, 252, 256, 262
articular surface of talus for, 250
Mammary artery, 324, 326
Mammary glands, 92, 98, 126, 414, 416
lactiferous ducts, 414
nipple, 414
Mammography, 414, 416
Mandible, 284, 388, 396
alveolar process of, 26

Mandible — *Continued*
angle of, 2, 20, 22, 30, 272
body of. *See under* Body(ies)
canal of, 2
condyle of, 278, 284, 392
coronoid process of, 2, 8, 10, 20, 22, 26, 28, 30, 32, 278
head of, 2, 6, 8, 10, 12, 18, 20, 22, 28, 30, 32, 38, 274
neck of, 2, 4, 8, 18, 20, 30, 32, 278, 392
ramus of, 2, 4, 6, 10, 14, 16, 18, 20, 24, 30, 32
with teeth, 2, 4, 6, 14, 16, 24, 26, 28, 34, 270, 276, 278
Manubrium sterni, 88, 92, 94, 96, 102, 112, 114, 126, 272, 324
Margin(s). *See also* Border(s)
of acetabulum, 196, 200, 202, 206, 318
superior part of, 176, 200
of foramen magnum, 24, 270, 278, 392
of kidney(s), lateral, 158, 164
of lobes of liver
lower
left lobe, 310
right lobe, 154, 162
of mandible, 282
of muscles of upper arm, 94
of obturator foramen, 302
of orbit, 2, 4, 6, 14, 16, 18, 22, 24, 26, 28, 30, 32
inferior, 2, 18, 22, 26
superior, 14, 16, 24, 26, 382
of psoas muscle, 158, 166, 304
lateral, 122, 124, 156, 160, 174, 304, 310, 376
medial, 124, 156, 338
of quadratus lumborum, lateral, 156
of scapula, 292
lateral, 106
of spinal cord, lateral, 402
of thoracic aorta, descending, 288, 290
of thymus, 108, 110
of tibia
distal end, 250
lower end, posterior, 244
of vena cava, superior, 354
of vertebrae, 290

Marker, radiological, 288
Marrow, bone, 204, 206
Mastoid air cells, 2, 4, 10, 12 14, 22, 26, 28, 30
Mastoid bone, 6
Mastoid process, 2, 20, 28, 30, 32, 278, 284, 388
Maxilla, 20
    with teeth, 2, 4, 6, 8, 16, 18, 20, 22, 24, 26, 28, 34, 36, 270, 278
Meatus
    auditory
        external, 8, 10, 18, 30, 32, 38, 284
        internal, 6
    urethral, external, 186
Mediastinum
    anterior, 92, 102
    posterior, 92, 98, 106, 112, 114
Medulla, of femur, 196, 208, 210
Membrane
    interosseous
        of forearm, 64, 66, 78
        of leg, 242, 248
    mucous, of stomach, 132
Meniscus, 220
Metacarpals (metacarpus), 64, 68, 70, 72
    epiphyses of, 82, 84
    fifth, 64, 68, 72, 74, 78, 82
        epiphysis of, 68
    first (of thumb), 64, 68, 70, 72, 74, 76, 78, 80, 82, 84
        epiphysis of, 68, 82, 84
    fourth, 72, 78
    second, 72, 74, 76, 78
    third, 72, 74, 76, 78
Metallic objects, on radiogram, 10, 34, 154, 332
Metaphysis, 222, 226
    of femur, inferior, 228, 230
    of fibula, 228
Metatarsal
    fifth, 246, 248, 256, 258, 260, 262, 264, 266
        epiphysis of, 264
    first, 246, 252, 254, 256, 258, 260, 262, 264, 266
        epiphysis of, 262, 264
    second, 252, 264
Molars, 20, 24, 30, 32, 34, 36
Mouth, 112
    cavity of, 38
Mucous membrane(s), of sto-mach, folds of, 132

Muscle(s)
    of abdominal wall, 124
        anterior, 160
        tissue of, 176
    of arm, flexor, 52, 54, 66
        carpi ulnaris, 64
    of foot, abductor digiti minimi, 266
    gluteal, 124, 194, 206
    of leg. See under Leg(s)
    of neck, 274
    postvertebral, 284, 312
    psoas, 150, 158, 300, 352
        margins of. See under Margin(s)
    quadratus lumborum, lateral margin of, 156
    quadriceps femoris, 224, 230, 236, 240
    soleus, 350
    sternocleidomastoid, 108
    tensor fasciae latae, 208
    of thenar eminence, 80
    of thigh. See under Thigh(s)
    trapezius, 108
    triceps, 52, 60
    of upper arm, 52, 54, 56, 60
        margin of, 94
        tissue of, 56, 64, 68, 70
Myelography, 402, 404, 406, 408, 410

Nates, 184, 204, 208, 320, 356, 372
Navicular bone
    of foot, 234, 242, 246, 248, 252, 254, 256, 258, 260, 262, 264
    of hand, 64, 68, 70, 72, 74, 78, 80, 82, 84
Neck
    anatomical, of humerus, 42, 46
    arteries of, 324, 388
    of femur, 170, 176, 184, 186, 194, 196, 198, 200, 202, 204, 206, 208, 210, 318, 320, 344, 356
    of fibula, 212, 214, 216, 230, 234
    of gallbladder, 150
    of mandible, 2, 8, 18, 20, 30, 32, 278
    muscles of, 274
    of radius, 50, 52, 54, 56, 60, 62, 64, 66
    of rib, 290
    skin of, 284
    soft tissues of, 402
    surgical, of humerus, 42, 44, 46, 48
    of talus, 246, 248, 252, 258
    of tooth, 34, 36
    of urinary bladder, 182

Needle lumbar puncture, 404, 406, 408, 410
Nephrogram, 156
Nerve(s), spinal
    foramina of
        eighth cervical, 284
        fourth lumbar, 296
    sites of emergence of, 402
Nervous system, central, 380–410
Nipple, 414
Node, lymph. See Lymphatic system
Nose, 2, 6, 10, 12, 16, 18, 22, 38
    bones of, 16, 18, 22, 28
        fetal, region of, 172
    cavity of, 34, 274
    floor of, 2
    septum, 2, 6, 10, 12, 14, 16, 20, 22, 24, 26, 28, 392, 396
    skeleton, 26
Notch
    acetabular, 194, 318
    intercondylar, 212, 216, 222, 228, 232
    radial, of ulna, 50, 54
    sciatic, greater, 164, 172, 174, 176, 178, 182, 184, 196, 200, 202, 302, 306, 308, 320, 356
    supraorbital, 6
    trochlea
        of ulna, 54, 60, 66
    vertebral, 292
Nucleus, caudate, 398, 400

Occipital bone, 6, 10, 12, 26, 270, 276
    basilar part of, 10, 12
Opening, cardioesophageal, 126
Orbit, 22, 28, 274
    cavity of, 8, 18, 20
    of fetus, 172
    margin(s) of. See under Margin(s)
Orifice, ureteral, site of, 164
Ossification, secondary centers of, 284

Palate, 4, 6
    hard, 14, 18, 20, 22, 24, 34, 38, 274
        posterior margin of, 28
    soft, 8, 18, 38, 274

Parenchyma, renal
  partially opacified, 160
  radiopaque material in, 156
Patella, 212, 214, 216, 218,
     224, 226, 228, 230,
     234, 240, 348, 358
  cartilaginous, 240
Pedicles, vertebral. *See specific*
     region under Vertebral
     column
Pelvic brim, 190, 316
Pelvic cavity. *See also* Bladder,
     urinary; Rectum; Ure-
     ter(s); Urethra
  colon, sigmoid, 136, 138, 140,
     142, 144, 146, 148
  seminal vesicles, 188
  uterine tubes, 190
  uterus, 124, 190
  vas deferens, 188
Pelvis
  female, 170, 178, 182, 190
    brim of, 316
    lymphangiogram of, 372
    in pregnancy, 320
  of kidney, 158, 160, 162, 164,
     166, 332, 338
  male, 174, 176, 180, 184,
     186, 188
    lymphangiogram of, 370
Penis, 370
  body of, 180, 186
  bulb of, urethra in, 186
Phalanges
  of foot, 256, 258, 260
    distal, 262, 266
    epiphyses of, 264
    intermediate, 262
    proximal, 258, 266
     epiphysis of, 262
  of hand, 68, 70, 76, 78, 80,
     82, 84
    distal, 78, 80, 82, 84
    epiphyses of, 68, 82, 84
    middle, 78, 80, 82
    proximal, 78, 80, 82, 84
Phalanx. *See* Phalanges
Pharynx, 38
  air in, 286
  oral, 8, 32, 284
  posterior wall of, 38

Phleboliths, 122, 158, 188, 190
Pisiform, 64, 68, 72, 74, 78, 80
Plantar aponeurosis, 266
Plate(s)
  antro-ethmoidal, 24
  cartilaginous, ossification of,
    178
  orbital, of frontal bone, 2, 4, 6,
    8, 14, 18, 24, 280, 384
  pterygoid, 18
  tympanic, region of, 30
Plateau(s). *See* Condyle(s)
Pneumoarthography, of knee, 220
Pneumoencephalogram(s)
  anteroposterior, 380
  lateral, 384
  posteroanterior, 382
Pons, 400
Popliteal surface, 216
Pregnancy, 316, 318, 320
  third trimester
    anteroposterior radiograph of,
     318
    lateral radiograph in, 172
    pelvis in, 320
    posteroanterior radiograph
     of, 316
Premolars, 20, 34, 36
Process(es)
  acromion, of scapula, 42, 44,
    46, 48, 104, 366
  alveolar, of mandible, 26
  articular, 174, 280, 282, 286,
    294, 300, 304, 404, 406
    of fourth cervical vertebra,
     inferior, 274
    inferior, 292
    joints between, 38, 178,
     182, 272, 284, 292,
     298, 300, 304, 312
    of lumbar vertebrae, 408
     inferior, 296, 298, 304
     superior, 296, 298, 304
    of sacrum, superior, 174, 308
    superior, 170, 292, 300
    of third cervical vertebra,
     superior, 274
  clinoid
    anterior, 4, 8, 18, 396,
     398, 400
    posterior, 4, 8, 18, 384
  coracoid, 42, 44, 46, 48, 90,
    108, 126, 354, 366
  coronoid
    of mandible, 2, 8, 10, 20,
     22, 26, 28, 30, 32, 278
    of ulna, 50, 52, 54, 56, 58,
     60, 62, 64, 66
  mastoid, 2, 20, 28, 30, 32,
    278, 284, 388
  nasal, of frontal bone, 18
  odontoid, 2, 4, 8, 14, 22, 26,
    28, 270, 276, 278,
    284, 286

Process(es) — *Continued*
  olecranon
    accessory ossification centers
     for, 60
    of ulna, 50, 52, 54, 56, 58,
     60, 62, 66
  spinous, vertebral
    of axis (C2 vertebra), 270,
     278, 284
    bifid
     of C2, 274
     of C4, 282
     of C6, 276
    of C3 vertebra, 278
    of C7 vertebra, 272,
     274, 280
    of lumbar vertebrae, 160,
     162, 172, 174, 296,
     298, 302, 304, 310,
     312, 352, 372
    of sacral vertebrae, 178,
     312
    of thoracic vertebrae, 114,
     288, 290, 292
  styloid, 2, 14, 28, 388
    of fibula, 214, 216
    of radius, 64, 66, 68, 70,
     72, 74, 76, 78, 80
    of ulna, 64, 66, 68, 72, 74,
     76, 78, 80
  transverse, vertebral, 122,
    124, 138, 156, 158,
    160, 162, 164, 166,
    170, 174, 178, 406
    anterior tubercle of, 276
    of cervical vertebrae, 402
     of atlas (C1 vertebra), 22,
      26, 270, 278, 392
     of axis (C2 vertebra), 270
     and vertebral artery, 392
     of C3 vertebra, 276,
      280, 286
     of C4 vertebra, 282
     of C5 vertebra, 272
     of C6 vertebra, 274, 284
     of C7 vertebra, 282, 402
    left side, 286
    of lumbar vertebrae
     of L1 vertebra, 294, 406
     of L2 vertebra, 296, 312,
      352, 372, 376, 404
     of L3 vertebra, 124, 156,
      300, 302, 304, 310,
      372, 376
     of L4 vertebra, 138, 160,
      162, 166, 178, 298,
      338, 404

Process(es), transverse, vertebral,
of lumbar vertebrae —
Continued
of L5 vertebra, 306
of thoracic vertebrae, 122
of T1 vertebra, 272, 280
of T3 vertebra, 290
of T6 vertebra, 288
of T9 vertebra, 292
xiphoid, region of, 92, 96
zygomatic, 30, 32, 382
Promontory, sacral, 172, 178, 304,
308, 312, 320, 410
Protuberance, occipital
external, 4, 276, 286, 384
internal, 8, 10, 12, 28, 284,
400
Psoas. *See under* Margin(s);
Muscle(s)
Pubis
body of, 170, 172, 174, 180,
182, 184, 188, 194, 196,
198, 200, 208, 316, 318,
320, 344, 368
rami of
inferior, 172, 180, 184, 194,
196, 198, 200, 208
superior, 124, 170, 172, 174,
176, 184, 196, 198, 200,
202, 208, 316, 318
symphysis of, 164, 170, 174,
176, 184, 188, 194, 196,
318, 342, 344, 356, 374
Pulp, of tooth, 34, 36
Pyelography
intravenous, 158, 160, 162,
164
retrograde, 166
Pylorus, of stomach, 126, 128,
130, 132, 134

Quadratus lumborum, lateral
margin of, 156
Quadriceps femoris, 224, 230,
236, 240

Radiopaque material
in canal of uterine cervix, 190
in common bile duct, 154
in deep veins, 356, 360, 362
in dorsal venous arch, of foot,
356, 360, 362
jet stream of, 164, 182
programmed injection of, 324,
326, 328, 330, 332, 334,
336, 338, 340, 342, 344,
346, 348, 350, 352, 392

Radiopaque material—*Continued*
in pulmonary vessels, 330
pumped into subcutaneous
lymphatic vessels, 372,
376
in renal parenchyma, 156
in subarachnoid space, 400,
402, 404, 406, 408, 410
in ureter(s), 160, 162, 164,
332, 338
in urinary bladder, 164, 166,
178, 180, 182, 184, 356
in vas deferens, 188
Radius
epiphyseal line of, 70
epiphysis of, 68
distal, 82, 84
head of, 50, 52, 54, 56, 58,
60, 62, 64, 66
neck of, 50, 52, 54, 56, 60,
62, 64, 66
shaft of, 50, 52, 54, 58, 64,
70, 78
styloid process of, 64, 66, 68,
70, 72, 74, 76, 78, 80
tuberosities of, 50, 52, 54, 56,
64, 66, 70
bicipital, 56, 60
Ramus (rami)
ischiopubic, 182
of ischium, 176, 180, 182, 186,
194, 198, 200, 202
of mandible, 2, 4, 6, 10, 14,
16, 18, 20, 24, 30, 32
of pubis. *See under* Pubis
Recess
cardiophrenic, 108
costodiaphragmatic, 302
costophrenic, 92, 108
lateral, 110
posterior, 112
Rectum, 130, 136, 138, 140,
142, 144, 146, 148,
178, 186, 188, 196
after barium enema, 140
contents of, 196, 312, 370,
372, 376
enema tube in, 136
gas in, 130, 178, 186, 188,
196, 306, 320
Renal sinus, 156
Rib(s), 42–48, 88–120, 290,
296, 312
angles of, 102, 296
eighth, 290, 334
eleventh, 122, 150, 162, 290,
294, 304, 334, 338, 352
fetal, 316, 318
fifth, 290
first, 42, 44, 46, 48, 88, 90,
100, 108, 272, 276,
280, 282, 288, 290,
324, 366, 402

Ribs — *Continued*
fourth, 290
neck of, 290
ninth, 290
second, 94, 96, 290, 402
seventh, 288, 290, 334
sixth, 290
tenth, 128, 130, 160, 290,
332, 334
third, 96, 290
twelfth, 124, 132, 134, 136,
142, 154, 156, 158,
160, 166, 290, 294,
298, 300, 304, 310,
316, 334, 372, 376
Ridge, supracondylar, medial
of femur, 216
of humerus, 52, 60, 62
Root(s)
lumbar, extension around
fifth, 408
third, 408
of lung, 92, 106, 108
of posterior horn, 400
of teeth, 34, 36
of tongue, 38
Root canal(s), 36

Sacroiliac joint(s), 122, 124,
138, 158, 164, 166,
170, 174, 176, 184,
188, 190, 194, 196,
198, 200, 202, 294,
300, 306, 308, 310,
316, 318, 340, 344,
356, 370, 372, 374
Sacrum, 136, 142, 164, 170,
172, 176, 182, 188,
194, 198, 294, 300,
308, 312, 320
alar of, 138
articular process of, superior,
174, 308
lateral mass of, 182, 190, 300
superior border of, 410
medial crest of, 172, 410
promontory of, 172, 178, 304,
308, 312, 320, 410
Scaphoid, 64, 68, 70, 72, 74,
78, 80, 82, 84
Scapula, 42, 44, 46, 48, 92,
100, 104, 106, 108,
126, 286, 366
acromion process of, 42, 44,
46, 48, 104, 366

Scapula — *Continued*
  angle of
    inferior, 42, 44, 46, 90, 96,
      326, 366
    superior, 42, 44
  borders of
    lateral, 42, 44, 46, 48, 96,
      106, 292
    medial, 42, 44, 46, 90, 366
    superior, 42, 44, 48
  coracoid process of, 42, 44, 46,
    48, 90, 108, 126, 366
  glenoid cavity of, 42, 44,
    46, 48
  lateral border of, 42, 44, 46,
    48, 96, 106, 292
  medial border of, 42, 44, 46,
    90, 366
  spine of, 42, 44, 46, 48, 110
  superior border of, 42, 44, 48
Scrotum, 180, 186, 370
  vas deferens in, 188
Sella turcica, 4, 8, 18, 38, 284,
    286, 384
  floor of, 14
Seminal vesicles, 188
Septum(a)
  fibrous, of mammary glands,
    414, 416
  nasal, 2, 6, 10, 12, 14, 16, 20,
    22, 24, 26, 28, 392, 396
  pellucidum, 380, 398, 400
Sesamoid bone(s). *See also*
    Fabella
  in foot, 256, 260
  in hand, 74, 76, 78, 80, 84
Shaft(s)
  of femur, 140, 176, 186, 194,
    196, 198, 200, 202, 204,
    206, 208, 210, 224,
    226, 228, 230, 238,
    318, 320, 346, 348,
    356, 358, 360, 368
  of fibula, 216, 224, 226, 228,
    232, 234, 236, 238, 240,
    242, 244, 252, 350, 362
  of humerus, 48, 50, 52, 54,
    108, 110, 326, 354, 366
  of radius, 50, 52, 54, 58, 64,
    70, 78
  of rib, 290
  of tibia, 216, 226, 228, 232,
    234, 236, 238, 240, 242,
    244, 252, 350, 362
  of ulna, 50, 52, 64, 70

Shields, lead, genital, 176, 202,
    206, 210, 226, 228,
    232, 358
Shoulder joint and region, 42,
    44, 46, 48, 96, 274
Sigmoid artery, 340, 342
Sigmoid colon, 136, 138, 140,
    142, 144, 146, 148
Sinus(es)
  cavernous, 394
    internal carotid artery and,
      386, 388
  confluence of, 394
  ethmoid(al), 16, 18, 22,
    24, 382
  frontal, 2, 4, 8, 14, 16, 22,
    24, 28
  frontal air, 18, 382
  maxillary, 2, 4, 6, 8, 14, 16,
    18, 20, 22, 24, 28, 30,
    32, 36
    lateral walls of, 16, 28, 34
    posterior edge of, 38
  occipital, 394
  paranasal, 14, 16, 18, 20,
    22, 24
  renal, area of, 156
  sagittal, superior, 394, 396
    groove for, 10, 12
  sigmoid, 8
  sphenoid, 8, 16, 22, 26, 28,
    38, 388
  sphenoid air, 4, 18
  straight, 394, 396
  transverse, 394, 396
    groove for, 12, 28
Skeleton, nasal, 26
Skin
  folds of, 376
    axillary, 48, 366
    buttocks, 180, 184, 204,
      208, 320, 356
    chin, 2, 110
  of head, 286
  of knee, 218
  of leg, 232, 234, 236, 238,
    240, 242, 244, 248
  of mammary glands, 414, 416
  of neck, 284
  of thigh, 182, 216, 222, 226,
    228, 230, 368
  of thorax, 112
  of upper arm, 48, 52, 54, 64,
    66, 80
Skull, 2, 4, 6, 8, 10, 12, 26, 28,
    110, 280, 282, 380, 382,
    384, 390, 392, 394, 402
  fetal, 172, 316
  sutures of. *See* Sutures
    (of skull)
  tables of, 2, 4, 6, 8, 12, 26,
    380, 382, 384
Space(s)
  diploic, 4, 8, 12, 26

Space(s) — *Continued*
  between maxilla and ramus of
    mandible, 16
  pulp, of tooth, 34, 36
  retropharyngeal, 38, 284
  retrotracheal, 284
  subarachnoid
    extensions around nerve
      roots
      lateral, 408
      proximal ends of, 406
      radiopaque material in, 400,
        402, 404, 406, 408, 410
Speculum, vaginal, shown in
    hysterosalpingogram,
    190
Sphenoid bone
  basal part of, 26
  body of, 10
  greater wing of, 2, 6, 14, 16,
    22, 24, 28
  lesser wing of, 6, 14, 24
  spine of, 28
Spinal cord
  lateral margin of, 402
  nerves of. *See* Nerve(s), spinal
Spine(s)
  iliac. *See under* Ilium
  ischial, 124, 158, 164, 170,
    172, 178, 194, 196, 198,
    210, 308, 312, 320
  sacral, fused, 308, 320
  of scapula, 42, 44, 46, 48, 110
  of sphenoid bone, 28
  of vertebrae
    bifid, of axis, 286
    fifth lumbar, 178, 308,
      320, 410
    fourth lumbar, 178, 308
    second cervical, 8, 286
    second lumbar, 294
    third lumbar, 300, 308
    third thoracic, 402
Spleen, 122, 156, 160, 162, 340
  blood supply of, 332, 334
  border of, 332, 334
Splenic flexure. *See* Flexure,
    colic
Sternebrae, 94, 112, 114
Sternum, 92, 94, 96
  angle of, 94, 96, 102, 112
  body of, 92, 96, 102
  xiphoid process of, 92, 96

Stomach, 130
  antrum of, 126, 128, 132, 134
  barium in, 98, 114, 128, 134
  body of, 126, 128, 130, 132, 134
  curvatures of, 132, 134
  fluid level in, 106
  fundus of, 106, 114, 126, 128, 130, 132, 134
  gas in, 106, 114, 132, 148, 292
  mucous membrane of, folds of, 132
  pylorus of, 126, 128, 130, 132, 134
Subcutaneous tissue, 64, 68, 238
  of mammary gland, 414, 416
Sulcus(i), cerebral, air in, 380, 382, 384
Sustentaculum tali, 246, 248, 254, 258
Sutures (of skull), 2, 4, 6, 8, 10, 12, 284, 380, 382, 384, 390, 392, 394, 396
  coronal, 2, 4, 8, 12, 384, 390, 394
    between frontal and parietal bones, 12
  frontozygomatic, 22
  lambdoid, 2, 4, 6, 8, 10, 12, 284, 380, 382, 384, 392, 394
  metopic, 6
  occipitomastoid, 26
  sagittal, 2, 6, 12, 26, 380, 382, 392, 396, 400
  zygomaticofrontal, 16
Sylvian fissure, 398
Symphisis of pubis, 164, 170, 174, 176, 184, 188, 194, 196, 318, 342, 344, 356, 374
Synchondrosis, ischiopubic, 208
Synovial joints, 272, 280, 282

Table, tilting, for use in myelography, 402, 404
Talus, 232, 234, 238, 240, 242, 244, 248, 262, 264, 266
  body of, 244, 246, 248, 250, 252, 258, 260
  edge of, 244
  head of, 234, 242, 244, 246, 248, 250, 252, 254, 256, 258, 260, 262, 264
    region of, 250

Talus — *Continued*
  for medial malleolus, articular surface for, 250
  neck of, 246, 248, 252, 258
  tubercles of, posterior, 246, 248, 254
  ossification center for, 252
Tarsal bone(s), 242, 244, 248, 252, 256, 258, 260, 262, 264, 266
Teeth, 2, 4, 6, 8, 14, 16, 18, 20, 22, 24, 28
  crowns, 34, 36
  deciduous, 20, 36
  dental films of, 34, 36
  dentures, 38
  of lower jaw (mandible), 2, 4, 6, 14, 16, 24, 26, 28, 34, 270, 276, 278
    canine, permanent, 20, 34, 36
    incisors, permanent, 20, 34, 36
    molars, 36
      deciduous, 20
      permanent, 20, 24, 30, 32, 284
    premolars, permanent, 20, 34, 36
  permanent, 20, 24, 30, 32, 34, 36
  pulp, 34, 36
  root(s) of, 34, 36
  root canal, 36
  unerupted, 6, 24, 36, 278, 284
  of upper jaw (maxilla), 2, 4, 6, 8, 16, 18, 20, 22, 24, 26, 28, 34, 36, 270, 278
    canines, 34, 36
    incisors, 36
      central, 20, 34
    molars, 34, 36
      third molar, 30, 32
    premolars, 36
Temporal bone(s)
  mandibular fossa of, 30, 32, 38
  petrous part of, 4, 6, 10, 12, 14, 16, 18, 24, 284, 286, 380, 384, 388, 394, 396, 398, 400
    aerated portion of, 398, 400
    apex of, 26
    superior border of, 2
  squamous part of, 26
Tendo calcaneous, 234
Tendon(s)
  of abductor pollicis longus, 82
  Achilles, 234
  of adductor magnus, 360
  of hamstring muscles, 234
  of hand, 74
  peroneus brevis, 262
  peroneus longus, 262
  of popliteus, 220

Tendon(s) — *Continued*
  of quadriceps muscle, 240
  rectus femoris, 230
Thenar eminence, 78, 80
Thigh(s), 204, 206, 208, 210
  lymphangiograms of, 368, 370
  lymphatics of, 368
  muscles of, 204, 208, 210, 216, 224, 228, 230, 236, 348, 358, 368
    anterior, 198
    lateral aspect, 204, 226
    medial aspect, 226
    posterior aspect, 230
  tissue of, 206, 222, 356, 358, 360
  skin of, 182, 216, 222, 226, 228, 230, 368
  soft tissues of, 194, 196
Thoracic cavity
  esophagus, 98, 102, 104, 106, 112, 114, 126, 134, 274, 292
  trachea, 26, 38, 88, 90, 92, 98, 100, 102, 106, 108, 110, 112, 116, 118, 126, 288, 292, 354
Thoracic wall
  anterior, 114, 416
  cardiophrenic recess, 108
  costophrenic angles of, 88, 100, 102
  costophrenic recess, 92, 108
    lateral, 110
    posterior, 112
  diaphragm, 88, 90, 92, 98, 116, 118
  vertebrae of, 114
Thorax, 88–118, 126. *See also specific structures,* e.g., Sternum; Trachea
Thumb
  first metacarpal of, 64, 68, 70, 72, 74, 76, 78, 80, 82, 84
  phalanges of, 68, 70, 76, 84
    proximal, 78
Thymus, 112
  lobes of, 110
  margins of, 108, 110
Thyroid
  arteries, 324, 326, 386
  cartilage of, 38, 274, 276
Tibia, 212, 214, 222, 246, 248, 250, 254, 258, 264, 266, 358

Tibia — *Continued*
  cartilage of superior epiphyseal, 226, 228
    site of former, 230
  condyles of
    lateral, 212, 214, 218, 220, 226, 228, 232
    medial, 214, 216, 218, 220, 226, 230, 232, 234, 348, 362
  distal end of, 250
  epicondyles of, 218
  epiphyseal line of, 220, 224, 250, 252, 348
    inferior, 232, 234
  epiphysis of, 252, 254, 264, 266
    inferior, 236, 238, 240
    superior, 222, 224, 226, 228, 236, 238, 240
  lower end of, posterior margin of, 244, 246, 248
  medial malleolus of, 262
  shaft of, 216, 226, 228, 232, 234, 236, 238, 240, 242, 244, 252, 350, 362
  tuberosities of, 212, 214, 224, 228, 230, 234
Tissue(s)
  of mammary gland, 414, 416
  muscular. *See under* Muscle(s) *and names of specific muscles*
  soft
    of ankle joint, 254
    of heel, 266
    of knee joint, 218
    of neck, 402
    of thighs, 194, 196
  subcutaneous, 64, 68, 238
Tomography, computerized, of brain, 398, 400
Tongue, 8, 274, 284
  dorsum of, barium coating on, 38
Tonsil, nasopharyngeal, 284
Tooth. *See* Teeth
Trabecula(e) of cancellous bone, 194
Trachea, 26, 38, 88, 90, 92, 98, 100, 102, 106, 108, 110, 112, 116, 118, 126, 288, 292, 354
  air in, 114, 272, 274, 280, 282, 284, 286, 328
  bifurcation of, 88, 90, 92, 98, 100, 104, 106, 112, 118, 126, 288, 292
  position of, 276

Trapezium, 64, 68, 72, 76, 78, 80, 82, 84
Trapezoid, 64, 68, 72, 74, 76, 78, 80, 84
Treitz, ligament of, 128
Tributaries, from lobes of liver, of hepatic ducts, 154
Triquetral (triquetrum), 64, 68, 72, 74, 76, 78, 80, 82, 84
Triradiate cartilage, 174, 176, 184, 200, 202, 310, 312
Trochanters of femur
  greater, 124, 170, 174, 180, 184, 194, 196, 198, 200, 204, 206, 318, 356
    ossifying, 208
  lesser, 170, 180, 184, 194, 196, 198, 204, 206, 210, 318, 320, 344, 356
Trochlea
  of humerus, 50, 52, 54, 56, 58, 60, 62, 64
  of ulna, 54, 60, 66
Trunk
  arterial
    callosomarginal, 386
    celiac, catheter in, 332, 334
    costocervical, 324
    pulmonary, 88, 98, 100, 108, 328, 330
    thyrocervical, 324, 326
  lymphatic, subclavian, 366
Tube(s)
  nasogastric (used in arteriography), 336
  T-tube, for radiopaque solution, in common bile duct, 154
  uterine, 190
Tubercle(s)
  adductor, 212, 216
  articular, 30, 32, 38
  genial, 20, 34
  of iliac crest, 318
  of intercondylar eminence, 226, 228
  quadrate, 198, 206
  of talus, posterior, 246, 248, 252, 254
  of vertebral column
    C1, posterior, 274, 286
    C3, anterior, 276
Tuberosity(ies)
  of humerus
    greater, 42, 44, 46, 48
    lesser, 42, 44, 48
  ischial, 140, 170, 172, 176, 180, 184, 194, 196, 198, 200, 204, 208, 210, 312, 318, 320
  of radius, 50, 52, 54, 56, 64, 66, 70
    bicipital, 56, 60
  tibial, 214, 224, 228, 230, 234
    position of, 212

Turbinate bone. *See* Concha(e)
Ulna, 56, 60, 62, 66, 68, 72, 74, 76, 80, 82
  coronoid process of, 50, 52, 54, 56, 58, 60, 62, 64, 66
  epiphyseal line of, 66, 70
  epiphysis of, 68, 70
    distal, 82, 84
  head of, 64, 66, 72, 74, 76, 78
  olecranon process of, 50, 52, 54, 56, 58, 60, 62, 66
  radial notch of, 50, 54
  shaft of, 50, 52, 64, 70
  styloid process of, 64, 66, 68, 72, 74, 76, 78, 80
  trochlea notch of, 54, 60, 66
Upper limb(s)
  arm, upper, 42, 44, 46
  elbow joint and region, 50, 52, 54, 56, 58, 60, 62
  fetal bones, 172
  forearm, 64, 66, 68, 70, 72, 78
  hand, 78, 80, 82, 84. *See also* Hand
  shoulder joint and region, 42, 44, 46, 48, 96, 274
  wrist region, 72, 74, 76
Ureter(s)
  female, 158, 160, 162, 164
  male, 186
    catheter in, 166
    radiopaque material in, 166, 332, 338
Urethra
  bulbous part of, 180, 186
  female, 182
  male, 180, 186
    external meatus, 186
    membranous part of, 180, 186
    penile part of, 180, 186
    prostatic part of, 180, 188
Urinary bladder. *See* Bladder, urinary
Uterine tubes, 190
Uterus, 124
  cavity of body of, 190
Uvula, 8, 38, 274

Valves, venous, 356, 358, 360, 362
Vas deferens, 188
Vein(s)
  anastomotic, 394
  axillary, venogram of, 354

Vein(s) — *Continued*
  azygos, 288
    position of, 88, 108
  basal, 394, 396
  basilic, 354
  brachial, venogram of, 354
  brachiocephalic
    left, 354
    right, 108, 354
  of brain, 394, 396
  cephalic, 354
  cerebral
    anterior, 396
    great (of Galen), 394
      region of, 400
    internal, 394
    middle, 394
      deep, 396
    superior, 394, 396
  cervical, transverse, 354
  deep, radiopaque material in,
    356, 360, 362
  femoral, 358, 360
    catheter in, 352
    lateral circumflex, 356
    tributaries of, 360
    valves of, 356, 358, 360
    venogram of, 356, 358, 360
  hepatic, 352
  humeral, circumflex, 354
  iliac
    common, 352, 356
    external, 356
    internal, 356
    superficial circumflex, 356
  innominate. *See* brachioce-
    phalic *above*
  jugular, terminal portion of, 354
  lumbar, 352
  muscular, 360, 362
  perforating, 362
  peroneal, 362
  popliteal, 360, 362
    tributaries of, 360
    venogram of, 358, 360, 362
  profunda femoris, 356
  pulmonary, 330
  renal, 352
  saphenous
    great (long), 356, 358, 360
      lymphatic vessels and, 368
      tributary of, 356, 360
    small, 358
  subclavian, venogram of, 354

Vein(s) — *Continued*
  suprascapular, 354
  thalamostriate, 394
  of thorax, 88, 90, 92, 100, 102,
    106, 108, 112, 288
  tibial, 358, 360, 362
Vena cava. *See also* Vein(s)
  inferior, 88, 90, 92, 100, 102,
    106, 112, 352
    venogram of, 352
  superior, 88, 90, 100, 108,
    288, 354
Venography, 352–362, 394, 396
Ventricle(s)
  of brain
    fourth ventricle, 398, 400
      lateral recess of, 398
    lateral, 380, 384
      anterior horn of, 380, 382,
        384, 398, 400
      body of, 398, 400
      inferior horn of, 380,
        382, 384
      posterior horn of, 384,
        398, 400
    third ventricle, 398, 400
  cardiac
    left, 88, 90, 92, 98, 100,
      104, 108, 110, 112, 116,
      126, 288, 328, 330
    right, 88, 100, 102, 104, 106
Vermis, cerebellar, 398
Vertebra(e). *See also* Vertebral
    column
  body of. *See under* Body(ies)
  fetal, 316
  superior surface of, 298
Vertebral column
  articular processes of, 170,
    174, 280, 282, 286, 294,
    300, 304, 404, 406
  joints between, 38, 178, 182,
    272, 284, 292, 298,
    300, 304, 312
  cervical region, 272, 274, 276,
    280, 282, 284, 286
    articular processes of, 280
    C3 vertebra, 274
    C4 vertebra, 274
    C1 vertebra, 38, 174, 178,
      284, 286, 312, 386, 394.
      See also Atlas
    C2 vertebra, 38, 274, 276,
      278, 284, 286, 386, 394,
      402. *See also* Axis
    C3 vertebra, 38, 272, 274,
      276, 278, 280, 282, 284,
      286, 386, 394, 402
    C4 vertebra, 38, 272, 274,
      276, 278, 280, 282, 284,
      286, 386, 402
    C5 vertebra, 38, 272, 274,
      276, 280, 282, 284,
      286, 324, 402

Vertebral column, cervical
    region — *Continued*
    C6 vertebra, 38, 272, 274,
      276, 280, 282, 284,
      286, 324, 402
    C7 vertebra, 108, 272, 274,
      276, 280, 282, 284,
      286, 325, 402
    myelogram of, 402
    odontoid process, of C2
      vertebra (axis), 274,
      284, 286
    pedicles of
      C3 vertebra, 278, 284
      C4 vertebra, 280
      C5 vertebra, 286
      C7 vertebra, 274
    spinous processes of. *See*
      under Process(es)
    transverse processes of. *See*
      under Process(es)
    tubercles of
      C1 vertebra (atlas), 274,
        286
      C3 vertebra, 276
    upper, 270, 278
    vertebral artery and, 390
  coccyx, 122, 124, 140, 172,
    176, 294, 306, 308,
    312, 374, 376
  fetal vertebrae, 172
  foramen of, 402
  intervertebral discs, 174, 178,
    284, 288, 290, 292, 296,
    298, 300, 302, 304, 308,
    312, 406, 408, 410
  intervertebral foramina, 276,
    284, 286, 292, 296,
    302, 304, 312
  joints between vertebrae, 2,
    38, 178, 182, 272
    280, 282, 284, 292,
    298, 300, 304, 312, 402
  lamina(e), 162, 270, 276, 290,
    294, 300
  lumbar region, 294, 296, 298,
    300, 302, 304
    articular processes of, 294,
      296, 298, 300, 302,
      304, 408
    extensions around roots of
      vertebrae, 408
    L1 vertebra, 122, 124, 128,
      132, 134, 136, 144, 154,
      156, 158, 160, 162, 164,
      166, 290, 294, 296, 298,
      300, 302, 304, 310, 312,
      332, 336, 338, 340, 352,
      372, 376, 404, 406

Vertebral column, lumbar
  region — *Continued*
 L2 vertebra, 122, 124, 132,
  134, 136, 138, 142, 152,
  154, 156, 158, 160, 162,
  164, 166, 294, 296, 298,
  300, 302, 304, 310, 312,
  332, 336, 338, 340, 352,
  372, 376, 404, 406
 L3 vertebra, 122, 124, 132,
  134, 136, 138, 152, 154,
  156, 158, 160, 162, 164,
  166, 294, 296, 298, 300,
  302, 304, 308, 310, 312,
  336, 338, 340, 352, 372,
  376, 406, 408, 410
 L4 vertebra, 122, 124, 132,
  134, 142, 152, 156,
  158, 160, 162, 164,
  166, 172, 176, 178,
  294, 296, 298, 300,
  302, 304, 308, 310,
  312, 320, 336, 338,
  340, 342, 352, 372,
  376, 406, 408, 410
 L5 vertebra, 122, 124, 132,
  134, 136, 140, 156,
  158, 164, 172, 174,
  176, 178, 182, 294,
  296, 298, 300, 302,
  304, 306, 308, 310,
  312, 320, 336, 340,
  342, 352, 372, 374,
  376, 408, 410
 myelograms of, 404, 406
 pedicles of, 294, 296, 298,
  300, 302, 304, 306,
  310, 312, 352, 372,
  406, 408, 410
 spines of vertebra, 178,
  286, 294, 300, 308,
  320, 402, 410
 spinous processes of, 160,
  162, 172, 174, 296,
  298, 302, 304, 310,
  312, 352, 372
 transverse processes of. *See
  under* Process(es)

Vertebral column — *Continued*
 lumbosacral region, 306, 310
 myelograms of, 408, 410
 pedicles of, 156, 160, 162,
  164, 174, 176, 178,
  182, 203
 sacral region, 308, 312
 fused spines of, 308
 S1 vertebra, 122, 124, 134,
  140, 164, 166, 172, 174,
  178, 190, 294, 296, 300,
  302, 304, 308, 310, 312,
  320, 336, 340, 342, 372,
  374, 376, 408, 410
 S2 vertebra, 122, 124, 140,
  172, 174, 178, 302, 308,
  310, 312, 374, 408, 410
 S3 vertebra, 122, 124, 140,
  172, 174, 178, 302,
  308, 310, 312, 374
 S4 vertebra, 122, 124, 140,
  172, 174, 178, 302,
  308, 310, 312, 374
 S5 vertebra, 122, 124, 140,
  142, 174, 178, 302,
  312, 374
 sacral canal, 172, 178, 302,
  308
 sacral cornu, 308
 sacral hiatus, 172, 178, 308
 sacrum, 308, 312
  spinous processes of, 178,
  312
 thoracic region, 288, 290, 292
 articular processes of, 292
 myelogram of, 404
 pedicles of, 292
  T1 vertebra, 326
  T5 vertebra, 290
  T8 vertebra, 288
 spinous processes of, 114,
  292
  T4 vertebra, 290
  T5 vertebra, 288
 T1 vertebra, 108, 272,
  274, 276, 280, 282,
  324, 402
 T2 vertebra, 108, 272, 276,
  280, 282, 288, 290,
  324, 402
 T3 vertebra, 108, 272,
  282, 288, 290, 324
 T4 vertebra, 108, 288, 290
 T5 vertebra, 108, 288, 290

Vertebral column, thoracic
  region — *Continued*
 T6 vertebra, 92, 108,
  288, 290
 T7 vertebra, 92, 108,
  288, 290
 T8 vertebra, 92, 108,
  288, 290
 T9 vertebra, 92, 108, 134,
  288, 290, 292, 334
 T10 vertebra, 92, 106,
  108, 134, 288, 290,
  332, 334
 T11 vertebra, 92, 106,
  124, 134, 136, 156, 160,
  162, 288, 290, 304,
  332, 334, 352, 404
 T12 vertebra, 92, 122,
  124, 128, 130, 134,
  136, 144, 148, 162,
  166, 288, 290, 294,
  296, 300, 302, 304,
  332, 334, 336, 338,
  340, 352, 376, 404
 transverse processes of. *See
  under* Process(es)
Vesicles, seminal, 188
Vesiculogram, seminal, 188
Vomer, 28
Vulva, 196, 316, 318, 356, 368

Wall(s)
 abdominal. *See* Abdominal wall
 of maxillary sinuses, 16, 28, 38
 of pharynx, posterior, 38
 of piriform fossa, 38
 of thorax, anterior, 114
White matter, 398
Wrist region, 72, 74, 76

Xeroradiograms, of mammary
  glands, 414, 416

Zygomatic bone, 14, 16, 22, 24,
  26, 28, 34